THE ULTIMATE BOOK OF WOMEN'S HEALTH

THE ULTIMATE BOOK OF WOMEN'S HEALTH

NAN KATHRYN FUCHS, PHD

Soundview Publications
Atlanta, GA

ISBN: 1-885385-01-3
Cover design by Elizabeth Bame

Additional copies of this book may be purchased from Soundview Publications. Please call for more information. Soundview Publications also publishes Nan Kathryn Fuchs' monthly medical newsletter, *Women's Health Letter*. To subscribe or obtain a free catalog describing all Soundview Publications' products, please call or write:

Soundview Publications, Inc.
Post Office Box 467939
Atlanta, Georgia 31146-7939
800-728-2288 or 770-399-5617

Acknowledgements

A health writer's information is only as good as her sources. I cannot give enough thanks to the practitioners, researchers, and writers I am privileged to call my friends. You have repeatedly given me your time and expertise so I could better understand the complicated subjects before me. Thank you, all.

Guy E. Abraham, MD; Susan Arima, OMD; Andy Bialek, MD; Mark Blumenthal; Hyla Cass, MD; Daniel Clark, MD; Ann Louise Gittleman, MS, CNS; Merri Harris, DC; Tori Hudson, ND; David Law; Jed Meese; Vesanto Melina, RD; Ingrid Naimen; Sharon Olson, DO; Janet Ralston; Uzzi Reiss, MD; Bill Sardi; Natasha Trenev; Terri Turner, DO; Melvyn Werbach, MD; Janet Zand, OMD.

Table of Contents

Introduction

Achieving and maintaining good health isn't easy. Our bodies are complex, and the effects of inherited genetic weaknesses, dietary assaults, and environmental toxins all take their toll. Information on how diet affects health is often conflicting and confusing. This is because in addition to being complex, our bodies are different. What works for one person doesn't work for another. I know this. I've seen it in over 23 years of clinical practice.

There's nothing that can compare with seeing patients year after year and reading scientific studies on nutritional therapies. This combination has given me an insight into disease prevention and reversal that few health writers can match. I've always been a detective, looking for the cause of a problem rather than focusing on a Band-aid solution. This book will help you find the bottom-line causes of your health problems, and make it easier for you to avoid many degenerative illnesses like arthritis, cancer, heart disease, and osteoporosis.

There are many causes of poor health. Part one addresses some of the most important ones like environmental toxins and dangerous household products. Then, with so much in the news about food poisoning, I'll help you understand the cause of food-borne illnesses and how to avoid them by taking simple precautions.

I maintain that you are not what you eat. You are what you eat, digest, and absorb. If you're eating nutritious foods, but not getting their nutrients into your cells due to poor digestion, you're headed toward illness. Poor digestion is a major cause of illness, and it's easy to correct.

Then there's the area of dangerous synthetic hormones that many doctors believe are killing women. I explain why they are harmful and suggest other alternatives so you can take anti-aging hormones safely. And since we are emotional beings as well as physical, I explain how toxic emotions can contribute to illness.

Part two deals with some of the most important health problems facing women today: heart disease, breast cancer, arthritis, osteoporosis, and diabetes. Reading this section, and making a few changes, can literally save your life. Some of the concepts I talk about, like emphasizing magnesium over calcium, I introduced to the public back in 1985. It was considered heresy at that time. It still is, by some. But now a number of companies are formulating supplements with equal amounts of magnesium as calcium — some with more magnesium than calcium. More than 15 years after I came out as a "magnesium advocate," this concept is becoming more mainstream. Still, many doctors and nutritionists are leading women down what I consider to be a dangerous path. This section will help you understand why I take the position I do, and help you reduce your risk of heart disease and osteoporosis with a single dietary change.

Part three tells you how to make the necessary changes in your diet and supplements to get healthier. Years ago I had a small herb business, so I'm very familiar with not only using them, but their interactions with vitamins and minerals. I like using herbs and other nutritional supplements when they're needed. I've seen miraculous changes in my patients and the patients of other doctors who have used the information I've uncovered. But I know that changing your diet comes first, and supplements come second.

There's no quick path to wellness, but in this book I've cleared the path for you and made it easier for you to get significant results. I know it's possible, because I've seen it happen with hundreds of my patients. The rest is up to you. Just know that I'll be by your side every step of the way through this book and other writings.

Nan Kathryn Fuchs, PhD

Section 1

The Causes of Poor Health

Chapter 1

Are Toxins Killing You Slowly?

As a child, my mother often said to me, "Stop being so sensitive!" I didn't know what she meant. Little things disturbed me profoundly, like the radio playing when I was trying to study or a harsh word that could bring me quickly to tears. To be less sensitive was not to be me.

Now we know there are biological explanations for these kinds of sensitivities. Some people's nervous systems react more strongly to less stimuli than others. A sensitive person can't will herself to be less sensitive.

The same goes for other sensitivities. Some people can eat sugar all day and feel fine, while others eat a cookie or even a baked potato and get exhausted. This may be caused by an insulin sensitivity. Certain foods trigger the pancreas to secrete insulin, lowering your blood sugar rapidly and causing fatigue. This response can differ from person to person depending on a genetic predisposition and your past history. Alcohol abuse and eating a lot of sweets over a long period of time, for example, can result in insulin sensitivity.

Thousands of women have silicone breast implants, and some have come down with devastating illnesses. Scientific studies say there is absolutely no link between breast implants and autoimmune diseases. Yet the women who have become sick, and who have died, would disagree vehemently with this conclusion. Science can't explain this phenomenon through its randomized, double-blind studies because if you're one in a hundred who is remarkably sensitive to silicone, it doesn't matter who else can tolerate the substance — you can't. And you can't stop being so sensitive.

We are all exposed to various toxins in the air we breathe, the water we drink, the foods we eat, and the chemicals we live with, from clothes that have been dry-cleaned to an artist's paints and glazes. But everyone's sensitivity is unique, and most of us have at least one substance to which we're sensitive. Is yours to a food, pollen, perfume, or polyester? Have you grown more sensitive over the years? A sudden sensitivity may be an early warning sign. Talk with your doctor or health practitioner about this. Perhaps your immune or digestive systems have become weakened.

There are a number of toxins we come in contact with everyday. You're probably aware of some of them, but others you might be surprised to learn about. So let's take a look at some of the toxins you may deal with regularly.

The Danger in Common Household Products

Household cleaners and synthetic pesticides may be harming your health.

If you suffer from chronic fatigue, extreme lethargy, breast cancer, Parkinson's disease, or symptoms your doctors can't trace back to any particular cause, the culprit may be a lifetime buildup of toxic chemicals. While your liver is a potent detoxifier, some substances are harder to eliminate than others. Detox formulas found in natural food stores may or may not work. Your best solution is to reduce your exposure to the toxins in everyday products.

Products you use in your kitchen, your bathroom, your garage, and garden can make you sick. They can attack your nervous system, put you at an increased risk for cancer, and contribute to a variety of health problems in you, your children, grandchildren, and pets. In addition, during their manufacturing they produce toxic wastes that further add to environmental pollution, continuing the cycle of toxic exposure. Truly, pesticides harm more than pests.

All Pesticides Are Not Alike

Pesticides include insecticides (which kill insects), herbicides (which destroy unwanted plants), and fungicides (which eliminate fungi). Unfortunately, they also upset the balance of nature and destroy the eco-system. In addition, using pesticides results in stronger strains of pests that are more resistant to pesticides. Synthetic pesticides are more toxic than natural ones, but all can affect your health. The EPA estimates that 280 million pounds of

---

Drugs Can Be Toxic Too

In a study by researchers at Boston's Brigham and Women's Hospital, tricyclic depressants such as Elavil, and benzodiazepine tranquilizers such as Valium and Halcion were found to increase the risk of ovarian cancer twofold. Women who used these drugs before age 50 had an increased risk of up to 3.5 times higher. This was a preliminary study, so more research on this will likely be underway soon.

Here are some other popular drugs that aren't nearly as safe as widespread use might lead you to believe:

Anti-Arrhythmics (drugs for irregular heartbeats). Research suggests most class 1 drugs in this category cause more deadly cardiac arrests than they prevent. A safer option might be up to 1,000 mg daily of magnesium, which helps regulate heartbeats.

Anti-inflammatories. These include aspirin, ibuprofen, and Naprosyn. It's estimated that their long-term use results in roughly 70,000 hospitalizations annually, mostly due to damage caused to the stomach lining. Alternatives include magnesium and vitamin B_6 supplements for headache relief.

Calcium Channel Blockers (including Procardia and Cardizem). The FDA based approval of these drugs on their short-term ability to lower blood pressure. With long-term use, however, study after study of persons taking various calcium channel blockers has produced a large number of unexplained deaths and other medical problems. Safer alternatives include weight loss, stress reduction, and magnesium supplements (up to 1,000 mg/day).

Serotonin Reuptake Inhibitors. These include Prozac and its close chemical relatives, Paxil and Zoloft. Initially, manufacturer Eli Lilly claimed that Prozac was nearly free of side effects. However, during a 10-year period, FDA reports associated it with more serious adverse reactions, hospitalizations, and deaths than any other drug. Non-drug solutions include amino acid therapy and nutritional therapies, as outlined in *Potatoes Not Prozac* by Kathleen Desmaisons, ($23 from Simon & Schuster).

pesticides are used in our homes, offices, schools, lawns, and gardens. Most homes, about 85 percent of them, in fact, contain three to four pesticides including bug foggers, cleaning agents, pest strips, flea collars, pet shampoos, and snail bait.

Sherry A. Rogers, MD, has written a number of books about chemical sensitivity and environmental illness. In *Tired or Toxic?* (Prestige Publishers, 1990) she explains how pesticides get stored in the body and are slowly released into the bloodstream over a period of months.

How Harmful Are They?

If pesticides and cleaning compounds are synthetic, the answer is, possibly very harmful — especially to women. The Environmental Protection Agency (EPA) has stated that 60 percent of herbicides, 90 percent of fungicides, and 30 percent of insecticides may lead to cancer. One classification of pesticides called

---

The Effects of Lead on Young and Old

If you are pregnant and believe you may have been exposed to lead from lead paint or from drinking water, you may want to have your blood lead-levels tested — preferably during your third trimester — according to a professor of dental research at Rochester University. He has found that the children of women exposed to lead tend to have more dental caries than children whose mothers are not exposed to it. The lead is transmitted through breast milk.

Women who were exposed had 10 times the levels of lead in their breast milk as women who were not. This suggests that at least some lead is concentrated in mammary glands.

Doctors who are studying this phenomenon are also looking at the possibility that lead may also impair salivary gland function, a condition that puts elderly people at a higher risk for dental problems. Salivary gland function is almost totally suppressed by diuretics, antidepressants, and beta-blockers. Lead, then, may be affecting the oldest and youngest people in our population. If you're concerned that you may have high levels of lead, consult a homeopath about a lead detoxification program.

Larkin, Marilyn. "Lead in mother's milk could lead to dental caries in children," *The Lancet*, vol 350, September 13, 1997.

organochlorines, used commercially in agriculture, act like estrogen and have been linked to breast cancer. Interestingly, 70 percent of women with breast cancer have no biological, hereditary, or behavioral risk factors for the disease. Recently, a study in *The Lancet* (December 18/25, 1999) found a correlation between exposure to organochlorines and pancreatic cancer.

In her book, *Chemical Sensitivity* (Keats Publishing 1995, $3.95), Dr Rogers explains that when pesticides break down, they produce substances called "metabolites." These metabolites are even more toxic than the neurotoxins and metabolic interrupters that kill pests. And because pesticides are so unstable, often they can't even be identified. "Pesticides are one of the main causes or contributors to the emergence of chemical sensitivity," she asserts.

Research oncologist Daniel Clark, MD, who advises hundreds of medical doctors worldwide on cancer protocols, agrees. He told me that many cancers start with exposure to environmental toxins. His mantra to the doctors who consult with him is: "Detoxify, and support the immune system." I would add to Dr. Clark's mantra: Reduce your exposure to all toxins in your home and yard.

A number of studies have shown a link between pesticides and

The Origin of Parkinson's Disease?

A family history of Parkinson's disease may be one cause for this condition, but researchers are finding that exposure to pesticides and herbicides may be another. Just about every study investigating the risk from chemical exposure has found that Parkinson's disease is increased three or four times when people who lived in rural areas or on farms were in regular contact with pesticides or herbicides.

The real connection may be a combination of these two factors. One hypothesis is that the herbicides and pesticides contain toxins that damage a portion of nerves, causing oxidation in cells known to be an element in Parkinson's. It seems very possible, say researchers, that there is a genetic defect in some people that prevents these toxins from being eliminated and allows them to damage cells. This would explain why Parkinson's runs in some families, and both how and why exposure to pesticides are involved.

Golbe, Lawrence. "Parkinson's disease: nature meets nurture," *The Lancet*, October 24, 1998.

childhood cancers — leukemias, lymphomas, neuroblastomas, and brain cancers. Children are exposed to pesticides by touching no-pest strips, walking on lawns sprayed with fungicides and herbicides, and getting into cupboards containing common household cleaning agents.

Peter Montague, writing for the Environmental Research Foundation, says there seems to be a strong link between brain cancers and products used to kill fleas and ticks — like pyrethrins (natural) and pyrethroids (synthetic pyrethrins: permethrin, tetramethrin, allethrin, resmethrin, and fenvalerate), and chlorpyrifos (known as Dursban).

Patricia Dines, author of *The Organic Traveler's Guide for Northern California* (Community Action Publications, 1998) suggests avoiding anything with chlorpyrifos, a widely used insecticide and neurotoxin banned by the EPA in June 2000 that can still be sold until December 2001. A survey of 1,000 people found that 82 percent of them had chlorpyrifos in their urine.

Adverse Drug Reactions

We have the Food and Drug Administration (FDA) to help regulate the safety of pharmaceuticals, but it cannot be fully responsible for keeping unsafe drugs off the market. You and your doctor need to help. Often there are side effects that are not reported to regulatory agencies like the FDA.

It's hard to believe, but true, that most drugs have been tested on only about 2,500 people before they're put on the market. Since we're each so different, this is a small sample of a population in need of a particular pharmaceutical.

Adverse drug reactions (ADR) are a major cause of death in our country, accounting for more than 100,000 deaths. This puts them right after heart disease, cancer, and stroke. Although some doctors are being more careful in monitoring drug doses, using multiple drugs could be causing this problem to remain high. About three-and-a-half percent of hospital admissions are due to ADRs, and 15 percent of patients in hospitals have to stay there longer because of adverse reactions.

Routledge, Philip, MD. "150 years of pharmacovigilance," *The Lancet,* vol 351, April 18, 1998.
Bonn, Dorothy. "Adverse drug reactions remain a major cause of death," *The Lancet,* vol 351, April 18, 1998.

Pesticides and Parkinson's

The connection between Parkinson's disease and pesticides is becoming stronger. A study out of Stanford University's School of Medicine looked at people who had recently been diagnosed with Parkinson's and their exposure to pesticides in their homes or gardens. The study of nearly 500 people found those who were exposed to insecticides in their homes were 70 percent more likely to get Parkinson's than those who had no exposure. The average amount of time of exposure was only 77 days — less than three months! Exposure of garden insecticides doubled a person's risk for developing Parkinson's. Herbicide exposure also increased risk for this disease. Exposure for 30 days resulted in a 40 percent increased risk for Parkinson's, while exposure for 160 days boosted the risk to 70 percent. Isn't this, alone, a good enough reason to move away from toxic products?

How to Identify Toxic Products

Look for the following words:
- Danger = the most toxic
- Warning = the next most toxic
- Caution = the least toxic — but still dangerous

Begin by replacing all products that say Danger or Warning with safer products.

Store all household cleansers and pesticides (synthetic or natural) where children and pets can't have access to them. Lock them up, if necessary.

Dispose all toxic products safely, through a Toxic Recycling Program in your area. Call your city hall to find out how and when you can do this. Do not bury them in your yard or put them in the trash where they can eventually pollute the water system.

What You Can Do

Stop buying products that say Danger or Warning. Replace them with safer products found in natural food stores as well as some supermarkets, hardware stores, and garden centers.

Become more aware. Read any book by Debra Lynn Dadd, such as *Home, Safe Home* (Putnam, 1997), for information about effective and safe alternatives to toxic products. For cleaning almost anything, I like the line of products made by Bi-O-Kleen (call 503-557-0216 for information on where these products are sold in your area). In addition to being non-toxic, they contain grapefuit seed extract that kills bacteria like E-coli. And they have no chemical smell of chlorine, ammonia, or artificial fragrances.

Buy and eat organic foods. Consumer's Union looked at the USDA's Pesticide Data program and found that the produce highest in pesticides included winter squash, peaches, apples, pears, grapes, green beans, spinach, and strawberries. Foods with low pesticide residues included bananas, broccoli, frozen peas, and corn. Use organic gardening methods to improve your soil and grow healthier plants. Read Dr. Sherry Rogers's book *Wellness Against All Odds* (Prestige Publishing, 1994) for information on how you can effectively detoxify these harmful chemicals from your body.

Chronic Fatigue and the Environment

An Australian research study conducted over a three-year period shows higher levels of organochlorines in the bodies of people with chronic fatigue syndrome (CFS) than in people who are not suffering from this condition. Whether these chemicals, which act like hormones in the body, are responsible for CFS or are simply adding to the toxic burden of the patient, is still unclear. High levels of organochlorines could be preventing the body from detoxifying or they may be collecting in the body as a result of an impaired detoxification system.

Toxic overload should, however, be considered as part of the treatment for any chronic condition. Whenever possible, organic foods should be eaten instead of those grown with chemicals. Pure, filtered water should be drunk regularly throughout the day. Stay away from tap water because chlorine is one of the chemicals that acts like estrogen in our bodies and may contribute to breast cancer and other health problems. Chlorine and other chemicals can be removed from shower water with a Hydro Spray shower head. (To order, call subscriber services at 800-728-2288.) And whenever possible, remember to use personal care and other household products that have the fewest chemicals.

Donohoe, Dr. Mark, MB, BS. *Our Toxic Times,* February 1996, p. 9. 406-547-2255.

What About the New Fruit and Vegetable Washes?

What about fruit and vegetable washes that claim to remove pesticides from food? First, they can't remove systemic poisons, only those applied externally. So organic is always best, but these washes may be valuable for anyone wanting to lower their exposure to toxins.

A representative from Proctor & Gamble, the company behind a fruit and vegetable wash called Fit, sent us an independent lab analysis that shows Fit actually does remove from 21-72 percent of pesticides that are not soluble in water. Bi-O-Kleen, a company with another produce wash made entirely from natural ingredients and sold in health food stores (Fit contains some synthetic chemicals), is in the process of getting laboratory tests to prove the effectiveness of its products in reducing pesticides. Both products do remove wax and bacteria such as E. coli.

Fluoride Alert!

Another common household product that could be damaging your health is fluoride. For many years now, fluoride has been one of the major additives to toothpaste and to the drinking water of many communities as a means to prevent dental cavities and help build strong teeth and bones. It's used more in toothpastes or given to children in liquid or tablets to keep their teeth strong and healthy.

But now, researchers are finding the reasoning for using this substance seems to be faulty. Not only does fluoride appear not to prevent dental decay or osteoporosis, it very likely contributes to cancer, gastrointestinal problems, and more.

Most people don't realize that sodium fluoride is a toxic waste by-product from aluminum manufacturing. Just as calcium was put on the nutritional map by the American Dairy Association when they were looking for a new way to market their products in the 1950s, fluoride came into our lives when the aluminum industry and fertilizer manufacturers needed a way to dispose of this toxic by-product. In fact, the original research indicating fluoride's benefits was funded by ALCOA and Reynolds Metals, as well as other aluminum manufacturing companies.

Just what is this elusive material called fluoride? It's any chemical containing fluorine, which is an irritating toxic gas. Fluorides are used in pesticides and fertilizers, the production of aluminum, Teflon, and in refrigerants such as freon. The most common fluorides used in drinking water (hydrofluosilicic acid and sodium silicofluoride) are toxic by-products from the manufacturing of phosphate fertilizers. They are added to drinking water without going through any refining process.

But Does Fluoride Really Work?

No, says a Canadian Dental Association panel, which came to the conclusion in 1987 that fluoride added to toothpaste and drinking water did not prevent tooth decay. They also found that fluoride often causes fluorosis, a condition that makes teeth mottled and brit-

---

Lead Toxicity and Hypertension

After I researched a recent article on hypertension, I came across this suspected link between exposure to lead and hypertension in women. One recent study of nearly 300 women in the Nurses' Health Study had blood tests and X-rays taken over a period of two years. The levels of lead that were revealed were compared with their blood pressure. The results indicated that there was, indeed, increased lead in women with hypertension — even after adjusting the data for a family history, dietary sodium, and other risk factors. The authors conclude that there is evidence that long-term, low levels of lead may lead to hypertension in women.

In my opinion: Low levels of lead can be absorbed by drinking wine out of a crystal glass or storing wine in a crystal decanter. Michael Murray, ND and Joseph Pizzorno, ND, in their book *Encyclopedia of Natural Medicine* (Prima Health, 1998, $24.95) point out that concentrations of lead increase with storage time. Environmental exposure may also be a factor and the only way to know if you have high lead levels is to be tested.

If you have hypertension or feel you're at risk for high blood pressure, ask your doctor to check you for high levels of lead. Bone lead concentrations help to identify chronic or past exposure. Concentrations in the blood can reveal acute or recent lead poisoning. A blood test could be a simple screening method that could identify your underlying cause for hypertension.

Houston, D.K. and M.A. Johnson. "Lead as a risk factor for hypertension in women," *Nutrition Review,* 57(9), 1999. From *Int'l Clin Nutr Review,* July 2000.

tle. Fluorosis is considered one of the most sensitive signs of fluoride poisoning. This year, the ministry of health and family welfare in India was so concerned over the danger of fluoride that they ruled that toothpastes containing fluorides need to carry a warning that children under the age of seven should not use them.

What about keeping bones strong? According to Dr. John Lee, a physician who has researched and written numerous articles about fluoride, there are more hip fractures in communities with fluoridated water than there are in communities with non-fluoridated water. Apparently, fluoride causes an inferior quality of bone formation which is weaker than bones which have not been exposed to fluoride. This means that while the bones may become more dense, they also become more brittle — and people are more prone to having bones break.

While a number of researchers have found increased hip fractures with levels of fluoride in drinking water exceeding one part per million (ppm), Dr. Lee has evidence that just one ppm fluoride caused more hip fractures in both men and women. The Environmental Protection Agency (EPA) raised the maximum amount of fluoride allowed in drinking water up to four ppm. It's not surprising to hear that pediatric orthopedists are now reporting more sports injuries — including stress fractures of the spine — in gymnasts and other active children.

All fluoride we ingest is not held in our bones or cells causing damage. Some is excreted. Adults excrete more fluoride than children and are holding more accumulated fluoride in their bones. I expect to see more children with brittle bones over the next decades. According to an Indian study, "Fluoride toxicity afflicts children more severely and after a shorter exposure to fluoride than adults, due to the greater and faster accumulation of fluoride in the metabolically more active growing bones of children."

Fluoride and the Cancer Connection

Fluoride has also been implicated in contributing to cancer. It damages chromosomes, says Dr. Lee, and inhibits proper enzyme function. When chromosomes have been sufficiently damaged, they can no longer regulate cell reproduction. While I can't say that fluoride causes cancer, it certainly appears to set the stage for rampant cell reproduction. A study at the University of Missouri indicated that just one ppm of fluoride in drinking water causes genetic damage.

In the state of Washington, studies listed in the appendices of a Department of Health and Human Services report showed a link between fluoridated water and cancer. Yet the two committees that reviewed this report stated, "There is no evidence of an association between fluoridation of water and cancer." Interestingly, the only people on these committees were dentists, doctors, and PhDs who were in favor of fluoridation. No fluoride opponents were asked to serve.

What You Can Do

Presently there is no control over how much fluoride a person is exposed to. In fact, by the year 2000, the Public Health Service is attempting to have 75 percent of all public drinking water fluoridated — despite 10 studies reviewed by the National Research Council showing no benefits from fluoride. The NRC even reviewed seven studies which showed evidence of increased hip fractures, but still concluded that four ppm of fluoride in water is acceptable.

To stop fluoridation of drinking water, you can write your senators and members of the House of Representatives, letting them know your views. If your town or city does not have fluoridated water, be alert and take action if you read or hear that it is being considered.

Mixing Prescription Drugs and Over-the-Counter Remedies

If you're seeing a doctor or other health-care provider, be sure to let her or him know about any herbs, over-the-counter remedies, or other self-care treatments you are using, since some of these shouldn't be mixed with prescription drugs. In some cases, such mixing can cause harmful interactions. For example, because of certain chemically based inhibiting properties, St. John's wort (an herb used for mild to moderate depression) shouldn't be used by patients taking anti-depressants such as Prozac.

It's bad enough that fluoride is in our toothpaste and drinking water, but that's just part of the problem. All canned foods that contain water produced in cities where the water is fluoridated contain additional fluoride. The more canned soups and juices you consume, the more fluoride you're adding to your diet unknowingly. In an article on fluoride in fruit juices published in the *Journal of Clinical Pediatric Dentistry* in 1991, white grape juice contained from three ppm to 6.8 ppm, while prune juice was around .26 and apple juice from .16 to 1.3 ppm. If you're regularly feeding juices to your child, look to see if it's reconstituted (meaning water has been added to a concentrate) or pure unreconstituted juice.

Condensed soups, if they were made with fluoridated water, should be avoided. When soups are condensed, water is boiled away, leaving all the fluoride. If your drinking water contains fluoride, you're adding back even more of this chemical when you reconstitute the soup. If you're not sure of a soup's fluoride content, contact the manufacturer and ask if the water they use in its preparation is fluoridated.

A Safer Environment?

When CFCs (chlorofluorocarbons) were found to contribute to the depletion of the ozone layer, other chemicals were substituted. HCFCs (hydrochloroflluorocarbons) are now used as a refrigerant for air conditioners, and in cleaning agents and industrial solvents and they don't harm the environment. The outer environment, that is.

But a recent study published in *The Lancet* indicates that people who worked around HCFCs and were exposed to very low levels frequently came down with a form of hepatitis and liver necrosis (necrosis means "death" or "dying"). Previously, HCFCs have been used in some anesthesias with few problems. Occasionally, someone who has been anaesthetized repeatedly with it will develop liver problems. It's the chronic low-level exposure that appears to be harmful.

The authors of this study urge that other substitutions for HCFCs be sought that are not carcinogenic to people or harmful to the environment. They also warn doctors to be on the lookout for liver diseases associated with this chemical, both in occupational settings and in the environment.

Hoet, Perrine, et al. "Epidemic of liver disease caused by hydrochlorofluorocarbons used as ozone-sparing substitutes of chlorofluorocarbons," *The Lancet,* August 23, 1997.

Teflon is also a fluoride. If you're cooking in Teflon pots or pans, stop. Never use the Teflon spray to re-coat them. Consider where the Teflon goes when it wears down. Most likely, in your foods.

By taking an active role in reducing the fluoride in your foods and beverages now, you can remain active with strong healthy bones later!

The Laxative Habit

Not to long ago, I received a heartbreaking letter from a subscriber about her sister who has had a lifelong habit of abusing laxatives. With the recent news that one of the ingredients of several popular laxatives, phenolphthalein, is carcinogenic, her sister was worried about getting cancer. (These products, including Ex-Lax, Evacu-U-lax, and Feen-a-mint, have since been reformulated.)

The sister has used laxatives for so many years that she can't have bowel movements without them. Many older persons, concerned with maintaining bowel regularity, also become laxative

Allergic to Your Cosmetics?

It's possible, even if you use a quality product, like Fruition Extra by Estee Lauder. This cosmetic was found to cause contact dermatitis on the eyelids or face of women in a number of countries. The culprit was a new synthetic compound used in some cosmetics called cystamine bislactamide, which first was used in the autumn of 1996. Estee Lauder has taken steps to remove this substance from their products, but other manufacturers may not be so quick to change their formulas.

We are alerting you to this situation because any cosmetic, even expensive quality items, may contain something to which you are sensitive. If your skin breaks out after using a particular product and stops when you stop using it, chances are there is something in that product you should avoid. Begin by contacting the manufacturer so they can take steps to follow up on your reactions with additional tests. If enough of us let them know we're getting rashes, instead of just not using their product, cosmetics will be reformulated.

Thank you, Estee Lauder, for being so quick to improve your product.

Borelli, S., et al. "Cystamine bislactamide: a cosmetic allergen," *The Lancet,* vol 351, June 20, 1998.

dependent. I'm worried about more health problems than cancer from relying on laxatives.

Why Women Use Laxatives

Some women use laxatives as a form of weight control. They think, erroneously, that by eliminating wastes in their colon they can keep their weight down. All they are doing is getting rid of the body's wastes more quickly. For women who have abdominal bloating, laxatives are tempting. They can often reduce bloating by reducing the bulk in their intestines. But bloating is often a sign of poor digestion. Perhaps digestive enzymes (either pancreatic or plant enzymes found in health food stores) would eliminate their bloating.

Some women use laxatives because they help them feel "empty and clean" inside, rather than full. One recent client of mine who abused laxatives was reluctant to stop them because she didn't want to feel full. She reduced her meal portions, took enzymes for a few weeks, and felt better without her laxatives than with them.

Then there are women who use laxatives because they're constipated. Often, constipation is a sign of a magnesium deficiency, and the only side effect of taking a lot of magnesium is soft, sometimes even runny, stools. I'll talk about using magnesium later. Constipation can also come from not eating enough fiber or not drinking enough water. Both are needed to bulk up and soften the stools so they can be easily eliminated. Exercise is another component if you're constipated. It's one way of tonifying all your muscles, including your intestines. Without tone, the intestines don't contract and push stools along to be eliminated.

Why the Laxative Habit Is Harmful

There are various kinds of laxatives, each having different properties. Some produce bulk, allowing the stools to become larger. As the stools touch the walls of the intestines, pressure builds up and they can be more easily passed — if there is tone in the intestinal muscles. Some laxatives are lubricants, which soften the stools. But the majority of the most popular laxatives — both over-the-counter and herbal — are irritants and stimulants. These act like sandpaper inside the colon, or repeatedly stimulate the nerves inside the colon. Taken occasionally, they should not cause any harm. Taken regularly, they irritate the lining of the intestines or cause a dependency on the stimulation. All laxatives reduce the natural tone in the muscles of the intestines and cause people to depend on them in order to have bowel movements.

Which Laxatives Do What?

Bulking agents like Metamucil and psyllium seed husks help the stools retain water. This, in turn, helps them get larger and often

---

Plastic Wrap for Foods

We've been wondering how long it would take before someone began to question the use of plastic wrap on foods. Some brands of polyvinyl cling wrap contain higher amounts of chemicals called endocrine disrupters, which leach from the plastic wrap into the foods and interfere with our hormones, than is considered safe. DEHA (di-(2-ethyl-hexyl) adipate) is one such chemical. This substance may contribute to cancer, reproductive problems, and some birth defects.

Consumer's Union, a group out of Washington, DC, tested the amount of DEHA in sliced cheese that had been wrapped in plastic at supermarkets. Nineteen pieces of cheese were analyzed, and seven, wrapped in PVC cling wrap, contained an average of 153 parts per million (PPM) of DEHA. Only 18 PPM is considered safe, according to the European Community's Scientific Committee for Food.

Children, with smaller bodies and a reduced tolerance for these chemicals, eat foods wrapped in plastic, and are probably at greatest risk. Eating more than 1 1/2 oz. of the cheeses with the most DEHA would exceed their safe daily dose.

In England, PVC wrap was replaced 10 years ago. I hope the FDA makes the same ruling in this country.

What about the plastic wrap you buy for home use? The CU tested seven brands. Reynolds Wrap contained DEHA. Other brands — Glad Crystal Clear, Duane Reade, Foodtown, Saran Wrap, America's Choice, and White Rose — did not. If you're using a safe brand, be sure you remove it before microwaving any food. High temperatures can transfer harmful chemicals into your food.

Stewart, Kim. "The future may not be in plastics," *Natural Foods Merchandiser*, March 1999, pg 22.

softer. But you need to drink plenty of water along with them. These bulk-forming laxatives can contribute to obstructions in the esophagus as well as the small and large intestines if the stools don't pass completely.

Many bulking agents contain sugar, which can cause an imbalance of friendly to unfriendly bacteria in your intestines (sugar feeds the bad guys). These bad bacteria, or pathogens, can contribute to gas and bloating.

Lubricants like mineral oil soften the stools, but they also can decrease your absorption of important oil-soluble nutrients, like vitamins A and E, and essential fatty acids. Large doses of mineral oil can also cause anal leakage, anal itching, and hemorrhoids.

Irritants and stimulants have a direct effect on the walls of the intestines, stimulating the nerves and blood vessels. Irritants act like sandpaper and can eventually reduce the sensitivity of these nerves, causing the intestines to lose their tone. Without tone, the muscles of the intestines can't contract on their own and help expel the stool without help.

Irritating laxatives include glycerin suppositories, castor oil, and two herbs — cascara sagrada and senna. Natural herbal laxatives are no safer than others. Any laxatives that are used regularly,

Safer Water

Nearly 75 percent of all drinking water in this country is chlorinated to kill bacteria. Unfortunately, chlorine by-products in water are carcinogenic. A group of 28,000 postmenopausal women in Iowa were evaluated for exposure to chlorine and a connection to getting cancer. The more chlorine they were exposed to, the greater their risk was for getting colon and other cancers.

Interestingly, the greatest exposure is not in the water we drink, but the water we bathe in. For that reason, if you get chlorinated city water or if you chlorinate your well water, I suggest you purchase an inexpensive shower de-chlorinator. This small attachment lasts for about a year and removes chlorine from shower water. It's a small price to pay to lower your risk for cancer. Plus it can get rid of itchy winter skin fast. To order one of these filters, call Subscriber Services at 800-728-2288.

Morris, Kelly. "Water, water, everywhere — but is it safe to drink?" *The Lancet,* August 23, 1997.

which cause irritation or stimulate the nerves in the intestines, can cause problems.

Safer Alternatives

Magnesium, especially magnesium citrate and oxide, helps attract water to the intestines, building pressure and allowing solid wastes to soften and be expelled more naturally. Overuse of magnesium, especially magnesium sulfate, could affect your fluid and electrolyte (sodium, potassium, chloride) levels. A number of alternative physicians believe the majority of people are magnesium-deficient.

Magnesium is found in nuts and legumes, as well as in whole grains. It is also a mineral our bodies need more of when we're under stress. I suggest taking enough magnesium to soften the stools, but not more than 1,000 mg daily, and only as much as you need for regular bowel movements. Be sure to drink plenty of fluids when you take magnesium.

Two kinds of fiber help with normal elimination — soluble and insoluble. Insoluble fiber, like wheat bran and the fiber found in celery, act like sandpaper. Don't overdo it. The idea is not to substitute Metamucil with wheat bran. Add soluble fiber, like rice bran (found in brown rice), oat bran (from oatmeal), and the skin on all beans, and you reduce the irritation in the intestines as well as increase the bulk of your stools. This means eating plenty of vegetables, beans (take Beano or other enzymes if they give you gas), whole grains (like brown rice and oats), and some fresh fruit with its skin.

Exercise helps you move all your muscles. As you move by walking, dancing, or swimming, even the muscles in your small and large intestines move. You want to tone your muscles, and this means more than firming up your biceps and triceps. It means bringing the ability to contract and relax back into your intestines after frequent laxative use. Get into the exercise habit, and work on your abdominal muscles to help firm out the outside of your tummy. Inside are your intestines. When you work your abdominals, you're toning your colon.

Psychological intervention is sometimes necessary for breaking a laxative habit, especially if it's related to body image, poor self-esteem, or other psychological issues. In such cases, laxative abuse is part of an eating disorder and requires developing a new outlook as well as new habits.

It seems harmless to use laxatives, but it's not. And bloating, gas, constipation, or infrequent bowel movements are often a sign that something's wrong. Look for the problem, then look for a natural solution. Modifying your diet, regular exercise, drinking more water, and perhaps taking digestive enzymes is the safest way to eliminate the problems caused by laxative abuse.

One of the Worst Toxins: Smoking

At her last public appearance, nutrition author Adelle Davis was wheeled onto the stage in a wheelchair at a national health convention to receive a lifetime achievement award. Her body was riddled with cancer. When asked why she had cancer, since all her

Ignoring Your Rights

The Environmental Protection Agency (EPA) and the United States Department of Agriculture (USDA) are putting out a brochure on pesticides. This brochure will talk about the benefits of these chemicals and their risks. But it may not address organic produce at all. Why? A number of powerful industry groups are asking the EPA/USDA to leave this out because it could confuse the public and cause people to question the safety of eating foods sprayed with pesticides. The groups that want to keep mention of organics out of the brochure are: The American Crop Protection Assn., American Farm Bureau Federation, Food Marketing Institute, Grocery Manufacturers of America, National Corn Growers Assn., National Food Processors Assn., and the United Fresh Fruit and Vegetable Assn.

So far, the EPA hasn't addressed organics, although I don't understand how this could have happened - except for strong lobbying groups like those mentioned above. Certainly, if this brochure doesn't mention organics, we can be sure the government is not interested in protecting our health. I'm looking forward to seeing the finished product.

Stewart, Kim. "Associations nix organics in consumer brochure," *Natural Foods Merchandiser*, October 1998.

writings were on nutrition, she said she didn't know. A friend of mine who had appeared on a TV show with her, and who was at this convention, was appalled. He knew she had been a chain smoker. Unfortunately, she was unable to admit it. That admission would probably have saved lives.

With all the news lately centered around the lawsuits brought against the tobacco industry, I don't have to tell you all the statistics proving how toxic smoking is to your health. In fact, I doubt many people believe that smoking isn't toxic — but they still smoke.

It's amazing to find out how many health conscious people still smoke. Whether or not you're one of them, chances are you know someone who is addicted to smoking and can't seem to stop. Since second-hand smoke has been found to be harmful, you have a strong interest in helping the people in your life break free from this addiction. And to do so, as in so many other areas we've looked at, the physiological and emotional aspects need to be addressed.

I spoke with a number of health-care practitioners who have an expertise in smoking and other addictions and came up with a three-point program unlike any you've heard of before that can help motivated people stop smoking. So use this program, or give it to a loved one who still smokes, and begin getting free of one of the most difficult addictions — nicotine.

Decide to Stop

First, get really clear and grounded in your desire to stop smoking. You have to want to stop smoking more than anything else. It is possible even if you've failed before. People fail because they don't want to stop, the technique they use is not right for them,

Higher Breast Cancer Risk for Smokers

A new study by the American Cancer Society indicates that a woman's risk of dying from breast cancer is 25 percent higher if she is a smoker. And that percent rises proportionally to the number of cigarettes smoked per day as well as the total number of years smoking. There is a 75 percent higher risk for women who smoke more than two packs a day.

or they didn't follow through. If you've tried one method and needed a combination of two or more, you probably failed. Be patient and decide now that you won't stop until you stop.

Prepare Yourself Emotionally

Spend the first two days paying attention. Think about how you feel now both physically and emotionally because you're smoking. Notice how often in the day your chest is tight or you can't breathe deeply. Notice your energy. The color of your complexion. Think about how you will feel when you're no longer smoking. You'll have more energy, more lung capacity. Your shortness of breath will lessen and disappear. Your circulation will improve and your skin will have a healthier glow. You'll slow down your aging process, both the visible and the invisible. Your heart and liver will get stronger and healthier, and your lungs will stop hardening.

For the next two days, look at the habits you've formed around smoking and change them. You smoke at specific times: after a meal, before a meeting, during a break. One friend who stopped

---

Women and Second-Hand Smoke

Women non-smokers living with partners who smoke are at twice the risk for coronary heart disease (CHD) as men in a similar situation, according to a new analysis of a study by the American Cancer Society. And these same women are 10 times more likely to die from heart disease than their female counterparts who are not living with smokers.

In the past, studies have shown that passive smoking does not increase CHD, but these studies, instigated by cigarette manufacturers, included people who had smoked at any time in their lives, not people who were currently smoking. If you're living with someone who used to smoke, but doesn't now, you're not at any increased risk for heart disease.

Often, studies are conducted or financed by vested interest groups and are not accurate. This is one case in point. It is now estimated that deaths from heart disease caused by passive smoke are 10 times more prevalent than deaths from lung cancer. Because children's lungs are more tender than adults,' they should not be exposed to a smoky environment. Just because you don't smoke doesn't mean you're not at risk for heart disease. Ask all smokers among your family and friends to smoke outdoors.

smoking noticed he would get to a regular meeting early and have a cigarette. Now he shows up a little late and has no time to smoke. If you smoke after a meal, substitute a cigarette for a sliced apple or chew on a toothpick. Better still, get up and take a 10-minute walk. You may feel uncomfortable for a while, but notice that discomfort and distract yourself. It's not easy, but it's possible.

Get Help

Psychologist Sheila Horowitz, MA, MFCC, says that studies show more success in stopping smoking when people join a support group. No support group in your area? Call a few friends and get together once a week to support one another. Give each other tips that have worked — even temporarily — and listen to their struggles and successes. Get a buddy you can call when the urge to smoke is greatest, and call her.

Use other resources like hypnotherapy. Look for a hypnotherapist in your area who has been successful with smokers. Make sure the person you work with has a good track record with this particular habit. My favorite resource to help change emotional habits is EMDR.

1-EMDR — The Quick Way

EMDR (Eye Movement Desensitization and Reprocessing) is a technique practiced by some psychiatrists and psychotherapists that actually reprograms your brain and changes how you feel. It helps remove mental or emotional obstacles that contribute to your desire to smoke so your craving or your stress response is forever changed. And it's done by using a simple tapping technique while you're thinking about the situation you want to change.

Some people are able to stop smoking through EMDR after only a few sessions. This technique is powerful. EMDR has been used successfully in numerous studies of people with post traumatic stress disorder. In some cases, only three sessions were needed to alleviate the devastating effects of trauma. EMDR is practiced by highly trained therapists and is a quick way of handling the emotional side of smoking without lengthy psychotherapy sessions. You can find a therapist who uses EMDR by calling the EMDR Institute, Inc. in Pacific Grove, CA (831-372-3900 extension 16). Or e-mail them at www.inst@emdr.com. I have personally found EMDR extremely effective for a lifelong nail biting habit. One single session, six months ago, eliminated over 50 years of biting my nails! If you don't want to use EMDR or hypnotherapy, look for another method for dealing with the emotions behind your habit of smoking.

Curbing the Craving

The nicotine patch: The media is filled with claims about the nicotine patch—that little band-aid-like device you tape to your arm. Because it slowly delivers nicotine through the skin there is less craving for cigarettes. If you're determined to stop, the patch can help you. But remember that nicotine is still getting into your body. While it won't hurt your lungs, it still affects your heart and bones. Nicotine is a poison used commercially as an insecticide. If you need to use it temporarily, by all means, do. The patch is better than smoking.

Acupuncture: Some acupuncturists specialize in using acupuncture to reduce the cravings of tobacco. But just putting needles in certain acupuncture points is not enough. Acupuncturist Leah R. Martino, O.M.D., L.Ac., who practices in a hospital in

---

Smoking and Appendicitis

As far-fetched as it may sound at first, researchers in Great Britain have found a strong association between exposure to tobacco smoke and incidents of appendicitis. The researchers took their information from over 5,000 people who were in a 1970 study that followed the lives of everyone born between April 5 and April 11, 1970, living in Great Britain. Study participants whose mothers smoked for five years or longer had significantly more inflammation of their appendix than those whose mothers did not smoke. The risk increased with adults who became smokers themselves and who smoked daily when they were 26 years of age. The researchers suspect that tobacco smoke disables an immune response, leaving the appendix more vulnerable to inflammation.

Montgomery, Scott M., et al. "Smoking in adults and passive smoking in children are associated with acute appendicitis," *The Lancet,* vol 353, January 30, 1999.

Northern California, has had extensive experience and success in helping people stop smoking using a five-step program she developed. This consists of an initial telephone consultation, providing the patient with initial information, the acupuncture treatments, herbal treatment, and a six-month maintenance program.

If you can find an acupuncturist in your area with experience in this area, give it a try. If you can't find anyone with experience you may want to send for Dr. Martino's protocol which indicates the acupuncture points and treatment protocol she has found to be effective. The herbs she has used, as well as where they may be ordered from, is included in this protocol. When I spoke with Dr. Martino she was overwhelmed with work and did not want to be contacted directly. But you can access her protocol through the Internet at www.accupuncture.com.

Homeopathy: Nico-End is a homeopathic formula found in natural food stores made by Enzymatic Therapy that reduces your cravings for tobacco. The people at Enzymatic Therapy are so convinced it will work that they offer a complete money-back guarantee if you're not satisfied with the results. When I talked with the

---

Mothers Who Smoke

The writers of an article in the *Archives of Pediatric and Adolescent Medicine* claim that "more young children are killed by parental smoking than by all unintentional injuries combined." This includes, but is not limited to, exposure to second-hand smoke. Another factor is due to the health problems that arise from pregnant women who smoke.

Women who smoke more than half a pack of cigarettes daily during pregnancy are four times more likely to find conduct disorders in their boy babies than women who don't smoke. Over 175 boys from 7-12 years of age were studied over six years. Those boys whose mothers smoked 10 or more cigarettes a day had significantly increased conduct disorders. I don't know what effect this has on girls, but I do know that when you smoke, you lower the amount of oxygen that gets to the brain of a fetus, and this can affect the way their brain neurons work. Don't take chances. If you're a smoker, stop during your pregnancy. And then, don't start back!

Moore, Peter. "Smoking in pregnancy linked with conduct disorder," *The Lancet*, vol 350, July 19, 1997.

people at Enzymatic Therapy they suggested you try it for at least three months. By itself, Nico-End may or may not be enough. But used with techniques that address the emotional aspects of smoking, it can be a huge help.

One box of 60 tablets of Nico-End costs around $13.50. You can take three a day, but the people I spoke with suggested you might need up to eight tablets a day at first. Don't be afraid to take this amount. Remember, there's a money-back guarantee.

Like all homeopathics, Nico-End should not be used half an hour before or after ingesting strong substances like mint (including toothpaste), garlic, caffeine. It's best to not eat anything half an hour before or after using homeopathics. While there have been no studies on the results from using Nico-End, the folks at Enzymatic Therapy discontinue products that people don't buy, and people are buying lots of Nico-End.

I know it's not easy to stop smoking, but of all the risk factors for serious degenerative diseases, smoking is at the top of the list. I urge you to use this integrated program that has a much better than average chance for success, rather try one method and hope it works. You've failed before. It's time to succeed now.

Overcoming Toxins

I started this chapter talking about how these and many other toxins can affect different people differently. You've probably seen some of these sensitivities in your own life. Funny thing is, I've seen people who smoked every day of their adult life who still lived to 100 and didn't even die of lung cancer or another disease associated with smoking. They just aren't sensitive to the smoke. But the truth is, the vast majority of smokers do die from complications arising from a constant exposure to smoke. So if you want to get healthy or stay healthy you have to get these toxins out of your life as much as you can.

Cigarette smoke is probably the easiest of the toxins to identify. Others, though, are much more difficult to identify. So if you have a sensitivity that's causing you some health problems, you need to look at your sensitivity as a gift and see what it has to teach you. While some children become less sensitive to allergens as they get older, adults tend to have more reactions. So what can you do?

Begin at the Beginning

Look back at the start of your symptoms, or, if they've become worse, when they worsened. What changed around that time? Were you under more stress? Stress causes your body to use up more nutrients (the B vitamins, zinc, and magnesium, for example) that support your immune system. Did you eat different foods? You may have eaten or done something that eventually created your problem.

Take responsibility for finding a solution and making changes. Don't assume it's all in your mind, or that you're mistaken. You know your body better than anyone else. This is the time to begin trusting your impressions.

We used to believe that doctors had all the answers. Now I see that the best doctors admit they don't have as much information as they'd like. As much as you'd like to go to someone who can "fix" you, you're in the best position to do it. You know even your most subtle symptoms. If you're willing to get better, you can sometimes tap into your body's innate intelligence and get information that even the best laboratory tests may miss — although they can be very helpful in confirming or denying the existence of a problem. I'm all in favor of checking everything out.

Identify the problem. Do you just get a reaction when you eat a particular food or do you get gas after eating anything? Do you have a digestive problem? Remember, chewing better can clear up a myriad of complaints, including allergies, by allowing you to better digest your foods. Are you getting sick more often than you used to? Perhaps your immune system needs a boost. Maybe you have been poisoned. Look at your work and home environment to find possible culprits. In some parts of the country, pathogenic bacteria, molds, and fungi are causing severe illnesses.

Research what you can do about your problem. The Internet is one place to look. Books by Sherry A. Rogers, MD, a physician who specializes in environmental illnesses, is another. These include: *Wellness Against All Odds* (Prestige Publishing, Syracuse, N.Y., 1994) and *Tired or Toxic?* (Prestige Publishing, 1990). For a list of other physicians who are familiar with immune problems, contact The American Academy of Environmental Medicine, P.O. Box 16016, Denver, CO 80216.

Finally, make whatever changes you can. Begin slowly, if necessary and don't be reluctant to seek out expert help if you feel stuck. Get whatever testing you can to show where you were when you started and how much you're progressing.

Most important, never give up! The solution to your health condition is the last thing you try. If you stop before trying it, you may miss out on how it feels to feel better.

One Final Suggestion: Detoxify Your Liver

Because your liver has more than 300 tasks it performs throughout every day, and because it is one place in your body where toxins that don't know how to be eliminated are stored, I recommend that you detoxify your liver. Simply take some of the chemical burden off the liver and your whole body functions better.

If you ingest foods with pesticides and insecticides, you might think they are just traveling through your body. But your body can only eliminate toxins when the usual channels, liquid waste, solid waste, breath, and skin are working optimally. Otherwise, the liver, along with fat cells and kidneys, ends up storing many uneliminated toxins.

In the past, people thought that fasting was the only way to detoxify. That isn't true. There are many ways to help the body release trapped substances that tend to break down, rather than build up, our health. Spring is the time of year when nature rejuvenates itself after a long winter, and it's also the best time of year to rejuvenate your liver (the Chinese call spring Liver Time). You should view this liver renewal through detoxification as a tune-up of sorts — one to do can do each and every spring. Some aspects of this detoxification plan you may be doing already. Others you may want to add.

Liquid Waste: Water helps move unwanted substances out of your body. How much is enough? Try drinking half a glass per hour, not two or three glasses at a time. Small amounts of water sipped throughout the day whenever your mouth is a little dry (pay attention — your body will tell you when it wants more liquid) will allow you to eliminate rather than store some unnecessary substances. Good, pure water is better than any other liquid for this purpose. If you drink coffee or tea, the caffeine acts as a diuretic. This means you need more water than I've suggested to replenish what the caffeine eliminates, and to help move out toxins. Many women say they can't drink more water because they don't like all the urinating that follows. That's the idea, though. Every time you go to the bathroom, you get rid of toxic substances and allow your kidneys to regulate your fluid levels. That's why drinking more water often gets rid of edema.

Cadmium Toxicity and Bone Loss

Cadmium is a toxic mineral, called a "heavy metal" that can cause serious health problems. Cigarette smoke, water pipes, storage batteries, dental materials, and some ceramics, contain cadmium.

A recent study in *The Lancet* indicates that even a low exposure to environmental cadmium may lead to the demineralization of bones, increasing their fragility. Cadmium has a 10- to 30-year half-life, meaning that environmental exposure is often higher than it seems, especially in industrial areas where airborne cadmium particles may be present. One way of determining lifetime cadmium exposure is through a 24-hour urine test.

Recently, over 1,000 people in Belgium were evaluated for cadmium levels and tested for bone disorders including osteoporosis (brittle bones) and osteomalacia (soft bones). The result showed that low to moderate environmental exposure to cadmium is linked to an increase in broken bones. The authors suggest that even a low degree of exposure can increase bone fragility. You may not live in or near an industrial site where cadmium gets into the air, but if you smoke, or are around second-hand smoke, this exposure to cadmium may be increasing your osteoporosis risk. Taking measures, such as more magnesium and weight-bearing exercise, to help keep your bones healthy are strongly recommended.

Staessen, Jan A., et al, "Environmental exposure to cadmium, forearm bone density, and risk of fractures: prospective population study," *The Lancet,* vol 353, April 3, 1999.Haas, Elson M., MD. Staying Healthy With Nutrition, Celestial Arts, Berkeley, CA, 1992.

Solid Waste: Before unfriendly bacteria, gasses, and toxic materials formed in the digestive process can be eliminated, you need a diet high in roughage. Not from Metamucil or psyllium husks, but from your diet. The fiber found in beans, fresh fruits, and vegetables helps move this unwanted debris out of your body.

Breathing: Even if you can't exercise for some reason, you can sit in a chair in an upright position and breathe deeply. Fill your lungs from the bottom, to the middle, to the top. Hold your breath for a few seconds and slowly exhale. Cleansing breaths may be combined with walking and other exercise, or done alone. Begin by breathing deeply for a few minutes. Increase gradually to 15-30 minutes. Done on a regular basis, the resulting health benefits can be impressive.

Skin and Lymphatic System: Your skin is the largest organ in your body, and your lymphatic system lies just underneath its surface. One sign that a cleansing program would be appropriate is having your skin break out for no apparent reason. Massage (whole body or feet only) and activities that produce sweating (such as exercise, steam rooms, and hot baths) are all ways to encourage your body to move out toxins, especially those near the skin surface. Ideally, your sweat-producing activity should be followed by a shower to completely remove any toxins remaining on the skin. This prevents the toxins from being reabsorbed.

You can give yourself a quick dry massage with a clean loofa sponge or natural bristle brush. This stimulates the circulation and eliminates dead skin from the surface of this huge organ. Vigorously drying all over (especially fatty areas) with a towel after bathing or showering has a similar effect and can be easily incorporated into your daily routine.

A Cleansing Diet: The first part of a cleansing diet is to eliminate toxic substances, which you should already be doing. This means there's less to eliminate on an on-going basis. Avoid chemicals and preservatives and any unnecessary drugs (of course, talk with your doctor before stopping any prescribed medications). Next, eliminate any foods to which you are allergic or sensitive. In many people, the first foods to eliminate would be wheat and dairy. However, not everyone has a problem with these foods. Foods that are deep-fried should be eliminated for now, and both refined foods (white sugar, white flour) and fats should be reduced. Concentrate on eating more vegetables and fruits with a little protein and starch. Hearty vegetables like winter squashes and potatoes can fill you up, allowing you to feel satisfied as you reduce the satisfying fats. Drink plenty of fluids in the form of diluted juices (1/2 juice and 1/2 water), soups, and herb teas. Also use a cleansing tonic.

For more detailed information on general, as well as special-

Environmental Estrogens and Your Health

For 15 years, the U.S. National Institute of Environmental Health Sciences has been looking at the effects of estrogen-like substances found in the environment on the people and wildlife. There is some concern that synthetic estrogens and the increased number of industrial products which have estrogen-like properties are contributing to breast cancer, endometriosis, testicular cancer, and low sperm counts.

It was found that while some estrogenic compounds show only slight estrogenic effects when they are tested alone, they may have significant activity when they are tested together. There are many chemicals, which have estrogenic activity, which are found in detergents, pesticides, herbicides, and toiletries. They are abundant in the commercially grown fruits and vegetables we eat and in our lakes and streams where they are affecting fish and wildlife.

We have seen an increase in some of these estrogen-like chemicals called organochlorines in breast tissues of women with breast cancer. Normal breast tissue contains fewer organochlorines than cancerous tissue. In addition, organochlorines are suspected to play a role in the increased incidence of lower sperm counts and testicular cancer in American men during the past 20 years.

While chemically created estrogen–like substances seem to contribute to a cumber of health problems, phytoestrogens found in plants have the opposite effect. They may actually be protective against cancer. Foods high in phytoestrogens include all beans and unrefined grains (brown rice, oatmeal, whole wheat). One participant at the most recent conference on estrogens and the environment, Kenneth Setchell of the University of Cincinnati, spoke of research that indicates that soy protein could both help treat and prevent breast cancer. With so many new soy-based foods on the market, from soy hot dogs, soy cheese, and braised tofu in sauces, it may be time for you to introduce them into your family's eating plan. Or just eat more bean salads, lentil soup, and fat-free burritos.

ized and specific detoxification and cleansing programs, read *Natural Detoxification: The Complete Guide to Clearing Your Body of Toxins* by Jacqueline Krohn, MD (Hartley & Marks Publishers, Vancouver, BC, 1996).

Putting It All Together

Okay. So it all sounds great. But where do you start and how long do you keep all this up?

Start by implementing three or more of the items below (which you are not currently doing), into your routine for the next 30 days:

• Every day drink around four ounces of water an hour whenever possible. (This should be a lifetime habit.)

• Increase dietary roughage, aiming for daily regularity. (This too, should be a lifetime habit.)

• Set aside 5-15 minutes daily for cleansing breaths. (For the next 30 days, then as desired.)

• Get a full-body or foot massage monthly, give yourself an optional overall dry loofa or brush massage weekly, and train yourself to towel dry vigorously after every bath and shower. (Can be continued indefinitely.)

• Induce yourself to sweat every third day using the method of your choice, exercise, hot bath, etc. (For the next 30 days, then as desired.)

• Follow the cleansing diet. (For 30 days, then as desired.)

As we take time to take better care of our bodies, we become more in tune with them. During the course of this 30-day program, headaches and other complaints can disappear, only to return. That can be a message to resume what you were doing. Experiment a little and you may discover it is one factor, or a combination, that can chase away a problem forever.

Even the simple urge to "spring clean" your house can be your body's way of telling you it actually wants cleaning. And an intensive cleaning of your house does, of course, include some of the same elements of a detox plan. It can work up a sweat, make you thirsty so you drink more water, and hours of scrubbing (no toxic cleaners, please) can produce deep cleansing breathing. Best of all, you don't have to wait for spring to start making changes. You can do them anytime. Just use spring as a time to evaluate and modify aspects of the detox program to fit your needs. You'll be glad you did.

Chapter 2

Is Your Food Killing You?

Most people don't consider their food to be a toxin, but it can be. As you'll see in the next two chapters, the food you're eating and the additives in your food could be causing your sickness. This doesn't mean you should be paranoid of all food, but it does mean you need to be aware of potential dangers and how to avoid them. Let's take a look at some of the things that could be keeping you sick.

What You Can Do About E. Coli and Other Food-Borne Illnesses

The most infamous type of toxin you'll find in your food is E. coli. E. coli and other bugs are the bacteria that cause food poisoning. Food poisoning, which sometimes results in death, is more common than you realize. The Centers for Disease Control receive about 40,000 diagnosed cases a year — 1,000 of them are fatal. Unreported cases could raise this number into the millions.

Food poisoning is caused by pathogenic (bad) bacteria that are found in meat, poultry, fish, eggs, tofu, corn, mushrooms, refried beans, and other vegetables. You can't escape these bacteria, but you can reduce their numbers and increase your body's ability to fight them off without your getting sick.

With the outbreak of E. coli in hamburgers in 1993, and more recently in unpasteurized apple juice, we are becoming more aware of one of the many disease-carrying bacteria that can affect our health. After children died from eating hamburgers tainted with E.

coli, the Food Safety and Inspection Service (FSIS), an agency in the U.S. Department of Agriculture, increased the guidelines for handling meat and poultry last year. But even the best procedures will not protect you and your family completely. Although you may feel helpless, you are not. There's a lot you can do.

Better Kitchen Hygiene

There are three ways you can become infected by bacteria and viruses on food: by handling raw meats, poultry, and fish; by eating these products raw or rare; and by contaminating other foods, like produce and bread through "cross-contamination," the most frequent cause of food poisoning. Here's how to avoid the above scenarios:

✔ Don't fix a salad on a kitchen counter that has not been properly cleaned.

✔ Don't let animal products sit and leak their juices on the counter.

✔ Bacteria on raw meat and poultry are not destroyed by cooking. When these foods are not refrigerated quickly enough, the bacteria can multiply. Refrigerate them quickly in a cold (40 degrees or colder) refrigerator.

✔ Don't let foods of animal origin sit on the kitchen counter either before preparing a meal or afterward. Refrigerate leftovers immediately after eating. The spores of some bacteria can survive cooking, and will multiply when the food reaches the proper temperature during the cooling process.

✔ Produce may have contaminants on them from the soil or unclean irrigation water and can be rinsed in a bath of Clorox and water (1/2 tsp. of Clorox in a gallon of water; allow produce to sit for 15-25 minutes, then rinse in clear water) or a citric acid product like BioCleanse or Citricidal. This, however, only destroys surface contaminants.

Further Precautions

✔ Avoid all raw animal products, including oysters, steak tartare, sushi, raw dairy, and raw eggs in breakfast shakes, Caesar salad dressing, and Hollandaise sauce. Don't buy or use cracked eggs.

✔ Put meat, poultry, or fish in another plastic bag while you're in the market to prevent their drippings (and bacteria) from getting on any other foods. Keep the food in these plastic bags until you're ready to use them.

✔ Refrigerate perishable foods immediately. Don't run errands if you have bags of groceries sitting in the car.

✔ Cook all animal products well, especially if your immune system is compromised, if you are pregnant, elderly, or making food for children. Egg dishes should not be runny or soft. Cook ground beef, ground chicken or turkey, and all sausages well. They are handled frequently, which can cause bacteria to grow throughout the meat.

✔ Wash your hands and kitchen utensils well in hot soapy water before and after handling animal products.

✔ Use a clean sponge to wash your dishes and counters. Disinfect them, regularly by soaking them for five minutes in a solution of nine parts water to one part of chlorine bleach.

✔ Use two cutting boards — one for meat, another for produce, and disinfect regularly.

✔ Microwaves don't cook evenly, so don't cook animal products in them.

Strengthen Your Body With Good Bacteria

Ultimately, the best defense against E. coli and other harmful bacteria in food is a strong immune system. This fact explains in large part why the fatalities from the E. coli-contaminated hamburgers in 1993, and the recently tainted apple juice were all children. Their immune systems are still developing, leaving them more vulnerable to pathogenic bacteria contamination. Persons with compromised immune systems are also especially vulnerable.

A strong immune system is based in the intestinal tract. It contains from 400 to 500 different species of microorganisms. Some are helpful, others are harmful pathogens. We're not born with these good bacteria. Babies pick up one, Bifidobacteria, from their mothers as they travel through the birth canal and by drinking breast milk. C-section babies who are not breast-fed, may become children who do not have sufficient beneficial bacterial to protect themselves from E. coli, salmonella, and other pathogenic bacteria.

The amount of friendly bacteria found in breast milk is affected by the amount in the mother's intestinal tract. Today, laboratory tests are showing numerous people with no beneficial bacteria in their intestines. (Your doctor can analyze the quantity of your friendly bacteria through Great Smokies Diagnostic Laboratory, 800-522-4762, one of the most accurate labs.)

After a child is weaned, another strain of microorganisms, Lactobacillus acidophilus, enters the intestines from food, the environment, and human contact. Eventually, balance is achieved, and colonies of Lactobacillus remain more prevalent in the small intestines throughout our life, while Bifidobacteria predominates in the large intestines. The average person with healthy colonies is carrying around several pounds of bacteria in his or her intestinal tract.

Antibiotics Contribute to Problems

Broad spectrum antibiotics or chemotherapy, destroy some helpful bacteria and leave places in the intestines for pathogens to grow. An article in the *Annals of Internal Medicine,* reported that the reason harmful bacteria, like E. coli, may be appearing in greater numbers in our bodies could be because they are becoming more resistant to penicillin. Antibiotics have been used for more than 40 years in factory-farmed animals like beef and dairy cattle to reduce pathogenic bacteria. But these harmful bacteria don't just cooperate and die off, they mutate into other strains, which may require stronger antibiotics. Over time, many harmful bacteria become better able to withstand the drugs designed to keep them in check.

Adding Friendly Bacteria

First feed the beneficial bacteria you already have. This will enable them to flourish, keeping the pathogens in check. Eat lots of fresh produce. Oligosaccharides, sugars found in vegetables and fruits, help beneficial Bifidobacteria grow in your colon. These bacteria aid in forming healthy stools, and improve the breakdown and utilization of fats. When you eat refined sugar from cookies, cakes, candies, and ice cream, you're feeding more pathogens and less of the good bacteria.

Include fermented milk products in your diet, like yogurt and kefir. While most people believe all yogurt is high in Lactobacillus acidophilus, it actually is higher in Lactobacillus bulgaricus — a bacteria that helps bifido and acidophilus thrive.

Sauerkraut and miso soup contain beneficial bacteria. If you like them, add them to your diet. Lactobacillus acidophilus and Bifidobacteria contain the highest potencies in the refrigerated section of health food stores. Tablets or capsules that do not need to be refrigerated are usually lower in potency. The strongest product I've found is Healthy Trinity, by Natren, Inc. (800-992-3323).

Which Variety Is Needed and When?

Bifidobacteria: Babies and nursing mothers need Bifidobacterium infantis, one of the predominant bacteria found in babies' intestines. Add it after any exposure to antibiotics, and use it with babies who are formula-fed.

Acidophilus: Children who show signs of deficiency of helpful bacteria, like thrush or colic, can take acidophilus as soon as they're eating solid foods. Consider using acidophilus after vaccinations.

Both: Women can increase their absorption of nutrients and protect themselves from getting infections by taking acidophilus regularly. Use it after any course of antibiotics to prevent vaginitis. Because acidophilus lives mostly in the small intestines and vagina, and Bifidobacteria lives in the large intestines, take both.

Take responsibility for living in an imperfect world swarming with bacteria — good guys and bad guys. With a little more effort, you and your family can remain healthy no matter what food-borne illness appears.

Fish: Is It Fit for
Female (and Male) Consumption?

Swordfish and shark taste great — especially grilled or broiled. Plus they're a low-fat source of protein and omega-3 fatty acids. But reports that these and some other large predatory fish may contain methyl mercury levels in excess of the Food and Drug Administration's one part per million (ppm) limit has dampened some fish lovers' appetites.

Adding to this newfound caution, scientists responsible for seafood safety are also concerned about the safety of eating these types of fish. Some experts believe the FDA's one ppm limit is too liberal, but the FDA contends that in general, fish is safe, provided it is eaten infrequently (no more than once a week) as part of a balanced diet. To date, safe levels of methyl mercury in fish have yet to be established for lack of research.

So what should you do? Before we answer that question, let's

Why You Crave Fats and Sugars

Many women crave high-fat foods because they have a need for essential fatty acids, specific fats that support the immune system and contribute to a healthy reproductive system (before and after menopause). These fats are found in highest quantities in flaxseed and raw walnuts. Try grinding one to three tablespoons of flaxseed in a seed or coffee grinder and adding it to your breakfast cereal or a glass of juice. Or add two or three walnuts to your cereal or salad. It may reduce your fat cravings. If you need more essential fatty acids, you may actually lose weight after you begin adding them to your diet.

Some people crave fats or sugar as a learned response. When fatty or sweet foods were given as a reward or just part of a normal everyday diet for years, our taste buds become accustomed to them. By reducing fats or sugars for a few weeks, often the craving goes away. But reduce fats and sugars in a diet high in whole grains, beans, and vegetables — high in nutrients. Then, if you have a favorite food that is high in fats, you're better off eating a little of it once in a while, and stick to a diet of low-fat natural foods for your daily regime. No low-fat, fat-free, or sugar-free fake food can take the place of the real thing.

take a look at a couple of general guidelines for fish consumption, along with the mercury levels of various fishes you're likely to encounter at the fish market. The FDA's contention that fish is basically safe is true, but it's important to minimize your risk of methyl mercury exposure — especially if you are pregnant or of child-bearing age.

The first guideline for consuming fish is that bigger is usually not better. Larger, predatory fish such as swordfish and shark tend to have the highest methyl mercury levels while smaller fish tend to have lower levels. Second, freshwater fish are usually lower in methyl mercury than marine, or saltwater, fish.

Mercury Is Everywhere

Mercury occurs naturally in the environment. And nearly all fish contain trace amounts of methyl mercury, some more than others. In areas where there is industrial mercury pollution, the levels in the fish can be quite elevated. This most frequently occurs in some large predatory fish, which are exposed to higher levels of methyl mercury from their prey. Certain species of very large tuna, typically sold as fresh steaks or sushi, can have levels over one ppm. (Canned tuna, composed of smaller species of tuna such as skipjack and albacore, has much lower levels of methyl mercury, averaging only about 0.17 ppm.)

FDA toxicologists say the one ppm limit for commercial fish is considerably lower than levels of methyl mercury in fish that have caused illness.

When humans are exposed to high levels of methyl mercury, poisoning and problems in the nervous system can occur. The types of symptoms reflect the degree of exposure. Paresthesia, a numbness or tingling sensation around the lips, fingers, and toes, is usually the first symptom.

A stumbling gait and difficulty in articulating words is the next progressive symptom, along with a constriction of the visual fields ultimately leading to tunnel vision and impaired hearing. Generalized muscle weakness, fatigue, headache, irritability, and inability to concentrate often occur. In severe cases, tremors or jerks are present. These neurological problems frequently lead to coma and death.

The best indexes of human exposure to methyl mercury are concentrations in hair and blood. The average concentration of total mercury in nonexposed people is about eight parts per billion (ppb) in blood and two ppm in hair. From Japanese studies, toxicologists learned that the lowest mercury level in adults associated with toxic effects (paresthesia) was 200 ppb in blood and 50 ppm in hair, accumulated over months or years of eating contaminated food.

Methyl Mercury and Pregnancy

Expecting mothers and women of child-bearing age who may become pregnant should take methyl mercury levels seriously. It is not clear what effect, if any, there is on fetuses who are overexposed, but FDA toxicologist Mike Bolger, PhD, explains, "During prenatal life, humans are susceptible to the toxic effects of high methyl mercury exposure levels because of the sensitivity of the developing nervous system." Methyl mercury easily crosses the placenta, and the mercury concentration rises to 30 percent higher in fetal red blood cells than in those of the mother.

"But none of the studies of methyl mercury poisoning victims have clearly shown the level at which newborns can tolerate exposure," says Bolger. "It is clear that at exposure levels that affect the fetus, adults are also susceptible to adverse effects. What is not clear is the effect, if any, on fetuses at much lower levels — those that approach current exposure levels through normal fish consumption."

The FDA and the National Institute of Environmental Health Sciences are supporting a study by the University of Rochester to gather conclusive data on the effects of long-term exposure to low levels of methyl mercury in the fetus and infant. The study is being conducted in the Seychelles Islands, off the coast of East Africa in the Indian Ocean.

Fish is the major source of protein for people in the Seychelles Islands. Begun about 10 years ago, the study focuses on the approximately 700 pregnancies that occur on the islands each year. It also tracks women from pregnancy to childbirth and monitors the babies' consumption of breast milk. As children grow older, they are followed for any signs of nervous system disorders. Reports from the Seychelles study are not ready for publication, but Bolger expects the results to make a significant contribution to the consideration of whether further regulatory controls or other actions may be needed.

How Much Is Too Much?

If you are pregnant or could become pregnant, the FDA advises you limit your consumption of shark and swordfish to no more than once a month. The first trimester of pregnancy appears to be the most critical period of exposure for the fetus. Dietary practices immediately before pregnancy would have a direct bearing on fetal exposure during the first trimester.

For all other persons, FDA toxicologists recommend limiting regular consumption of fish species with methyl mercury levels around one part per million (ppm) to about seven ounces per week (about one serving). For fish with levels averaging 0.5 ppm, regular consumption should be limited to about 14 ounces per week. Current evidence indicates that nursing women who follow this advice do not expose their infants to increased risk from methyl mercury.

For the top 10 seafood species, making up about 80 percent of the seafood market — canned tuna, shrimp, pollack, salmon, cod, catfish, clams, flatfish, crabs, and scallops — methyl mercury levels are all less than 0.2 ppm. The suggested weekly limit of fish for this level of methyl mercury contamination is 2.2 pounds.

The FDA's action level of one ppm for methyl mercury in fish was established to limit consumers' methyl mercury exposure to levels 10 times lower than the lowest levels associated with adverse effects (paresthesia) observed in actual poisoning incidents to date. FDA toxicologists are developing a more complete database for addressing low-level methyl mercury exposures from fish; however, they consider the one ppm limit to provide an adequate margin of safety.

Still, not everyone agrees about what advice to provide to consumers. This is particularly evident in lack of uniformity in sport fishing advisories provided by states around the country. Adjoining states may even provide different advice about fish from the same bodies of water. But federal efforts are underway to increase uniformity.

Sport-caught predator freshwater species like pike and walleye sometimes have methyl mercury levels in the one ppm range. Other freshwater species also have elevated levels, particularly in areas where mercury levels in the local environment are elevated due to pollution. When in serious doubt, you can always call local fish and game authorities and ask whether ppm levels have been tested for a specific species and what was the result.

The Hidden Dangers of MSG

If you simply can't get well and have tried just about everything, I may have important news for you. You may be reacting to the MSG (monosodium-glutamate) occurring in many manufac-

Artificial Sweeteners Kill Brain Cells

Artificial sweeteners like aspartame and flavor enhancers like MSG (monosodium glutamate), may cause brain damage by killing brain cells, according to Russell Blaylock, MD, neurosurgeon and clinical professor at the University of Mississippi Medical Center. In science circles, these substances are called excitotoxins and are known to overstimulate brain neurons in a way that leads to their self-destruction several hours later. In adults, this can eventually contribute to the development of such neurological diseases as Alzheimer's disease, Huntington's chorea, Parkinson's disease, amyotrophic lateral sclerosis, seizures, strokes, migraine headaches and AIDS dementia. In children, it can cause developmental brain defects including learning disorders, autism, hyperactive behavior and schizophrenia. Excitotoxins are also able to pass through the placenta to the fetus, and possibly cause irreversible fetal brain damage.

To make matters worse, these additives are not required by the FDA to be listed on ingredient labels unless they are used in their pure forms. Ingredients that usually contain MSG include products on which labels may merely say: broth flavoring, natural beef or chicken flavoring, natural flavoring, bouillon, malt extract, seasoning, stock, spices or flavoring. Your best line of defense against ingesting these substances is to carefully read labels and select the least processed foods available.

tured foods during their processing. MSG-reactivity is more than the Chinese restaurant syndrome, a condition that leaves you with a headache or burning feeling after eating Chinese food. And it affects 30 percent of people in this country. That's right. A full third of our population may be reacting to MSG in processed foods.

MSG Reactions

Whether foods with MSG cause these symptoms or aggravate an underlying problem is not known for certain. But here are a number of symptoms that people with MSG-sensitivity have reported after eating foods containing the manufactured form of free glutamic acid, which is a man-made form of MSG. This information comes from Truth in Labeling Campaign (P.O. Box 2532, Darien, IL 60561; phone 312-642-9333).

The symptoms include: swelling, muscle stiffness and achiness, joint pain, rapid or irregular heartbeat, sudden drop in blood pressure, angina, depression, dizziness, disorientation, anxiety, sleepiness, migraines, nausea, diarrhea, stomach cramps, irritable bowel, bloating, shortness of breath, chest tightness and/or pain, runny nose, sneezing, rash, flushing, extremely dry mouth, blurred vision, and difficulty focusing.

Now, before you point a finger at MSG as being a causative factor for everything that is or could ever be wrong with you, remember that these are symptoms that occur in people only after they eat foods containing processed glutamic acid. While it's true you may be eating foods with this chemical every day, the amount of MSG ingested may be responsible for any symptoms. You may not react to a small amount of MSG, but only to a larger quantity. This amount can vary from person to person You may want to look at the foods and ingredients you eat that contain MSG and see if your symptoms — or those of any member of your family —can be associated with their ingestion.

MSG Reactions From Processed Foods

Why processed foods? To answer this, we first need to look at just what MSG is. It is a form of free glutamic acid — a naturally occurring chemical found in protein — that is found in many processed foods. Naturally occurring glutamic acid is different from the glutamic acid found in processed protein foods. This difference is significant. People sensitive to MSG have adverse reactions to the glutamic acid in processed foods, but not to the glutamic acid found in unprocessed proteins. And what's more, these reactions may be immediate or occur up to two days after you've eaten foods with MSG.

All Glutamic Acid Is NOT Alike

Unfortunately for us, the consumers, the FDA does not differentiate between these two forms of glutamic acid. In fact, they say the two are functionally and chemically identical. But that's not true. Bear with me while I explain why. This simple lesson in biochemistry can keep you from getting sick!

Natural glutamic acid found in unprocessed proteins is L-glutamic acid. The manufactured glutamic acid is a combination of L-glutamic acid with several other forms of glutamic acid. Does this look to you like two chemically identical products? Of course not. But the FDA, which is highly influenced by special interests, plus overworked and understaffed, can't afford to address the reality of MSG, so it appears that they're sweeping it under a rug so no one will see it. Meanwhile, millions of us are getting sick without knowing why!

Processed Foods Containing MSG

MSG is always found in calcium caseinate, sodium caseinate, gelatin, texturized protein, hydrolyzed protein, yeast extract, yeast food, and yeast nutrient.

MSG is often, but not always, found in the following: malt extract, barley malt, bouillon, carrageenan, maltodextrin, whey protein, whey protein isolate or concentrate, pectin, enzymes, natural flavorings, seasonings, soy sauce, soy protein, soy protein isolate or concentrate, anything fermented. It can even be found in the milk solids added to low-fat milk products!

Even some soaps, shampoos, hair conditioners, and cosmetics that are hydrolyzed or contain amino acids may cause sensitive people to have an MSG-reaction. Fillers and binders used in prescription and over-the-counter drugs, as well as nutritional supplements, may contain MSG.

Why "No MSG" on Labels Means Nothing

Right now, there are no regulations that say MSG must be labeled if it is in a product. Some manufacturers put "No MSG" or "No MSG Added" on their labels even when their products contain ingredients like hydrolyzed protein or yeast. They can get away with it because the FDA is no longer coming after the manufacturers. Remember, this agency is really overworked and understaffed. Unfortunately, we can't rely on them alone for the safety of our foods — especially when the consequences are not life-threatening. The FDA is busy hunting down sources of deadly bacterium in foods which may kill several hundred people a year, rather than scrutinizing the thousands of products that could be making millions of people sick, but not sick enough to die.

Any product that has a little bit of protein in it and has been exposed to heat, enzymes, or hydrochloric acid during manufacturing, can contain MSG. The amounts may not be significant, but they could add up. Remember, people who are sensitive to MSG often react in a dose-dependent way: the more they ingest, the worse they feel.

MSG Is Everywhere — What Can I Do?

I'm not trying to frighten or overwhelm you, but the sad truth is that products containing MSG are, indeed, everywhere — from the foods we eat to the shampoo we use and the vitamins we take. Not all, of course, but MSG is in some of them. We just want to alert you to a substance that is so common it just may be the reason you can't get well.

If you'd like to see whether or not an MSG-sensitivity is responsible for any of your health problems, begin by using the least-processed foods, supplements, and cosmetics you can find. If necessary, write to the manufacturer of your favorite natural products asking them to show you documentation that the finished product they're selling you does not contain MSG. That is the only way you can know for sure that the product is MSG-free. (Hint: Many large companies have 800 numbers. Call 800 information — 800-555-1212 — to see if you can locate the company you want information from.)

Get back to basics with the foods you're eating. Stop eating any processed foods for two weeks. If you've been using protein powders, switch to eating tofu, lentils, split peas, and beans. Instead of buying instant or canned soups, make them from scratch. Cooking beans isn't time-consuming if you use an electric crock pot.

A diet based on whole grains and beans, a little animal protein if you like, plenty of fresh vegetables, and a little fresh fruit is not so difficult. Especially if it can help you identify or eliminate a potential problem like MSG-sensitivity. We know that MSG is almost everywhere. But we're also aware of how many people suffer from the many symptoms that could be due to the exposure to too many products containing this chemical that is formed during the manufacturing process.

Support Truth in Labeling

For more information on MSG, or for a list of selected references showing how MSG can harm people, send a donation and

Check Your Oat Milk

A respected colleague of mine, Dr. Guy Abraham, pointed out to me that most, if not all, commercial oat milk products contain tricalcium phosphate, a substance that can cause kidney stones and other calcification. This substance should be avoided in oat milk and any other foods. Read all labels carefully.

If you like the taste of oat milk, it's easy enough to make at home. Combine organic oats (as in oatmeal) with pure water, blend it thoroughly, and strain it through a strainer or cheesecloth. Refrigerate your oat milk, and use within a few days. If you like, you can add a little honey, maple syrup, or stevia to sweeten it.

your request to Truth in Labeling Campaign, P.O. Box 2532, •
Darien, IL 60561. They are a non-profit organization, so a contribution of even a few dollars (tax-deductible, of course) is as appre-
ciated by them as the information is by you.

Are Genetically
Altered Foods Safe?

Some people call them "Frankenfoods," and Europeans are
shouting a resounding "No!" to them. I'm talking about genetically engineered foods, called GMOs for genetically modified organisms, and they're beginning to pop up in supermarkets across the
country and in countries around the world. I've been following
this story for years and feel it's time for you to understand what's
going on behind the scenes, and take action if you choose to.

Seeds and strains of grains and produce are being altered to
contain natural pesticides or to have a longer shelf life. Basically,
these changes are being made to increase the profitability of foods,
not because they're healthier. In the early 1990s, the U.S.
Department of Agriculture (USDA) gave the okay to Calgene, Inc.,
a biotechnology company, to come out with the Flavr Savr tomato,
a tomato that takes longer than usual to rot. The Campbell Soup
Company was going to market the new tomato since it financed
some of Calgene's development of the Flavr Savr. Campbell's
decided against it because the image of Campbell's foods is one of
wholesomeness, and GMOs are getting a tainted reputation.

Scientists in Newfoundland have been attempting to create a
salmon that can live in below-freezing waters where salmon cannot
survive. But what happens when these fish find themselves in other
waters after a flood or hurricane? We don't know. We do know that
when a non-native fish is introduced into an ecosystem — and
genetically altered fish are non-native — there have been changes
in the ecosystems. This domino effect can ultimately change the
balance of nature. The bottom line is, we don't know the effects
GMOs will have on our bodies or on the environment.

How Safe Are GMOs?

For people with severe allergies, GMOs can be devastating. They can trigger an allergic response if the food contains genes from an allergen. Recently, there have been recalls of candies that do not contain peanuts, but were manufactured in plants that make candy with peanuts. Some people with severe peanut allergies can go into anaphylactic shock if they eat anything that has even touched peanuts! Well, GMOs can contain minute amounts of genetic material from plants and foods other than those on the label. What's more, these altered foods do not have to be tested for safety and require no labeling to inform you of adding other genetic material to the original food.

Pioneer Hi-Bred, an agricultural seed company, spliced a gene from Brazil nuts into soybeans to make them taste nuttier. The odds of this gene causing an allergic reaction to people with nut allergies were so low that the company felt certain their product was safe. But researchers were amazed when three separate tests indicated that people with allergies to Brazil nuts were definitely affected. For people with severe food allergies, the consequences could be fatal.

GMOs are so widespread that I'm saying you're already eating them unless the foods you eat are all organic. Soybeans and corn have been modified since 1996 with bacterial, viral, and other genes that are not native to human food, says an article published in the *Santa Rosa Press Democrat.* If you're eating anything with corn or soy added to it, you're eating GMOs.

Concerns are growing from studies showing that GMOs are contaminating crops grown in adjacent fields, and are killing beneficial insects and butterflies needed for the integrated pest management programs used by growers of organic produce. There has not been adequate testing to show the environmental consequences of GMOs, says Craig Winters, executive director of The Campaign to Label Genetically Engineered Foods in Seattle, WA. He is one of a number of people lobbying Congress for a law that would require all foods containing GMOs to be labeled.

What does the Food and Drug Administration (FDA) say? In

a 1992 policy paper, it claimed that GMOs are equivalent to conventional food. But scientists within the FDA have admitted that the subject is so complex that we really can't predict what GMOs will do to people. Whatever they do to adults, they will do to a greater degree to the small bodies of infants and children.

I don't believe GMOs are necessarily safe; in fact, I think some of them are potentially very dangerous. There's a growing concern about their safety in this country. This seems to be one arena where your opinion may help shape the form that food takes as we enter the 21st century.

It's Time to Take Action

Just a few years ago, in 1996, people in the Natural Law Party called a summit meeting to discuss this potential problem. Thirty people attended and five scientists presented their information. This year, a second summit meeting was held at the Capital Hilton Hotel in Washington, DC with 140 attendees, 20 scientists and experts, and a dozen European government officials (who called in by phone).

Concerns are not only coming from a small group of activists in this country. German Chancellor Gerhard Schroder placed the subject of GMOs on the agenda of the G8 Summit in Cologne this year under the listing of "Global Threats," calling it one of the greatest threats facing the new century. French President Jacques Chirac wrote the original initiative against the use of GMOs that brought the seriousness of this problem to Schroder's attention. Not all world leaders see GMOs as a problem. British Prime Minister Tony Blair and President Bill Clinton support them. We're not surprised. GMOs are big business.

Laura Ticciati, former executive director of Mothers for Natural Law, and now part of the Natural Law Party, told the second summit meeting that she wants to see all genetically altered foods labeled. Mothers for Natural Law estimates that 60 percent of foods on grocery store shelves contain some genetically engineered material.

What You Can Do

Where people have protested, changes have been made. In England, GMOs are not being used by Kentucky Fried Chicken, Pizza Hut, and Burger King. Even McDonald's agreed to stop using GMOs when anti-GMO activists protested. However, it has not said it would stop using GMOs in this country. Why not? We haven't complained enough.

Gerber Baby Foods has stopped using GMOs. After being contacted by Greenpeace, Gerber decided to eliminate any GMOs in its baby foods, saying that it didn't want mothers to worry about the safety of its products. J.J. Heinz and Healthy Time Natural Foods have joined Gerber in supplying products without GMOs.

If you see signs in supermarkets that say Genetically Modified Organisms, now you'll know what the pretty label means. It means the food may or may not be safe for you and your family. Want to take a chance? I don't!

Eating Grapefruit Could
Be Dangerous to Your Health

Chock full of vitamin C and potassium, grapefruit and grapefruit juice are a healthy way to start your day, right? Not if you're taking particular prescription drugs. They could, in fact, be very dangerous to you.

Are you taking the popular herb St. John's wort for depression? Here's another potential danger to your health. If you're taking certain medications, you could be putting yourself at great risk.

You probably know that some medications react unfavorably with others. One drug may interfere with the action of another or it may even increase its potency. In either case you can end up with serious side effects. That's right. Some drugs lower the potency of another drug while others make them stronger — too strong to be safe. Many times you don't know that the various drugs you're taking are having these interactions.

These same kinds of dangerous and potentially dangerous

drug-to-drug interactions exist between grapefruit or grapefruit juice, or St. John's wort (*Hypericum perforatum*), and a number of prescription drugs. Most people don't consider that there's any interaction between foods or herbs and their medications. But all have chemical components that have the potential to change a drug's action.

If you're using any of the prescription drugs mentioned in these pages, stop eating grapefruit or drinking grapefruit juice immediately. Stop taking St. John's wort for depression, even if it's helping you. Then, pick up the phone and make an appointment to talk with your doctor as soon as possible about any of these interactions. Don't resume taking St. John's wort or having grapefruit in any form until you get an "all clear" from your doctor.

How and Why This Interaction Occurs

There is an enzyme called CYP3A4 that is part of the cytochrome P450 enzyme system. This system has a job: to break down some drugs in your intestines. That's just part of what it does. The dosage of any drug your doctor prescribes takes this enzyme's activity into account when it's a drug that's affected by this enzyme system.

Grapefruit and grapefruit juice contain substances called furanocoumarins, along with a bioflavonoid called naringin, that attach themselves to the CYP3A4 enzyme and prevent it from reducing the absorption of these particular drugs. This means that you're getting a greater effect from your drug than your doctor intended — in some cases up to 50 percent more! Just imagine what it would be like if you took one-and-a-half times as much of a drug as your doctor prescribed. Or from three to six times as much. Unthinkable? Well, you may just be doing this by increasing its potency when you combine some medications with grapefruit or St. John's wort.

Joe and Theresa Graedon, authors of *Deadly Drug Interactions* (St. Martin's Press, 1997) point out that you don't have to combine grapefruit with your prescription drug during the same day. You can drink a glass of grapefruit juice one day and increase the potency of a drug taken the following day. Interestingly, no other forms of citrus have these drug-altering substances, so you can still safely drink orange juice or eat strawberries and kiwi. And we don't know of other herbs that have this same interaction, although in time, as they're studied more closely, we may find some.

St. John's wort, used extensively as a natural antidepressant, appears to have the same action on the CYP3A4 enzyme as grapefruit. So as you read this article, consider that all symptoms known or suspected to be due to a grapefruit/drug interaction may also be applied to St. John's wort.

Which Drugs Are Affected

Grapefruit in any form, along with St. John's wort, could increase the potency of a number of drugs used for hypertension, heart disease, organ transplants, cancer, AIDS, and allergies. Basically, any drug that inhibits CYP3A4 (or the cytochrome P450 enzyme system) can be affected. Let's take a look at various categories of drugs and see which ones St. John's wort or grapefruit could possibly affect.

Calcium-channel blockers for your heart: If you're taking Plendil, be extra careful. Grapefruit increases the levels of some drugs by 50 percent, but it's known to increase the levels of Plendil in your blood stream from 300-500 percent! This increase in absorption can cause even healthy people to feel faint, lightheaded, and to flush. If you have a heart condition — one reason you may be taking Plendil — your side effects could be much more serious. Other calcium-channel blockers that are affected by grapefruit (and probably St. John's wort) include Adalat, Procardia, Nimotop, Sular, Calan, Isoptin, and Verelan.

Antihistamines for allergies: Hismanal, when taken along with grapefruit, can produce serious side effects in people who have normal heart rhythms. No one knows whether or not Claritin or Allegra fit into this category. To be on the safe side, eliminate the herb and fruit until sufficient studies show them to be completely safe, or until your doctor says it's safe for you.

Organ transplant drugs: Grapefruit juice is known to increase blood levels of Cyclosporine, a drug commonly used in organ transplant recipients, from 300-500 percent. Side effects may include diarrhea, high blood pressure, seizures, and kidney problems. Is grapefruit safe to take with other transplant drugs? Only if they don't become absorbed along the same CYP3A4 pathway. Check with your doctor or pharmacist to see if the medication you're taking falls into this category.

Cholesterol-lowering drugs: A number of the "statins," drugs used to lower cholesterol, are affected by grapefruit. Both lovastatin (Mevacor) and simvastatin (Zocor) may be increased in absorption up to 15 times. This increase could cause muscle pain, muscle weakness, or impaired kidney function. Interestingly, not all statins are affected by grapefruit. Pravastatin (Pravachol) seems to be unaffected by this fruit. However, to be safe, we suggest that if you're taking any statin you might be wise to eliminate grapefruit, grapefruit juice, and St. John's wort.

Drugs for people with HIV, AIDS, or cancer: Grapefruit affects protease inhibitors, drugs used for people with HIV and AIDS. But instead of increasing the drug's action, as it does with statins and other medications, in this case it actually lowers the availability of one protease inhibitor, Indinavir. In fact, grapefruit reduces Indinavir to levels that are low enough to lead to drug resistance or even treatment failure. People on any protease inhibitors should stop taking St. John's wort and eliminate grapefruit unless their doctor says otherwise. Some other immunosuppressive drugs and cancer agents also affect the CYP3A4 enzyme. If you are taking any medications for these conditions, check with your doctor or pharmacist before continuing to use either of these substances.

Hormone therapy: Grapefruit increases the amount of estradiol (Estinyl, Estrace) in your blood and causes its effects to continue nearly one-third longer than normal. Because excessive estrogen has been implicated in other health problems, so you want to take the lowest amount your doctor believes will give you the results you're looking for, no more. If you're combining estradiol with grapefruit or St. John's wort, you may be getting much more hormone activity than you think. Susan E. Brown, PhD, in her excellent book *Better Bones, Better Body* (Keats Publishing, 1996) points out that too much estrogen can increase your risk of gall-bladder disease, lupus, and endometrial cancer. Used properly, and if it's determined that you actually need it, the right amount of estrogen can be helpful. But don't increase your levels unknowingly by combining it with grapefruit or St. John's wort.

Other drug, food, and herbal interactions: Grapefruit increases the potency of Propulsid, a heartburn medication. Increased activity of this medication can place you at risk for an irregular heartbeat. Don't exchange one health problem for another. While you may not be eating grapefruit if you have heartburn, you could be taking St. John's wort. The heart medication Digoxin, as well as the blood thinner Coumadin, also have increased potency when taken with grapefruit in any form.

What's Next?

Because some grapefruit and St. John's wort increase the absorption of certain drugs, I expect to hear about researchers who are looking for ways to use the active ingredient in either of them to enhance the effectiveness of various medications. Using this enzyme-inhibiting factor could reduce the cost of many pharmaceuticals in the future by lowering the amount of the actual drug in

---

Loss of Libido? The Culprit May Be Candy

Your man's low libido affects your life just as PMS affects him. If your partner has a low sex drive, I have one question: Does he eat a lot of licorice? Licorice in tea, herbal supplements, and candy lowers testosterone and can lead to sexual dysfunction. The active ingredient, glycyrrhizic acid, is the culprit. One study we found showed that men taking seven grams of licorice a day with 0.5 grams of glycyrrhizic acid had altered sex hormones.

How can you measure this amount of licorice? You don't have to. Just ask your partner to stop eating licorice for a month or two and see if there is any improvement. If not, a session or two with a good psychotherapist, or a weekend away together, might be in order. In any case, you need to get to the cause of the problem — which could simply be licorice candy.

Alan R Gaby, MD, Licorice affects testosterone metabolism, *Townsend Letter or Doctors & Patients*, June 2000.

a formula while boosting its bioavailability many times over.

Expect, also, to hear more about drug-herb-vitamin-food interactions. As people mix more of these substances and report their side effects to their doctors, we'll learn more about which are safe to combine and which we would be better off avoiding. Just because a substance is natural, like the herb St. John's wort or the common grapefruit, doesn't mean it's safe for everyone, especially in combination with pharmaceuticals.

Your Responsibility

Talk with your doctor and tell him or her about every vitamin, mineral, herb, and other supplement you're taking. Share this information with your local pharmacist who may be even better informed in the subject of interactions. Consider buying one or two reference books on this subject to have on hand in case you or your loved ones are given a prescription without a complete understanding of it interactions. These books can save your health and possibly your life. I like both the Graedon book and the *A-Z Guide to Drug-Herb-Vitamin Interactions* (Lininger, Schuyler, W., Jr., DC, editor, Prima Publishing, 1999).

Do not, under any circumstances, use St. John's wort or grapefruit in any form to enhance the use of any of the drugs mentioned here. The amount of active ingredients that can affect these drugs may vary according to the variety of grapefruit, and the fluctuations in growing conditions for both the fruit and herb. Be safe today.

Beyond Ensure

They're fast. They're tasty. They're filled with vitamins and minerals. And you can buy them by the case almost anywhere. So what's wrong with drinking Ensure, Resource, Boost, SlimFast, and other similar canned meal replacement drinks? It's better to drink one and get plenty of vitamins than to skip a meal, isn't it?

I don't think so.

Meal replacement drinks were designed to get calories into hospital patients who could not eat solid food, or people in convalescent homes who were unable to eat properly. They consist of lots of sugars, water, and protein with inexpensive vitamins and minerals added. The problem with inexpensive nutrients is that they're poorly absorbed. Take Ensure, for example. It may say it contains 25 percent or more of the Recommended Daily Allowances of a vitamin or mineral, but the amount found in a can of Ensure isn't the amount that gets into your body.

Ensure contains such minerals as potassium chloride, calcium phosphate, and thiamine chloride, for example. The chloride, phosphate, and hydrochloride forms of nutrients are not as well absorbed as the citrate, malate, fumarate, aspartate, or gluconate forms. This is because our body contains citrate, malate, fumarate, aspartate, and gluconate, and it recognizes and uses larger amounts of the minerals, which are bound to these chemicals.

So don't compare vitamins and minerals in mass market drinks like Ensure with those in health food company drinks like Recovery, Naturally Complete, Vigoraid, and Balanced. They may look the same, but they don't perform as well. Technically, they

Diet Causes Constipation, Colon Cancer

We've talked about a high-fiber diet and magnesium as solutions to constipation. Now we find that frequent constipation can be a marker for colon cancer. In a study of over 800 people, half of whom had colon cancer, it was found that those who were chronically constipated had a higher risk for getting colon cancer. For people who were constipated more than 52 times in a year, the risk quadrupled. Using laxatives did not contribute to colon cancer, say the researchers. It's the production of cancer-causing chemicals, released during fermentation in the intestines that sit around too long when a person is constipated.

Still, if you've been constipated over a period of time, you do want to check with your doctor to rule out any problem. In the people participating in this study, colon cancer followed after two years of constipation. Many people are constipated much longer than this.

A high-fiber diet and taking extra magnesium is a good way of moving food through the intestines. So is regular exercise and drinking water throughout the day.

Jacobs, E.J. and E. White. "Constipation, laxative use, and colon cancer among middle-aged adults," *Epidemiology* 9 (4), 1998. From *Int'l J Clin Nutr*, April 99, 111.

may have the same amount of a nutrient, but the amount your body can use varies tremendously.

Is Cancer in the Mix?

This is the difference between a good quality product and a cheap one. But it's not what alarms me. I'm very upset that many of the mass market drinks, including strawberry and orange cream flavored Ensure, contain food dyes like red dye number 3, which is a known carcinogen that has been shown to promote the growth of breast-cancer cells! More than that, this food coloring, like many pesticides, is estrogenic. For women who want to guard against breast cancer, repeatedly ingesting drinks with red dye number 3 is totally counterproductive.

While you might argue that there's not much of any dye in a single can of Ensure, we suggest you take a look at the majority of people using it. Sick people. Infirm people. People with cancer, AIDS and other weakened immune systems, children who don't eat much variety of food and need more calories, and even women recovering from breast cancer. In our opinion, these people can't afford to be eating any amount of dangerous products. They need all the help they can get. They need the best quality nutrients in a product that's easy for their bodies to absorb.

Food dyes are in everything from candies to hot dogs, lunch meats, and snack foods. And just because a particular dye hasn't been found to cause breast cancer or other problems doesn't necessarily mean it's safe. It could mean it hasn't been thoroughly tested. Our suggestion: Read labels carefully and pass up those products with dyes and other artificial ingredients.

These original supplemental drinks (Ensure, Resource, Boost, and other mass market drinks) served their purpose. They brought our attention to the needs of busy and sick consumers who need a fast way to get calories and vitamins. Now their popularity has driven a number of health food companies to come out with products made with healthy ingredients and nutrients the body can more easily absorb. So stop buying chemicals-in-a-can. There are healthier choices.

The best of the best, in our opinion, are products called Recovery Power Foods, made by the same people who founded Earth's Best Baby Foods more than a decade ago. Their products include the ready-made drinks, packets you can mix with water, drink mixes, and supplemental nutrition bars. All of them come with information on fruit, starch, and fat protein exchanges for diabetics and people on other restrictive diets, including those who simply want to lose weight.

They have a ready-to-drink liquid supplement in 8 oz boxes. Each serving contains 270 calories, 10 grams of protein, and six grams of fat. But not just any fats. Recovery drinks have a variety of essential fatty acids (to boost the immune system) and medium chain triglycerides (fats that are easily digested). Made from rice and whey protein, these beverages are low in lactose and contain no soy — a protein some people have difficulty digesting, especially when they're elderly or sick. The sweetener, fructose, has no corn protein in it, so if you're sensitive to corn, you can still use these products. The vitamins and minerals are expensive, high-quality nutrients chosen for their ability to be well digested and absorbed. This is a very sophisticated line of products that work. If you can't find them in your health food store, call the company, Great Circles, at 800-872-0611.

Westbrae Natural has a new product called West Soy VigorAid made from organic soybeans. The company has added 50 mg of isoflavones, nutrients found in soybeans that protect against breast and prostate cancer, boosting the nutritional value of their beverages. These drinks also contain essential fatty acids to help the immune system, and are lactose free. From 240 to 260 calories per serving, with 50 calories from fat, three 8 oz boxes (choose vanilla or chocolate) sell for about $3.99. You should be able to find them in health food stores around the country.

Pacific Foods' answer to Ensure is called Naturally Complete, 8 oz and 32 oz boxes of a drink made from whole grains and soybeans with added vitamins and minerals. An 8 oz box will give you either 170 or 200 calories (chocolate has 30 calories more than vanilla), and sells for around $2.99 for a set of three. The larger box costs from $3.49-$3.99.

Balanced, which comes in 11 oz cans, is made by American Natural Snacks from organic soybeans and contains no lactose. It's higher in calories than the two above (230 with 25 calories from fat), but a little lower in nutrients. But remember, these are still better absorbed than the nutrients in mass market drinks. Their quality far surpasses Ensure. For more information, call them at 800-238-3947.

Whether you're using these drinks as a meal replacement for a weight-loss program, a way to boost your nutrients with a healthy snack, or looking for a drink to help a sick person, the elderly, or the very young get high-quality nutrients, you are no longer limited to using Ensure. Leave dangerous food dyes and poorly absorbed nutrients behind.

Finally, if you think a meal replacement drink can truly take the place of a nutrient-dense meal made up of whole foods — it can't. A better name for these beverages might be meal supplement drink. When circumstances permit, it's always better to return to eating whole-food meals, rather than continue using these drinks.

Aspartame: The Toxin That Destroys Brain Cells

Weight control is the single greatest challenge for millions of women. And no matter how bad a weight loss aid is for us — like fen-phen, for instance — if it helps us lose weight, we tend to use it.

The problem is that unless a substance is found to be life threatening, it tends to stay on the market and remain in our foods, giving us the illusion that it's safe. If it were dangerous, we rationalize, the FDA wouldn't allow us to use it, right?

Not necessarily. Take aspartame, for instance.

Aspartame, or NutraSweet, is an artificial sweetener made by combining aspartic acid (a non-essential amino acid) with phenylalanine (an essential amino acid). It's used on a regular basis by more than 100 million people in this country alone. Amino acids are compounds that are building blocks of protein.

So what's the problem? Ask neurosurgeon Russell L. Blaylock,

MD, and he'll tell you he's convinced that aspartame is an excitotox-in — a brain toxin that destroys brain neurons. In small quantities, it may be harmless. But when you eat foods and drink sodas laced with aspartame, you're getting a dangerous dose, he claims.

Dr. Blaylock is the author of an impressive book, *Excitotoxins: The taste that kills* (Health Press, 1997). In it, he discusses the vast research that leads him to implicate both aspartame and MSG (monosodium glutamate) as harmful substances in our foods. He is seeing evidence linking these two excitotoxins to Parkinson's disease, Alzheimer's disease, Huntington's disease, and ALS (Amyotroophic Lateral Sclerosis — Lou Gehrig's disease). He is also convinced they contribute to brain tumors, seizures, and other brain-related dysfunctions.

How It Works

Aspartame is made from aspartate, phenylalanine, and methanol (otherwise known as wood alcohol). In your body, more methanol is formed. The methanol then becomes formaldehyde, a poisonous immune-suppressant. What about the methanol in beer, wine, and other alcoholic beverages? Are they just as dangerous? No, because alcoholic beverages also contain ethanol, and ethanol just happens to be an antidote for methanol! So … it may be safer to drink an alcoholic beverage than a diet soda. In fact, in his book *Maximum Immunity* (Simon & Schuster, 1987), Michael A. Weiner, PhD suggests that the only way to keep aspartame from breaking down into formaldehyde is to drink alcohol at the same time. This suggestion is not likely, healthy, or advisable.

Aspartate is a neurotransmitter that is normally found in your brain and spinal cord. In small amounts, it's safe. In larger amounts, Dr. Blaylock says it can cause specific neurons linked to aspartate or glutamate receptors (found in MSG) to degenerate and die. These receptors are found in the area of your brain that affects the brain diseases we've mentioned.

There are a small number of people in the world who can't handle the amino acid phenylalanine. They have PKU, phenylke-tonuria, a genetic disease that can cause headaches, dizziness, mood swings, and insomnia. But in the 1980s, Dr. Richard J. Wurtman studied phenylalanine and found that even people without PKU could have these symptoms, depending on how much phenylalanine an individual can handle. Nutritionally oriented physician Elson M. Haas, MD, advises his pregnant patients to avoid all aspartame during their pregnancy, believing it can affect the fetus adversely.

How Much Is Too Much?

No one knows really. Dr. Wurtman discovered someone with night twitches, severe headaches, and grand mal seizures (epilepsy) who drank four or five glasses of diet drinks a day. Other people he studied drank a liter or more with no side effects. Because it's thought of as being safe, some women drink half a dozen diet drinks or more a day or regularly eat foods with aspartame. Other people eat foods with MSG along with some that contain aspartame. The total amount of excitotoxins in your body, as well as your particular sensitivity to them, determines your reactions. Children may be most susceptible to the negative effects of these excitotoxins since their bodies are smaller.

Q. I recently bought a diet soda that contains Sunette's sweetener, acesulfame potassium. Is it safe? — *C.D., Bronx, NY*

A. Acesulfame potassium, or Acesulfame K, was approved as a sugar substitute to be used in some products back in 1988. But Michael F. Jacobson, PhD, executive director of the Center for Science in the Public Interest, thinks it could be very dangerous. In the book *Safe Food,* which he co-authored with Lisa Y. Lefferts and Anne Witte Garland (Living Planet Press, 1991), Jacobson found that acesulfame K has not been tested adequately. And the test that were done showed that it causes cancer in animals.

Additionally, when acesulfame K breaks down in the body, it creates a chemical called acetoacetamide. This chemical affects the thyroid in laboratory animals. In one case, using acesulfame K for three months caused nonmalignant thyroid tumors in rats. I join Michael Jacobson in his concern that if a substance can cause tumors in rats in just three months, it could cause problems in humans when it's used over long periods of time. Of three sugar substitutes — aspartame, saccharin, and acesulfame K, Jacobson lists acesulfame K as the very worst.

Combining Excitotoxins

The damage caused by excitotoxins is multiplied when you have more than one type in your diet. You need to look at how much MSG you've consumed over the years as well as the amount in your present diet. Hydrolyzed vegetable protein, for example, contains glutamate, aspartate, and cysteine. So if you're eating foods made with hydrolyzed vegetable protein and drinking diet sodas, you're getting a hefty dose of excitotoxins.

Other Consequences

Headaches are the complaint most often reported from people using aspartame. While the makers of NutraSweet conducted studies that failed to show an association, Donald R. Johns, MD, report-

---

To Look and Feel Your Best, Spring Clean Your Body

Springtime is when life begins to renew itself once more. Plants that have been dormant in winter begin to sprout. We think of spring cleaning our homes, perhaps as an unconscious way of complementing the changes occurring in nature. However, we often forget that we are part of nature, and spring is the perfect time to clean our bodies as well.

Janet was a college student who came to see me complaining of fatigue. Her family has a history of breast cancer, so I was especially concerned when she told me she had time to eat only fast foods and frozen dinners. Many of these foods are heavily processed (luncheon meat sandwiches) and high in fat (French fries and cheese). She ate few vegetables and drank enough coffee and soft drinks for a small family. All of this explained why she was fatigued, but her diet was doing something much worse. It was turning her body into a toxic-waste dump and increasing her risk for breast cancer.

I told Janet she needed to do some spring cleaning. She looked puzzled until I explained that the body needs to be cleaned and maintained just like our homes. Janet's face lightened, and she agreed to eat more salads, less fried foods, and reduce her coffee intake for two weeks. She drank flavored mineral water instead of sodas and made fast nutritional meals for herself like fat-free refried beans and corn tortillas piled high with salsa and sprouts.

Janet soon realized that the fatigue was gone and life was enjoyable once again. Her increased energy convinced her to continue eating better, and she understood the long-term benefits of spring cleaning.

ed a connection between aspartame and migraines in a patient two hours after she drank sodas with aspartame. She had a headache and upset stomach that stopped when she stopped these drinks. Dr. Johns then gave her tablets containing 500 mg of aspartame. Her headache reappeared. While the association between migraines has not been definitively established, we suggest it may be another case of an individual's sensitivity to aspartame as well as how often it's been consumed over the years.

Brain tumors in rats ingesting aspartame have been observed, but we don't know if this translates into humans. If it does, we still don't know how much aspartame or combined excitotoxins are dangerous. The possibility for this connection exists, however.

Do you have chronic urinary tract infections (UTI)? Aspartame lowers the acidity of your urine and can increase your susceptibility to UTI. This may be why drinking cranberry juice has not been sufficient to eliminate these infections.

If you're taking plenty of antioxidants in your diet and supplements (vitamins C, E, A, selenium, coenzyme Q10, etc.) and drinking diet sodas, you may be canceling the beneficial effects of your nutrients. Antioxidants fight free radicals, while aspartame can stimulate the production of enormous concentrations of free radicals.

What You Can Do

Reduce the total load of excitotoxins in your diet: MSG and aspartame. Add an inch or two of pure fruit juice to a glass of sparkling mineral water instead of drinking diet sodas. Choose foods with low amounts of fructose, barley malt, or rice syrup rather than sugar-free aspartame-ladled foods. Even sugar may be safer for you than aspartame.

Magnesium raises the threshold for seizures. Keep your magnesium levels higher than your calcium intake for added protection. Magnesium and zinc both block the effect of excitotoxins in some glutamate receptors, and zinc is normally found in high levels in your brain's temporal lobes. Take 15-30 mg of zinc in your multivitamin mineral and eat foods high in zinc (whole grains, brewer's yeast, and pumpkin seeds).

Chapter 3

Obesity and Poor Digestion Are Major Causes of Illness

M ost people don't consider their food to be toxic, but it can be — especially when taken in extremely large doses.

New studies are coming out all the time showing that obesity is a major precursor to common diseases. In fact, many of the diseases I'll discuss in Section 2 can be caused by eating too much food, even when those foods are healthy foods. But the health problems are worsened considerably when the foods you consume are unhealthy foods.

Recent studies have connected obesity to heart disease, hypertension, stroke, cancer, diabetes, gall-bladder disease, arthritis, pulmonary abnormalities (such as asthma), and endocrine abnormalities (i.e., hormone imbalances, which I'll discuss in the next chapter), to name just a few.

According to Dr. Michael Blumenkrantz, a recognized authority in the treatment of obesity-related disorders, "The major health risks of obesity increase in a curvilinear relationship, with prevalences increasing progressively and disproportionately with increasing weight. Weight increases beginning during adulthood and continuing for many years have the greatest adverse affects." So the older you get and the more weight you gain, the more likely your weight will cause health problems. In fact, if you are more than 100 pounds overweight, the likelihood that you'll have some type of health problem related to your weight more than doubles.

As a result, Dr. Blumenkrantz says, "The trend toward increasing levels of obesity in the industrial world has to be reversed. Public health measures including education, counseling, and possible legislation similar to that done with smoking are necessary to counteract this serious disease."

I agree completely, so instead of spending more time expounding on the problem, I'm going to do my part in the educational field to help you lose those unwanted pounds, and possibly add a number of years to your life.

How to Lose Weight and Keep It Off

Everyone's looking for the perfect weight-loss program — one that can help take weight off and keep it off.

Obviously, if there was one such program everyone would be doing it, and we'd all know just what to do. But each of us is different emotionally, and our bodies are different physiologically. For example, your body's sensitivity to insulin production accompanied by fluctuating blood-sugar levels can cause you to crave sugars and starches when someone else on a similar diet won't.

I believe the only successful weight-loss program addresses the specific emotional and physical aspects of weight loss for each person. You need to understand, and work with, the physical and emotional causes for your food cravings and overeating patterns. When you do this, holidays, birthdays, anniversaries, and other celebrations won't be an excuse for eating lots of fatty or sweet foods, or binging on starches, resulting in still more weight gain.

Books on weight loss usually concentrate on emotional eating. In *Feeding the Hungry Heart* (Plume Books, 1993), Geneen Roth calls bingeing purposeful acts that signal something is wrong, and you're not getting what you want. What she's talking about is a lack of intimacy, relationship or work problems, and other psychological needs. But I've found that both physiological needs and nutritional deficiencies also can trigger bingeing.

For instance, we often crave foods we're allergic or sensitive to, setting off a never-ending bingeing cycle. A need for magnesium can cause chocolate cravings, because chocolate is very high in this important mineral. Many psychologists and registered dieticians

(RDs) still concentrate on behavioral modification techniques and understanding psychological needs to control weight. But there's more to overeating or eating foods that are counterproductive to your health and weight goals than your emotions. And you probably know by now that it's not just a matter of self-control.

In 1989, I wrote a book, now in its third printing, called *Overcoming the Legacy of Overeating* (Lowell House, 1999). It was the first book addressing the need to look at both the emotional and the physical sides of eating disorders. The physical aspects address why some people crave sugar, chocolate, and other "trigger" foods (foods that cause bingeing), and what can be done to balance the body so that these cravings disappear. The emotional reasons suggest that solutions to eating patterns that may have worked for us in the past can sometimes work against us now. This would include experiencing hunger before eating for people who were brought up to eat constantly. I was amazed to learn some people don't know what it feels like to be hungry!

In more than 23 years of clinical practice, I've found that a permanent weight-loss program consists of:

Another Anti-Obesity Drug Fails

This time, a pharmaceutical company has withdrawn its FDA application for approval of an anti-obesity drug, orlistat (under the name of Xenical), before it has caused problems. Orlistat blocks fat absorption in the intestines, but may be associated with breast cancer in women who took the drug. The number of women who got breast cancer was minimal, and Roche Holdings, the pharmaceutical company behind this new drug, insists that orlistat doesn't stimulate or enhance tumor growth. The question is whether or not there is an indirect effect that hasn't been identified as yet.

I think obesity is one of the toughest conditions to address. It's not simply a matter of eating less. Inborn metabolic differences cause some people to burn fat more slowly, and obesity itself places limitations on fat-burning exercise that would eventually lower the weight of many obese individuals. Still, when I look at the importance of such fat-soluble nutrients as vitamins A and E, along with essential fatty acids, I cannot agree with a solution that blocks the absorption of all fats. It can't result in good health.

Ault, Alicia. "Newest anti-obesity drug fails to pass FDA muster," *The Lancet,* March 21, 1998.

• Addressing the physical and emotional reasons for overeating or choosing problem foods (like sugar and fatty foods).
• Eating the proper amount of the right foods.
• Exercise.
• Using supplements safely to increase your metabolism and reduce hunger.

Genetics Are Important

Some people have always been heavy and always will be. They come from families that are heavy, so losing weight is a struggle. But even people who have genetic tendencies to be obese can trim down with the right program that helps them burn more calories faster by speeding up their metabolism safely. And the right program is not a starvation diet or eating just one meal a day, as these actually slow down your metabolism so you burn *fewer calories.*

You might want to read more about this type of program and consult with a health practitioner who works with weight loss for information that's specific to your body's physical and emotional needs. Let's start at the beginning and see what you may have missed:

The Physiological Aspect

It takes more than willpower to stop eating chocolate. Chocolate is high in magnesium, a mineral important to the heart and bones that I talk about often. Magnesium helps all muscles relax. It helps carry calcium into the bones. And magnesium, found in nuts, seeds, and legumes (beans) in abundance, is excreted in higher-than-usual quantities when you're under stress. This is why so many women crave chocolate before menstruation, a time when magnesium levels are lower due to physiological stress. When magnesium levels are increased, chocolate cravings decrease.

To stop eating sugar and refined starches, it's often necessary to look at blood-sugar levels and insulin sensitivity. If your body produces more insulin than it needs, or produces it inappropriately, your blood-sugar levels will bounce around and you'll crave sugar, fruit, or fruit juice. Or you might crave potatoes and corn which are high carbohydrate foods that turn quickly into sugar. A low-carbohydrate diet with protein at each meal, along with extra chromium and frequent small meals, can often reduce sugar cravings. Willpower may work for a while, eventually though, your physiological need for specific foods or nutrients will win and you'll be back in your bingeing cycle again.

The Psychological Aspect

We eat because we're lonely, bored, or want to avoid doing something. We use food as a substitute for love, to cover up feelings, and as a reward. We then think we have to be on a perfect eating program, so we begin eating healthy foods in smaller quantities

Orlistat and Weight Loss

In an effort to find the perfect, or at least a good solution to obesity, we report the findings of a two-year European study using 120 mg of Orlistat three times a day in over 700 obese people. On first glance, the results sound encouraging.

During the first year of the double-blind study, people on Orlistat lost more weight than people who took the placebo — 10 percent vs. six percent weight loss.

The second year, the Orlistat people maintained a greater weight loss than the controls. Statistically, Orlistat is a success. But what else do we know from this study?

Orlistat works by lowering the body's absorption of dietary fat by 30 percent. You can get the same effect, without taking anything and without any side effects, by putting yourself on a low-fat diet. The authors of this study are aware that Orlistat can reduce the absorption of fat-soluble vitamins like vitamins D, E, and beta carotene, noting that some participants needed additional supplementation.

People who took Orlistat had less weight gain than the placebo group. But more significant, we think, is the sentence in the study: "Cessation of orlistat therapy resulted in a market rebound effect." Is it safe to take indefinitely? No one knows. Will you gain weight if you stop taking it? Most likely. Is it worth the risk for a temporary weight loss? You be the judge.

Sjostrom, Lars, et al. "Randomized placebo-controlled trial of orlistat for weight loss and prevention of weight regain in obese patients," *The Lancet,* vol 352, July 18, 1998.

and give up when we fail to reach our impossible goal of perfection. I have a sign in my office: "Forget perfection. Aim for excellence."

Be easier on yourself. Understand the emotional side of over-eating or eating poorly, and learn how to deal with your feelings. Your emotions may not be entirely responsible for your weight problem, but they do enter into the equation and need to be addressed.

The Best Foods to Eat

Some people gain weight when they eat a low-fat, high-carbohydrate diet. We're now seeing that this type of food plan, once considered ideal, is not necessarily best for many people with weight problems. Nor is a diet too low in certain fats. Essential fatty acids (EFAs), fats from fish, raw nuts and seeds, flax oil, evening primrose oil, and borage seed oil, actually speed up your metabolism, enabling you to burn calories faster.

Emphasize protein from fish, tofu, chicken, and small quantities of beef throughout the day, not just at one meal. Keep portions of carbohydrates low, and when you eat them, make sure you include beans of all kinds. Beans have both protein and carbohydrates. By adding protein powder to your cereal, you can increase your protein at breakfast. Or try a few Boca Burger Breakfast Patties, fat-free, soy-based sausage-like patties high in protein.

What about the Atkins diet? In my opinion, an opinion shared by numerous physicians and nutritionists, it offers only temporary weight loss. Much of the weight lost on this program is water. What's more, your body needs carbohydrates to feed your brain. You need almost twice as much protein as carbohydrates to get enough glucose to feed your brain. Without carbohydrates, your brain uses up to 200 grams of muscle protein a day, causing a loss of muscle. Most important, a high animal protein diet doesn't change your struggle, it just causes a momentary diversion. Be smart. Keep some carbs in your diet, like beans and small amounts of grains.

How Much Food Do You Need?

Most people eat until their stomach is full and they feel pressure. This may be more than you need. Try eating when you're hungry and stop when you're no longer hungry. Then wait 20 minutes. Why? Because it takes twenty minutes for a message to travel from your stomach to your brain, telling you that you're no longer hungry. After 20 minutes, if you're still hungry, eat a little more. Additional tips for recognizing hunger and dealing with portions can be found in my book, *Overcoming the Legacy of Overeating*.

Exercise Is Essential

Eating more calories than you burn causes weight gain. If you're postmenopausal, especially if you're taking hormones, weight loss is a bigger challenge. But it is possible. Find some activity you enjoy doing — walking briskly through the mall, walking or biking with a friend, or gardening (weeding and digging can burn up plenty of calories). If you like going to a gym or working with a personal trainer, fine. If not, there are plenty of other ways to be active. But you're not going to lose the weight you want without regular exercise. Four to five times a week, for half an hour or more, is ideal. But forget about perfection. Just start today. And I don't mean tomorrow!

Supplements

Herbs and other nutrients can help speed up your metabolism, helping you burn extra calories. Some are safe, but others are not. The safe ones include:

Caffeine, especially before exercising, helps increase your metabolism and reduces hunger. Try a cup of green tea, which is an appetite suppressant and has healthful antioxidants. If you avoid caffeine because it makes you anxious, consider taking an anti-anxiety herb, such as kava, along with it. It will take the edge off any anxiety, whether it's from caffeine or just an underlying emotion.

Many weight-loss supplements on the market contain caffeine because it's so effective. But it's very important to avoid those with ephedra (*ma huang*), which has caused serious side effects, including hypertension, tightness in the chest, and even death. Green tea or just caffeine extract are much safer.

Garcinia cambogia (Malabar tamarind) is an herb that reduces sugar cravings, blocks fat storage, and suppresses the appetite. CitriMax™ is the brand name of tamarind extract and is used in some weight-loss formulas. The recommended dosage is from 250-1000 mg before meals. Use the lowest amount you need, and begin by taking a small amount for five days before gradually increasing it.

5-HTP (5-Hydroxyl-Tryptophan) is a precursor to the amino acid tryptophan. It helps regulate moods by helping your body produce serotonin, a "feel good" hormone, in your brain. Since low-level depression is often a cause for overeating, this supplement could address one of the causes for being overweight. It also helps regulate your appetite. From 50-100 mg three times a day appears to be sufficient. St. John's wort is an herb used for depression. If you're not taking any medications, it may be safe for you. But studies have shown this herb interferes with the absorption of numerous drugs, so check with your doctor before taking a supplement with this ingredient.

Low **chromium** levels are often found in people who crave sugar. This mineral aids in blood-sugar regulation and helps your body use carbohydrates rather than store them in fat tissues. Chromium has been found to help diabetics and people with low blood sugar (hypoglycemia) when taken in quantities of 200 mcg, two or three times a day, so you may need to take extra chromium in addition to your multivitamin/mineral.

Bulking agents taken before a meal can cut back on your food intake by reducing hunger. Glucomannan and apple pectin are two high-fiber substances added to some weight-loss formulas for this purpose. You could also mix a tablespoon or two of ground psyllium seed or oat bran in a little water and drink it before your meal. Or simply add more vegetables to your diet.

Green tea: The proof of green tea's ability to promote weight loss came in an article published in the *American Journal of Clinical Nutrition*. Green tea extract contains a high amount of catechin polyphenols, which may work with other chemicals to increase levels of fat oxidation and thermogenesis (where the body burns fuel, such as fat, to create heat). This increase in energy expenditure is probably the mechanism causing weight loss. Green tea is a safe alternative to traditional pharmaceuticals because, reported Dr. Abdul Dulloo, of the University of Geneva in Switzerland, "green tea is not accompanied by an increase in heart rate."

Cayenne: While cayenne isn't the best fat metabolizer in the group, it does help oxidize fat and decrease your appetite. The best attribute of cayenne is its ability to increase thermogenesis. If you've ever eaten a chili pepper, you know from first hand experience the heat these herbs can produce. And, by increasing thermogenesis, cayenne also increases your metabolism.

L-Carnitine: Studies have shown that carnitine is essential for a healthy heart and it plays an essential role in fat metabolism. It helps the body convert fat into energy while sparing the use of glucose and protein for energy production. That means it promotes fat burning for energy and leaves the protein for muscle building. It also allows an increased supply of glucose to travel to the brain, which reduces your appetite.

The Genetics of Bulimia

Researchers at the University of Pittsburgh Medical Center's Western Psychiatric Institute and Clinic are looking at a possible genetic link with people who have bulimia (eating and purging with laxatives or by vomiting). In a preliminary study, psychiatrist Walter H. Kaye, MD, found that women who had recovered from bulimia had abnormal amounts of serotonin in their brain. In theory, alterations in serotonin production can cause anxiety and obsessive behavior, as well as affect appetite control.

Dr. Kaye and his colleagues found that the women who had suffered from bulimia in the past had more moodiness and obsessions with perfectionism than those who had normal eating habits. Other brain chemicals were normal in the women who had been bulimic. In his reference book, *Nutritional Influences on Mental Illness,* psychiatrist and author Melvyn R. Werbach, MD, mentions that a vitamin B_6 deficiency may be correlated to bulimia. Since this B vitamin affects serotonin production and supports the nervous system, I wonder whether or not additional vitamin B_6 should be considered for bulimics past and bulimics present.

News release, University of Pittsburgh, October 14, 1998.

Werbach, Melvyn R., MD. *Nutritional Influences on Mental Illness,* Third Line Press, Tarzana, CA, 1991.

L-Tyrosine: This is a little-known amino acid that is a building block for hormones that enhance fat metabolism, increase the body's metabolism, and decrease appetite. It also supports thyroid function, along with iodine, which is important for maintaining a healthy metabolism.

Lipotropics are substances that improve liver function and fat metabolism. If your liver is working well and making bile to help break down the fats in your diet, you may find that your weight drops a bit. Of course, limiting fats is important. But digesting those you eat is even more important. Michael Murray, ND, suggests using a lipotropic formula with 1,000 mg of combined choline, betaine, inositol, and methionine each day.

Garcinia is the fruit of a plant indigenous to India and Asia that has been used as a natural appetite depressant. It contains a

---

Effective Weight Loss

If you're overweight and have exercise equipment at home, or are disciplined enough to go to a gym regularly, we have good news for you. A study published in the *Journal of the American Medical Association* (vol. 282, no. 16, 1999) shows that exercising briefly throughout the day gives the same results as one longer daily session.

Nearly 150 women were given treadmills and were divided into two groups. One group was told to exercise once a day for 20 minutes, then 30 minutes, and eventually 40 minutes. The other group was told to exercise for just 10 minutes at a time, but the total time they exercised was the same as the first group, gradually increasing to four 10-minute sessions rather than one longer one. All women exercised five days a week for 18 months.

The difference in weight loss between the two groups was negligible. The answer to weight loss through exercise seems clear: You need to exercise regularly-five times a week. The good news is that you can break up your individual sessions rather than one longer one. This dispels the old view that an hour a day or more is needed for weight loss. Get your exercise bike or treadmill out of storage, or dust it off. It's time to work on your exercise routine before summer! Just 10 minutes at a time, three to four times a day will do it.

Jakicic, J., C. Winters, W. Lang, and R. Wing. "Effects of Intermittent Exercise and Use of Home Exercise Equipment on Adherence, Weight Loss, and Fitness in Overweight Women," *JAMA* 282:1554-60, October 1999.

compound called hydroxycitric acid (HCA), that helps balance blood sugar and tells your brain you're not hungry.

One product that contains cayenne is Thermo-Nutrients Plus, which is a Women's Preferred product. You can order it by calling 800-728-2288.

Pyruvate and Ciwujia: Are They Worth Taking?

These substances are among the most recent to hit the airwaves. They sound absolutely marvelous. Are they? You'll have to decide for yourself. But before you can, you need more information than what you'll read about in most articles or hear from people selling them. What are they? What are we told they will do? And what's the truth behind the claims?

Pyruvate is being called the latest breakthrough in weight loss and fat burning. And maybe it is. *Maybe.* Pyruvate is made from pyruvic acid, a chemical the body uses to produce energy. Pyruvic acid is chemically unstable and can cause digestive problems and nausea. Pyruvate, made by combining pyruvic acid with sodium or other salts or amino acids, appears to be safe.

Studies have shown pyruvate helps you burn fat, increase muscle during weight loss, and lose weight. Sounds great. So what's to argue? Well, pyruvate (PYR) combined with another chemical, dihydroxyacetone (DHA) is what has been used in most studies. And most studies have been on laboratory animals, not humans. Those done with humans have been with very small numbers (12-18) of obese people on liquid diets of 500-1,000 calories/day in a hospital setting.

The amount of pyruvate used in animal studies is equivalent to 75-100 grams a day; in human studies they used 28-36 grams daily. The amount being touted for weight loss is 3-5 grams. The primary researcher, Dr. Ronald T. Stenko at the University of Pittsburgh, theorizes that lower amounts will work as well as higher amounts. But we don't know. The research done on pyruvate alone used sodium pyruvate, which is high in sodium. Other forms have not been studied. Nor have smaller amounts on people who are overweight, but not obese, and who eat food, not limit themselves to a low-calorie, liquid diet. Until better human studies have been done, it's too early to jump on the expensive pyruvate bandwagon.

Ciwujia is the root of a Chinese herb that is being sold to enhance exercise performance and increase fat metabolism — resulting in weight loss. I always look for the botanical name of herbs when I research a product. Ciwujia is *Acanthopanax senticosus,* a name that looked suspiciously familiar to me. That's because it's also called *Eleutherococcus senticosus*, or Siberian Ginseng, an herb that helps the body adapt to stress and protect against radiation. The fact that a company is promoting it under a different name and pushing the claims in the direction of weight loss makes me suspicious of their motives. Call it what it is. *Eleutherococcus* is a valuable herb. You may feel better while you exercise if you take it. You might even burn more fat. And you might not.

Losing weight and maintaining it is best accomplished by working with both your emotional and physical needs. The people I've worked with in the past 23 years are no longer struggling to eat healthier foods or to keep their weight lower. Life shouldn't be a struggle. Neither should losing weight.

Improve Your Digestion; Improve Your Health

Consider the possibility that those extra five pounds you're carrying around may not be fat at all. They could be a sign of bloating caused by poor digestion. If you're bothered by a puffiness around your stomach that gets bigger after you eat, you may be able to eliminate your problem within a week or two — forever!

Time after time, I consult with women in my practice who have trouble losing their last few extra pounds, or with women who are overweight, but who bloat and appear like they weigh even more than they do. This bloating is uncomfortable as well as unsightly. And it's completely unnecessary.

Some of the most dramatic changes I've seen in my patients' health in 22 years of practice as a nutritionist have come from their making one small adjustment in their eating habits. No single other change has resulted in such profound improvements. I've seen reductions in allergy symptoms, malnutrition, and constipation.

I've seen the elimination of gas, bloating, heartburn, and other digestive complaints. I've watched nutrient deficiencies become normalized. I've seen energy levels rise and blood-sugar levels normalize. I've seen people who struggled with overeating suddenly find they are eating normally and not bingeing.

This technique costs nothing. All you have to do is to change a single habit. You can't buy any supplement that will do as much as this little change does to improve your health. I'm talking about chewing your food well — just like your mother told you to when you were a child. The health and function of your entire digestive system is dependent upon whether or not you chew your food well enough for it to break down into the size particles your body can handle. Until you chew everything you eat well, your digestive problems can only be kept under control, at best.

You Are Not What You Eat

The old adage, "You are what you eat" is not true. You are what you eat, digest, and absorb. Unless you can digest your foods, you can't get all their nutrients into your cells. You can take antacids to get relief from digestive discomfort, but antacids neutralize the hydrochloric acid (HCl) your stomach makes to break down proteins. Without enough HCl, you can't completely digest meats, fish, beans, tofu, or other soy products.

What happens to partially digested foods? Your body identifies them as foreign invaders and they can lead to food sensitivities and fatigue. Your stomach needs sufficient acid to begin digesting calcium, magnesium, iron, and other minerals. Taking antacids is a sure way to continue having digestive problems — and nutrient deficiencies, as well.

You can take digestive enzymes with or without HCl every single time you eat and let a supplement help your body work properly. But you may need to take them for years and years, and good quality enzymes are expensive. Plus, you have to remember to take them. Isn't it better to have your body function on its own?

Step One: Chewing Well

The first stage of digestion for all carbohydrates (starches and sugars) begins in the mouth. But unless these carbohydrates are mixed well with saliva, you may miss some of the digestive process. This is because saliva contains an enzyme called amylase that breaks starches down into smaller sugars. These sugars are more digestible than when they're larger. In fact, the larger starch molecules fight with proteins to be digested in your stomach. If you don't break down your carbohydrates by chewing well, you're setting the stage for painful and embarrassing gas.

Protein digestion, on the other hand, begins in the stomach. This could give a false impression that you don't have to chew your chicken or beans well. Nothing could be further from the truth. Chewing breaks everything into smaller particles, and since all food stays in your stomach until it's partially liquified, the better you chew proteins, the easier they are to digest.

When you chew, your taste buds give a signal to produce other digestive juices, like HCl, pancreatic enzymes, and bile. Bile is a substance that helps break down fats. So all foods are broken down into more usable particles when you chew your food thoroughly.

We know that different foods contain different amounts of various vitamins, minerals, fatty acids, and other nutrients. Somehow we think that because we eat foods that contain these nutrients, they automatically get into our body and provide us with nourishment. Unfortunately, this is not the case. Unless foods are well digested, some of their nutrients will not be freed from fibers and other material and these nutrients can't be used. If you're not

---

Diets and Eating Disorders

Eating disorders have a direct relationship on dieting, according to a proclamation issued by the British Nutrition Society. The more women there are who diet in any country, the higher the percentage of women with eating disorders like bingeing, anorexia, and low self-esteem. Our emphasis should be on health, not on weight, which varies according to genetics and age as much as with eating patterns.

chewing your food well, you could be malnourished, even if the foods you're eating are healthy!

Step Two: Reduce Sugar

When you eat foods that contain a lot of sugar, you're upsetting the balance of friendly bacteria (called "probiotics") that help you digest proteins, lactose (milk sugar), and other substances. Beet sugar and cane sugar feed harmful, or pathogenic, bacteria like *Candida albicans. Candida* is a yeast that can become a fungus, and sugar is its only food.

Fructose, or fruit sugar, actually feeds the good bacteria. You can still eat sweet foods at times, but make sure that some of them are sweetened with fruit juice. There are excellent, tasty cookies available in natural food stores that even the fussiest eater can enjoy. Try some made by Pamelas. While they're a bit high in fats (limit yourself to one or two) they taste like bakery cookies.

In the past, people have been told to avoid eating protein with starches to improve their digestion. And it can help, because your body will digest fats and proteins before starches and sugars. But this way of eating means you can never eat a sandwich again, and it simply isn't practical. I believe it's better to improve a weak digestive system than to support the weakness without strengthening it. You can take a burden off your digestive system by waiting an hour or more after a protein meal to eat anything sweet.

Step Three: Don't Drink Large Amounts of Liquids With Your Meals

If you sip a glass of water or another beverage with your meal, it's probably fine. But more than that may dilute the hydrochloric acid produced in your stomach to digest proteins. As you grow older, it becomes more important to reduce drinking large quantities of liquids with meals because our bodies tend to produce less hydrochloric acid with age. Many older people suffer from gastrointestinal complaints simply because their bodies can't digest the foods they are eating. If you drink a lot with meals because you're thirsty, be aware that thirst is a sign that you're already dehydrated. It's best to sip water throughout the day and not wait until you sit down to a meal.

Step Four: Watch What You Eat Late at Night

If you like to eat a snack before going to bed, you need to know that many snack foods, such as high-fat nuts, ice cream, and chips, are hard to digest. If you're not ready to give up your favorites, at least reduce their fat content and chew them well! For a few weeks, switch to non-fat ice cream or frozen yogurt, and fat-free corn chips or potato chips. Temporarily avoid nuts.

Eat fewer snacks made with sugar. Instead, find fruit juice-sweetened cookies (some are non-fat as well), muffins, and cereals. Make low-fat or air-popped popcorn, and be sure to chew it well. Fresh fruit, carrots, or slices of jicama (a sweet, crunchy root vegetable that's eaten raw) make good snacks that feed your friendly bacteria as well as your taste buds.

Make a pot of herb tea — something with chamomile, passion flower, or skullcap — and drink a few cups of tea instead of eating. These herbs will relax you and give you something to do with your mouth at the same time.

Step Five: Increase Probiotics

You've probably heard of lactobacillus acidophilus, and possibly bifidobacteria bifidus, as well. They are two of the most common types of probiotics, and the most studied. Acidophilus concentrates on the small intestines while bifidus lives in the large intestines, or colon. Both of them produce enzymes that help digest foods. These enzymes also help ferment fiber found in beans and other carbohydrates into fatty acids. One of these fatty acids is called butyric acid. It's used in your colon as a fuel. Interestingly, butyric acid is low in many people with digestive diseases like colitis, colon cancer, and irritable bowel disease.

Acidophilus and bifidus both acidify your intestines. Since minerals need acid in order to be absorbed in the small intestines, adding acidophilus to your diet can help you absorb more of the minerals in your foods. Bifidus creates an environment in your large intestines that kills pathogenic bacteria like staphylococcus and E. coli. Many people who get food poisoning from foods that contain harmful bacteria have low levels of probiotics. This is why food poisoning tends to affect children and older people the most. These populations, due to a high-sugar diet or years of poor eating, often have insufficient friendly bacteria to handle pathogens.

Bifidus also manufactures many of the B-complex vitamins. Since vitamin B_{12} is absorbed in the large intestines, taking bifidus supplements could increase your B_{12} levels if you are a vegetarian, or if you have a B_{12} deficiency anemia.

There are two ways of increasing probiotics. The first is to eat more foods that either contain them (like sauerkraut, yogurt, tofu, miso, and tempeh), or feed them. By the way, although yogurt contains acidophilus, it's usually a very small amount. Don't depend on yogurt to solve your low-probiotic problem. It's just a good addition to your diet for additional support. A substance in fruit sugar (fructose) and grains called fructooligosaccharides feeds friendly bacteria. Eat one or two servings of fruit every day to feed your friendly bacteria.

The second way to increase probiotics is to take them in supplement form. If you decide to take supplements, be aware that many of the products on the market are low in potency. Acupuncturist Janet Zand, co-author of *Smart Medicine for Healthy Living* (Avery Publishing, 1999) suggests you buy probiotics cultured from "super strains," and only purchase those products that are refrigerated and have an expiration date. We have found only two companies whose products consistently contain high levels of probiotics: Culturelle and Natren. Natren's Healthy Trinity tops the list. But it's expensive, so you may want to begin by using a bottle of natren's acidophilus and then follow it with a bottle of bifidus — unless you have reason to believe your condition warrants the highest levels available.

How long should you take probiotics? It all depends on the health of your intestines and on your diet, and how quickly you feel a difference in your ability to digest your foods. But health care practitioners frequently suggest a three-month course of any supplement. After three months, see if you notice a decline in your digestion when you discontinue taking probiotics. They are safe to take for any length of time.

Step Six: Check With Your Doctor

If the above is not enough, it may be time to seek out professional advice. Always check with your physician if you have problems that don't clear up quickly to rule out more serious conditions. Any imbalance, when caught early, is easier to correct than when it has persisted.

Many health care professionals can assess you for intestinal permeability (or leaky gut syndrome), intestinal parasites (through stool samples), and a need to take hydrochloric acid or enzymes with meals.

One over-the-counter digestive aid is worth trying if grains,

Evaluating Weight-Loss Drugs

Some people seem to be drawn to pharmaceuticals to help them lose weight. Two relatively new anti-obesity drugs, orlistat and sibrutramine were found to be effective, but for a limited time only, and when accompanied by a diet lower in calories than the one that contributed to obesity in the first place.

Orlistat, which works for about two years, blocks fat absorption (including fat-soluble vitamins). Sibrutramine has a one-year effectiveness track record and helps you feel satisfied by providing a bulking agent. Apple pectin does the same thing, but without side effects of headaches, dry mouth, anorexia, and possible high blood pressure. Orlistat causes only oily stools, gas, and a need to use the bathroom quickly and frequently.

Perhaps the most important fact to remember is that all anti-obesity or weight-loss drugs require a lowered fat and total calorie intake. Without a change in diet, these magic bullets lose their magic. Our suggestion: Begin choosing better foods with higher fiber and lower fats, increase your exercise, try more natural products with fewer side effects, and then start looking at medications. Chances are, you won't need them.

"Better than slim chances for orlistat and sibutramine to promote weight loss," *Drug & Therapy Perspectives,* 15(12):1-6, 2000.

vegetables, and fruit cause you to bloat. It's called Beano, and it helps you digest all the above, not just beans. You can find Beano in most pharmacies, many grocery stores, and in health food stores. If you would like to try Beano for free, call 800-257-8650 or send your name and address to AkPharma, Inc., P.O. Box 111, Pleasantville, New Jersey 08232, and tell them you would like to receive a free sample of Beano.

Digestive problems may be a sign of a more serious condition. If you don't get significant improvement after implementing these ideas, by all means check further with your doctor. But whether your intestines need a little help, or further treatment, when you pay attention to your digestion your health will improve. Sometimes the biggest changes can occur with small steps you can take on your own.

Is Candida Keeping You Sick? Identifying and Understanding Candida Overgrowth

If you've been struggling with a chronic illness for years and have tried everything — allopathic medicine and alternative medicine — but still can't get well, you may have overlooked a secondary imbalance that's keeping you sick. You may have an overgrowth of a yeast called candida.

It's important to understand that you will never "get rid of" candida. It's one of more than three hundred bacteria that coexist in our digestive and vaginal tracts, keeping one another in balance. You can, however, reduce the colonies of pathogenic, or "bad" bacteria, like candida, when there are too many of them.

Some women are familiar with candida as being a cottage-cheese-like vaginal discharge accompanied by itching and irritation. This form of overgrowth often comes from taking antibiotics that kill off the friendly intestinal and vaginal bacteria, which keep candida from overmultiplying. It is also common in women with diabetes. Vaginal candida is rarely a long-term problem. It is often controlled with vaginal suppositories or anti-fungal medications, both natural and allopathic, along with eliminating sugar (its favorite food) for a few days.

It is estimated that 90 percent of Americans have either a minor or major overgrowth of candida, which often prevent them from clearing up numerous health problems. These include digestive disorders like bloating and gas, chronic fatigue, chemical sensitivities, difficulty concentrating, eczema, headaches, migraines, panic attacks, sore throats, weight gain, and many more.

Yeast or Fungus?

Candida begins in the digestive tract as a yeast. When it grows out of control, it is able to change from a yeast into a fungus, just like a caterpillar changes into a butterfly. As a yeast, it is encapsulated in the intestines, unable to push its way through the intestinal lining. But as a fungus, its long, root-like structures can break through the intestines, get into the bloodstream, and cause allergies and other problems. This is called systemic candida, and is most often found in people with severe, chronic health problems. Withholding food from the fungus is only one step in its control. It also may be necessary to take an antifungal medication — either pharmaceutical or natural — to kill off some of the overgrowth.

Now, there's one additional factor to consider with systemic candida overgrowth: the immune system. Usually, our white blood cells recognize the foreign substances in candida called antigens and kill some of them off. Dr. William Crook believes some people with candida overgrowth may have a genetic weakness in their immune response to this organism. Others may simply have an immune system that's been suppressed over the years through illness. This is why, with systemic candida, the immune system needs a great deal of support.

One type of support is to eliminate foods to which a person is allergic, since these foods also produce antigens that require more white cells to kill them off. It's a vicious cycle.

Confusion Over Candida Treatment

Candida was first brought to our attention by two doctors who specialized in allergies, Drs. Orian Truss and William Crook, in the early 1980s. Their patients — who had systemic candida — were put on extremely restrictive diets: nothing with yeast in it (this eliminated most breads and baked goods, as well as foods with vinegar), no sugar of any kind, no wheat or dairy, and almost no carbohydrates. Few people could stay on this diet long enough to effect changes.

What few people realized was why Drs. Truss and Crook devised such restrictive and difficult-to-follow diets. It came out of their specialty as allergists. And in their individual practices, Dr. Truss and Dr. Crook noticed that their allergy patients with chronic illnesses seemed to remain sick because of an overgrowth of candida.

Remember now, these were allergy patients. People who had allergies severe enough for them to seek out experts in the field. And these two eminent doctors found that if their patients stopped feeding the yeast and took anti-fungal medications, they still didn't get better because their allergies suppressed their immune system. Their bodies couldn't establish enough friendly bacteria to keep the disease-causing bacteria under control. So Drs. Truss and Crook took their allergy patients off the foods they were most frequently allergic to: molds and fungi (like mushrooms, vinegar, and foods with yeast), dairy products, and wheat.

At the same time, they lowered carbohydrates and eliminated sugar, because these foods fed the candida. They also put their patients on anti-fungal medications like nystatin and nyzerol. Patients who tried alternative medicine were put on another anti-fungal like garlic or caprylic acid. But many of these medical and alternative treatments didn't work because candida albicans is a wily critter. Try to kill it and it mutates. By the late 1980s, there were hundreds of species of candida, and many were resistant to the anti-yeast and anti-fungal medications.

Alternative health practitioners heard about Drs. Truss and Crook's work with candida, and began diagnosing this overgrowth in almost all of their patients. They used some of the same protocol with the exception of medications. Garlic, caprylic acid, or other "natural" anti-fungals were used instead of prescription drugs. So was the restrictive diet. Some patients got better, many more didn't. Instead, they grew more discouraged and more frustrated.

What was missing?

The diets most people were put on to control candida were often unnecessarily restrictive, causing people to "cheat" and feed their candida, rather than kill it off. And not many practitioners addressed the issue of probiotics — friendly bacteria — which naturally keep candida from flourishing.

Identifying Candida and the Treatment That Will Work for You

For some people, just knowing that candida may be contributing to ongoing illness is enough. Others may want a laboratory test that says, "Yes, this is a problem for you." I know of one excellent laboratory, Great Smokies, that does a Comprehensive Digestive Stool Analysis that's extremely accurate. This Great Smokies panel is a combination of 18 tests that identify bacterial and yeast overgrowths and even show which treatments, allopathic and natural, will work for your specific overgrowth problem.

If you have taken nystatin, nyzerol, fluconozol, or other anti-fungals and still have your original problems, your Candida overgrowth may be one that responds to garlic or caprylic acid instead. And, of course, the reverse is true as well. You may need pharmaceuticals to control your candida. Garlic may just not work against your particular strain.

Your doctor can contact Great Smokies Diagnostic Laboratory (800-522-4762) for the necessary information and kits. This comprehensive analysis, which evaluates digestion, absorption, intestinal functions, and microbial flora, as well as giving therapeutic information on what will correct these imbalances, costs around $200. Ask your doctor to get the pre-paid customer price for you. If you pay when you send in your sample, and do your own insurance form filing, the price can be considerably lower.

Controlling Candida:
A Comprehensive Approach That Works

There are many causes of candida overgrowth.

The most common cause of an overgrowth of candida albicans in either its yeast or fungal form seems to be the overuse of antibiotics. Antibiotics kill off large colonies of beneficial bacteria in the intestinal tract that keep candida in check. Allowed to spread, candida mutates from a yeast into a fungus, producing toxic by-products that cause allergy symptoms and digestive tract disorders.

Additionally, these medications create antibiotic-resistant strains of microbes that make it virtually impossible to restore the body's intestinal flora to its original, healthy, balanced state.

It is not, however, only antibiotic use that is contributing to candida overgrowth. Some antifungals are having the same effect. In an article published last year in the *American Journal of Medicine,* Victor Yu predicted we will be seeing more candida problems with strains other than the most common candida albicans. Already, in four teaching hospitals in the U.S., other strains of candida are appearing that seem to be resistant to fluconazole, one of the most popular new antifungal medications. Resistance to fluconazole has, in the past, been seen only in cases of thrush in AIDS patients. Now it is being seen in other patients, as well.

Poor digestion is another factor in candida overgrowth, since the presence of hydrochloric acid in the stomach helps kill off many types of unwanted fungi. As we get older, our stomachs naturally produce less hydrochloric acid. Some people have almost none. Others neutralize or inactivate their hydrochloric acid when they take antacids such as TUMS and Rolaids. In addition to not being able to digest your food properly, colonies of candida and other fungi can proliferate when your body is not producing sufficient gastric juices. Numerous degenerative diseases like arthritis, lupus, and other autoimmune diseases have connections to fungal overgrowth.

Any change in hormone balance can also contribute to an overgrowth of candida, including pregnancy, the use of birth control pills, and hormone replacement therapy. A diet high in sugars, especially lactose (milk sugar), contributes to high amounts of candida, since all fungi thrive on sugars. This includes alcoholic beverages, which need to be eliminated completely for a while.

Reducing Candida Overgrowth With Diet

Diet is a key in controlling candida. There's no way around it. If you continue to eat foods high in sugar, it doesn't matter what else you do. You won't get well. All the antifungals in the world won't help you. You can't kill off a yeast while you're feeding it and expect to get better. Candida overgrowth is stimulated by feeding the yeast or fungus. You simply have to starve it. This means eating a diet higher in protein (fish, chicken, tofu, beans) and lower in all sugars and starches. A diet high in carbohydrates, such as starchy vegetables, grains, pasta, bread, fruit, and fruit juice, and refined sugars, is not a healthy diet for someone who has an overgrowth of any yeast or fungus. Concentrate on eating lots of vegetables and protein with small amounts of fruit. People often need to be on this diet for three to six months to get results.

Because a suppressed immune system makes it difficult to control a fungal infection, you'll also want to boost yours by eliminating any foods to which you are allergic or sensitive. These may be "good" foods that impair your immune system. This means they're not good for you at this time. If you get sleepy after eating corn products (tortillas, corn chips, polenta), eliminate corn from your diet temporarily. If chicken makes you feel mentally foggy or tired, don't eat chicken for now. You're better off with a limited diet that allows you to get better than with eating a wide variety of foods that prevent you from healing.

Medications and Supplements That Work

S. Colet Lahoz, RN, author of *Conquering Yeast Infections: The Non-Drug Solution,* is a nurse and acupuncturist in Minnesota who has found a comprehensive solution to candida overgrowth. She includes a four-part colon cleansing program using Caprol, an antifungal oil; bentonite, a fine clay used as an intestinal cleanser; psyllium, as additional fiber; and implanting acidophilus. I believe her approach in thoroughly cleansing the colon and repopulating it with beneficial bacteria is a key to controlling this overgrowth.

Lahoz has her patients on the colon cleansing program twice a day for three months. In my experience, a lengthy program is essential in getting the results you're looking for. Just eating better and taking a little acidophilus for a few weeks won't accomplish anything.

For repopulation, I would suggest using Natren brand probiotics (friendly bacteria). It's one of the strongest I have ever seen and it's available in most health food stores. The best of Natren's products is a formula called Healthy Trinity, which consists of three types of friendly bacteria each suspended in an oil base (so they won't compete with one another and lose their potency). Although more expensive than any other formula, Healthy Trinity out-performs all others in my opinion and in the long run is no more expensive than any other good brand. Because it is super-strong, you may need to take only one capsule a day. If you have problems finding it, call Natren at 800-992-3323.

Individualize your antifungal treatment by getting a Comprehensive Digestive Stool Analysis from Great Smokies Laboratories (800-522-4762). It will indicate which natural and pharmaceutical antifungals will work to control the particular form of candida you have. Without this information, you're shooting blindly in the dark. With it, you can get excellent results.

Some particularly helpful antifungals include:

Caprylic acid: A fatty acid found in coconut oil, this antifungal works in the intestinal tract. It is similar in effectiveness to nystatin, a pharmaceutical that can adversely effect liver function, but is very safe to use.

Citricidal and other citrus seed extracts: In addition to being effective as antifungals in the digestive tract, citrus seed extracts also kill off parasites like giardia and blastocystis hominis. If you take them an hour before or after meals you can avoid any upset stomach it might cause.

Flax oil and fish oils: These oils contain essential fatty acids, which boost the immune system. They are also antifungals.

Garlic and onions: Natural antibiotics and antifungals used for centuries. You can use deodorized garlic oil capsules if you want to avoid garlic breath.

Tanalbit is a non-prescription intestinal antiseptic used by many health-care practitioners instead of nystatin and caprylic acid. It is made from natural tannins (resins found in tea) and zinc.

Drug therapy: If you use any medications, be sure your forms of candida will respond to the drug you're taking. And to avoid drug-resistant strains of candida from mutating, ask your physician to rotate your drugs frequently. If possible, include natural antifungals as well as pharmaceuticals.

When Candida Can't Be Controlled

If you've done everything possible to control an overgrowth of candida and still are unable to get well, there may be an underlying problem you haven't addressed: intestinal permeability, also known as leaky gut syndrome. When the fungal form of candida works its way across the intestinal mucosa it makes larger holes in the intestinal walls, allowing particles of food or bacteria to "leak" across this barrier. Food allergies also enlarge the lining of the intestines, making it more vulnerable to harmful particles.

Leaky gut syndrome will not get better by itself or with a simple change in diet and a few antifungals. It can be diagnosed by laboratory tests and treated by doctors familiar with it. In the article that follows this one, I'll talk about what you can do to identify and correct leaky gut syndrome, which often leads to autoimmune and bowel problems. Please read it carefully, and if necessary, tackle leaky gut syndrome before beginning an anticandida regimen. Otherwise, your candida eradication efforts will be thwarted by a leaky gut syndrome.

Treating Leaky Gut Syndrome and Irritable Bowel Syndrome

If you haven't paid attention to your diet and digestive tract for some time, two problems you likely could encounter are leaky gut syndrome and irritable bowel syndrome. I consider these "syndromes" to be warning signs that worse diseases are on their way if you don't do something quickly. Many of the steps involved in fixing these problems were addressed earlier, but I'd like to spend a little more time on each of these conditions.

Leaky Gut Syndrome

For more than 50 years, doctors and folk healers alike have said that good health begins in the colon. Now we're finding out they were right. Not only are the intestines the tubing through which nutrients are absorbed into our bloodstream, they are designed to allow only those particles we need for cellular health to get through, while keeping out larger particles that could lead to disease.

Food allergies, Candida overgrowth, and parasites (like Giardia) all contribute to increased permeability of the gut lining, otherwise known as leaky gut syndrome. What this means is that larger spaces between the cells of the lining of the intestines develop. Although these spaces are microscopic, they are still larger than they should be. These larger spaces allow undigested food particles, toxins, and bacteria to "leak" through the intestines (the "gut"). The result can be a myriad of complaints from food and chemical sensitivities, autoimmune diseases, headaches, inflammation, joint pain, constipation alternating with diarrhea, gas, bloating, or cramping. Over a period of time, leaky gut syndrome can lead to irritable bowel syndrome, Crohn's disease, arthritis, or celiac disease (a sensitivity to gluten, a sticky substance found in many grains).

A well-designed program that first identifies this problem and its causes, and then helps heal the lining of the intestines, is needed to correct this imbalance. It won't ever correct itself or just go away. If you've been experiencing some of the above symptoms and can't find their cause, you may want to explore the possibility of intestinal permeability, or "leaky gut."

Diagnosis: Leaky Gut Syndrome

There aren't many laboratories that diagnose this condition. The best we know of from numerous medical doctors is the

Intestinal Permeability Test from Great Smokies Diagnostic Laboratory (800-522-4762). This test measures the ability of two sugar molecules, mannitol and lactulose, to permeate the intestinal walls. Low levels of these sugar molecules in urine indicate there is a malabsorption problem. High levels indicate intestinal permeability. This test is highly predictive of leaky gut syndrome.

What Causes a Leaky Gut?

Intestinal permeability allows particles that should stay in the intestines to leak through its lining. In our bloodstream, there are cells that protect us from unwanted particles. When they see a food particle, they attack it by manufacturing antibodies that will destroy this foreign invader. But when these cells make antibodies to eliminate food particles, these antibodies can attach themselves to any organ in the body and cause numerous diseases. Arthritis is one such disease, caused when these antibodies attach themselves to joint tissues, causing substances to be made that result in inflammation, swelling, and pain.

One of the most common causes of leaky gut syndrome is non-prescription, over-the-counter medications called non-steroidal anti-inflammatory drugs (NSAIDs) like Motrin, Aleve, Advil, and aspirin. Although they are called anti-inflammatory drugs, they actually inflame the intestinal lining, causing the spaces in the gut to widen. Chemotherapy drugs have also been shown to affect intestinal permeability and contribute to malnutrition in cancer patients.

Anything that continually irritates the intestines can cause leaky gut. This includes caffeine and alcohol. Partially digested food particles fall into this category. This means we should improve our digestion by chewing more thoroughly and by taking pancreatic enzymes and/or hydrochloric acid if our body is not producing sufficient digestive juices. As we age, we produce less and less digestive juices. If you are over 50, you may want to try taking some pancreatic enzymes with meals.

Upsetting the balance of good and bad intestinal bacteria, called dysbiosis, contributes to intestinal permeability. An overgrowth of candida, a yeast that grows in the intestines, can cause inflammation in the gut lining. So will continued overgrowth of other organisms like Giardia lamblia and Helicobactor pylori (H. pylori is associated with inflammation of the stomach as well as stomach and esophageal cancers). Taking sufficient friendly bacteria is one step in correcting this imbalance.

Any condition that increases bowel inflammation contributes to leaky gut syndrome. This includes Crohn's disease, celiac disease, inflammatory joint disease, food allergies, and alcoholism. In addition, the aging process contributes to a lack of integrity in the intestinal walls.

Correcting Intestinal Permeability

A number of substances can be used to reduce inflammation and the size of the intestinal wall openings.

Quercetin is a bioflavonoid from plants that reduces permeability caused by food allergies. It can be found in health food stores alone, or combined with vitamin C.

Glutamine is an amino acid that prevents and reverses damage to the intestinal lining. It is the principal fuel used in the small intestines, and decreases bacterial overgrowth, as well. In a double-blind study conducted back in 1957, 92 percent of ulcer patients had completely healed their ulcers after taking 1.6 grams of glutamine a day for a month. Glutamine is sold in health food stores in 500 mg capsules. Be sure any glutamine you buy is labeled "pharmaceutical grade" and consider taking one capsule on an empty stomach three times a day for a month or two.

Ginkgo biloba is an herb best known for its ability to improve memory due to aging. Ginkgo increases circulation. But it also protects the intestinal lining. If you are taking ginkgo for memory, 40 mg three times daily is the amount found to be helpful. This amount can also be used to repair the intestines.

Gamma-linolenic acid (GLA) is a fatty acid found in borage seed oil that prevents and treats intestinal lining inflammation. It protects against inflammatory damage from alcohol and aspirin, as well as from chemotherapy and radiation.

Probiotics are friendly bacteria. Flooding the intestines with good quality acidophilus, bifido, and bulgaricum l.b. is essential to establishing the proper ratio of good to bad bacteria.

Digestive enzymes and hydrochloric acid. If you're not digesting your food, large particles are passing through your intestines contributing to inflammation, permeability, and food sensitivities. Consider taking two pancreatic enzyme tablets or capsules with each meal, and talk with your health provider about the advisability of including hydrochloric acid, as well. If you're not producing the necessary digestive juices to break down your foods into small enough particles to be absorbed correctly, you may need help for a while.

Enzymes and hydrochloric acid should never be taken by anyone with an ulcer. If you're not sure, check with your doctor before using these products.

Irritable Bowel Is Not Indigestion

If you're one of the many people who reaches for an antacid whenever you get stomach pains or bloat after a meal, I've got news for you. You may not have simple indigestion or need an antacid at all, even if an antacid makes you feel better temporarily. You could be one of the 15 percent of Americans who suffers from irritable bowel syndrome (IBS). Other IBS symptoms include diarrhea and/or constipation. And while IBS is rarely life-threatening, it's uncomfortable and can drain your energy.

The problem with taking an antacid or other medication that offers symptomatic relief is that you never get to the source of your problem and eliminate it. You just find a Band-Aid approach and cover up the discomfort. The only time to take an antacid is if a medical doctor has determined that your body is making too much acid. Taking any unnecessary medications can lead to other problems. They all have side effects, including antacids.

Stomach acids like hydrochloric acid are important to your digestion. They help you break down the foods you eat into small enough particles to be absorbed. Antacids neutralize them, making it difficult for you to thoroughly digest your food. So you begin by missing out on some of the vitamins, minerals, proteins, and fats your body needs that are in the foods you eat. But that's not all. Partially digested foods often ferment in the intestines causing more gas. They also upset the balance of friendly bacteria needed for a healthy immune system and to guard against vaginitis, candida, and pathogenic bacteria like streptococcus and E. coli. They can also contribute to colon problems.

Find Out What You've Got

Frequently, stress and food sensitivities cause irritable bowel syndrome, which puts it more in your control than your doctor's. Other more serious colon problems like colitis and Crohn's disease are forms of chronic relapsing inflammatory bowel disease, and may require medication as well as lifestyle changes. These more-serious illnesses may be genetic or could be caused by an auto-immune problem. Don't confuse them with IBS, which can respond well to stress management and dietary changes.

Begin by having an examination from your doctor and rule out the more serious problems like colon cancer, colitis, and Crohn's disease. Then, if you are told you have IBS, prepare to change your life before reaching for a medication that may only control symptoms. Ask your doctor or other health care practitioner to monitor you as you make some lifestyle changes.

Diet and Stress — Common Causes of IBS

Have you been under stress for three months or longer? Studies show that digestive disturbances occurring after prolonged stressful periods of our lives are usually symptoms of IBS.

Not a lot of stress in your life? Then it's time to look to your diet and begin to make some changes. IBS can be caused by food allergies or food sensitivities, by causing an irritation to the intestinal lining. Try avoiding a food or foods completely for two to four-weeks, and then reintroducing them into your diet. This will let you know whether or not a particular substance is causing your digestive complaints without having to get expensive tests.

Stress Management Works

It may be that IBS isn't caused by stress, but its symptoms are more likely to be present when you're under stress. This is because stress often leads to poor digestion. When you're anxious, your body doesn't make enough digestive enzymes and acids to break down the foods you eat, leaving partially digested foods to ferment and cause IBS symptoms. Any technique or tool that breaks your stress cycle can calm down your intestines and help you feel better.

One method that has been documented as giving great results with IBS-associated stress reduction is hypnotherapy. In a study of 33 patients with IBS, two-thirds got relief within a month and a half of weekly hypnotherapy treatments. Group treatments worked as well as individual ones, and the benefits lasted for three weeks after the treatments ended.

If you want to try hypnotherapy, look for a licensed psy-chotherapist who also practices hypnotherapy technique. This person is better able to evaluate the origins of your stresses and how they are impacting your life. A trained therapist can be a strong support for you as you make changes. You may need more than a lay person who has studied hypnotherapy. Ask to have a tape made for you that you can play at home each evening. This way your treatment can continue past your hypnotherapy sessions. Other methods of stress reduction include biofeedback, meditation, or relaxation exercises. If they're not enough, look to your diet for the next step.

Dietary Irritants — And Solutions

Food allergies always cause a negative reaction; food sensi-tivities cause problems periodically — when you eat too much of a certain food, when you're under stress, or when your body's out of whack (like an imbalance of friendly bacteria in the intestines, or a suppressed immune system, for instance). Any food can contribute to IBS, but some are more commonly associated with it than others.

The foods most commonly associated with IBS are: wheat, corn, dairy, coffee, tea, and citrus. If you crave any of these, look out. Craving a certain food is often a symptom of a problem.

Many people have sensitivities to more than one of these foods. If you eat wheat, corn, or dairy daily, stop eating one or all of them — 100 percent — for two full weeks. Read all labels carefully and ask questions when you're eating out.

Some prepared foods, like veggie burgers, for instance, have wheat or flour (made from wheat) in them. Cornstarch, corn oil, and high fructose corn syrup are ingredients you need to avoid when you're eliminating corn. And to completely avoid dairy products, shop for foods marked "vegan" in health food stores. Vegans are vegetarians who don't eat eggs or dairy.

The more processed the foods you eat, the more likely you are to find some of these ingredients lurking in them, so simplify your diet for a few weeks. Rice is rarely a problem for people with IBS. Use it as your primary starch. You can find rice crackers, rice cereals, rice bread, and even rice noodles (these can be found wherever Asian foods are sold).

Instead of dairy, use rice milk or soy milk in your cereal, beverages, and cooking. A number of delicious frozen desserts that resemble ice cream include: Sweet Nothings (their non-dairy fudge bars are remarkable!), Rice Dream, It's Soy Delicious, and Ice Bean. Avoid those with a lot of sugar like Tofutti. Sugar can upset the intestinal flora and cause diarrhea.

Keep your refined sugar intake very, very low. Use fruit-juice sweetened foods instead. Beware of the unrefined cane sugar found in a lot of "health foods" these days. We have not seen enough studies to convince ourselves that it doesn't cause at least some of the bowel problems associated with refined sugar like gas and diarrhea.

At the end of two weeks, have a small amount of the food you've been avoiding: a piece of bread, a little milk or cheese, some baked corn chips. If your symptoms reappear, you need to avoid the offending food longer.

Helpful Supplements

Three supplements are key in reestablishing balance to your intestines: fiber, probiotics and peppermint oil. If you're constipated, increase your fiber by eating more whole grains and vegetables.

Because adding more fiber increases your need for water, drink water throughout the day. Half a glass an hour, whenever possible, is ideal, and better than drinking two or three glasses at a time, which can cause bloating.

Probiotics are friendly bacteria, like Lactobacillus acidophilus and bifido bacteria. Adding these to your diet daily for two or three months is important for keeping large enough colonies of "good" bacteria present, which fight disease-causing bacteria. One sign you don't have enough probiotics is vaginitis and systemic Candida, caused by an overgrowth of pathogenic Candida bacteria.

Enteric-coated peppermint oil capsules have been found to relax the smooth muscles in the intestines and prevent the cramping some people get with irritable bowel syndrome. They work by blocking the intestines' ability to utilize calcium. Calcium causes muscles to cramp; magnesium and peppermint oil cause muscles to relax. The first step you take might be to remove large sources of calcium from your diet (dairy products) and supplements. Next, if you are constipated, consider taking a little extra magnesium. It causes looser stools and helps muscles relax. If you have loose stools or diarrhea, try Enzymatic Therapy, or another brand of enteric-coated peppermint oil found in many health food stores.

A Final Comment

I support your desire to take more responsibility for your health and to use more natural methods of achieving it whenever possible. But I caution you to first get a diagnosis from a health care practitioner to rule out any serious problem and help you decide what options are open to you. Next, look for the simplest step to take first. In the case of IBS, perhaps you can begin by simply chewing your food better and eating when you're relaxed. This has a great effect on your body's ability to digest.

Keep a food diary and see if certain foods seem to trigger your symptoms. Most importantly, don't oversimplify and automatically reach for an over-the-counter or prescription medication that alleviates symptoms without addressing the cause of your problem. Irritable bowel is not indigestion, and antacids are not its solution.

But it may be just as easy to eliminate or control as daily stress reduction and a change in your diet.

The only way to correct any health condition is to find the source of the problem. While it takes time and effort to correct your problems, it can be done.

Chapter 4

Can Negative Emotions Be Toxic?*

Have you ever been upset with a doctor who told you, "There's nothing wrong with you. It's all in your head," when you knew you weren't feeling well physically?

Whether you've ever had difficulty getting a specific diagnosis or not, your past or present illnesses probably got started or were helped along by toxic emotions. Most people don't realize that chronic and severe illnesses usually have an emotional component.

Toxic emotions make you feel tired, depressed, listless, and upset. They lower your immune system and help cause bothersome and serious illnesses. Most of all, they waste your time. They waste your life.

Anger, resentment, hate, bitterness, impatience, unkindness, negative thinking, and vindictiveness are all toxic emotions. When you hold on to them and live with them day in and day out, they create a great deal of stress. This constant stress lowers your immune system, contributing to illness.

Positive emotions, like love, enthusiasm, and happiness, cleanse your system and give you energy. They heal your body, mind, and spirit. They are responsible for serious illnesses going into remission and for your body's ability to heal itself more quickly.

Where It Begins

As I mentioned in the previous chapter, our illnesses are rarely all physical or all emotional in origin. We've known this since the

---

*Portions reprinted from *The Giant Book of Women's Health Secrets.*

1950s when Dr. Hans Selye, a biochemist, began writing about the effects of stress hormone activity and illness in his classic book, *The Stress of Life*. And in 1977, Kenneth Pelletier wrote *Mind as Healer, Mind as Slayer*, in which he described some of the diseases caused by stress: from heart disease and cancer to migraines and arthritis.

Today, the mind-body connection is accepted by more physicians, psychotherapists, and other health-care professionals. Decades of scientific studies have shown that our minds do, indeed, control our bodies' chemistry, and that negative thoughts produce destructive chemicals that can harm us. It's time to take a closer look at your toxic emotions and your health, because the thoughts you think and the feelings you have can either help you become and stay healthy or can literally kill you.

I don't want you to assume that all you need to do to be healthy is to eliminate your toxic emotions and take a positive attitude toward life. Although that approach certainly has its merits. First, get a diagnosis of any physical symptoms you are experiencing from one or more doctors, so you know what you're dealing with. Then look at some of the emotional aspects of your problem and address it.

Psychological and Physiological Aspects of Stress

Just saying that emotions are toxic is not enough. We need to understand their physiological consequences. Toxic emotions lead to prolonged mental stress — and stress can kill us.

As far back as the 1930s, Harvard physiologist Walter Cannon believed our bodies regulated themselves according to our needs. This balance, or homeostasis, was affected by our blood pressure, body temperature, heart rate, blood sugar — and by stress. Cannon saw that when we were in particularly stressful conditions, our bodies adapted by working overtime to try to restore us to balance. He called this the "fight-or-flight" response. What this means is that when we're surprised by a bear in the woods we're either going to fight it, or run like crazy. This fight-or-flight response is affected by chemicals secreted in the brain that send a signal to the adrenal glands (glands that produce hormones like cortisol and adrenaline).

The adrenal hormones affect your nervous system and muscles. They are responsible for the shakiness you feel when you barely avoid an accident or are suddenly surprised by someone sneaking up on you. They give you superhuman strength to lift something far heavier than you could ordinarily to save someone from being crushed, and they give you the energy you need to run faster than you thought possible when you feel you're in danger.

This stress response was, most likely, the way many of our ancestors survived difficult situations, and in itself is not necessarily toxic. But we encounter stressors much more often in our daily lives, and although they may not be life-threatening, they overwork our glands, organs, nervous system, and brain. Our bodies can deal with a little stress. High levels of stress over prolonged periods of time, however, can be toxic — more than our bodies can handle.

Decades after Walter Cannon's work, Dr. George F. Solomon, a psychiatrist at Stanford University, decided that stress and emotions not only set off our fight-or-flight response, they also affect our immune systems. He began to experiment with the hypothalamus, a tiny part of the brain where hormone secretions associated with stress responses begin. Solomon, and an immunologist, Alfred Amkraut, found that when the hypothalamus in rats was damaged, their immunity decreased. This was the beginning of the scientific study of the mind/body connection — and examination of the effects of toxic emotions.

What Happens When You're Under Stress

There are two areas in your body that are activated by stress. These are the autonomic nervous system, which is involuntary, and the endocrine system. The autonomic nervous system has two components, which are called the sympathetic and the parasympathetic nervous systems. The sympathetic system causes your involuntary muscles to tense up, and it activates your endocrine system. The parasympathetic system dilates your smooth muscles, causing you to relax.

When you're under stress, your sympathetic nervous system is activated; blood leaves your hands, feet, and stomach and starts to go to your head and torso. You get cold hands, chills, a knot in your stomach. Your muscles get tight — shoulders, neck, throat. You are feeling the effects of the fight-or-flight response.

The sympathetic nervous system works with your endocrine system when you're under stress. Your endocrine system — pituitary glands, thyroid, parathyroids, islets of Langerhans in your pancreas, and adrenal glands — become activated and secrete hormones inappropriately. Two of the most important ones in the stress response are ACTH (adrenocorticotrophic hormone) and TTH (thyrotrophic hormone), both released by the pituitary gland, which cause you to sweat, feel nervous and shaky, have a rapid heartbeat, and feel exhausted. These are the same kinds of feelings you would get from food poisoning. It's just a different kind of toxic reaction.

The sympathetic system also stimulates your adrenal glands to make adrenaline, and you may feel an adrenaline "rush." Adrenaline also sends a message to your liver to release glucose (sugar) for quick energy. It causes you to burn carbohydrates faster, opens up the arteries to your heart so you breathe faster, and raises your temperature. If your fight-or-flight response occurs only when you're facing a bear in the woods or escape an accident, your immune system won't suffer. That's what it's for. But if you are under stress constantly, your immune system may lose its ability to protect you from microorganisms and disease.

Stress and Immunity

Joseph Pizzorno, ND, founding president of Bastyr University, the first accredited university of natural medicine in the country, and author of *Total Wellness* (Prima Publishing, 1966) says, "In general, the degree of immunosuppression is proportional to the level of stress." So the more stress you're under, the weaker your immune system is likely to be.

Stress overactivates the sympathetic nervous system. Your immune system works best when the para-sympathetic nervous system is up and running and when the sympathetic system is not stimulating the production of adrenal hormones. These hormones have a toxic response in your body by lowering your white blood cells —

your body's defense system — and they actually shrink your thymus gland. Your thymus is the gland that rules and supports your entire immune system.

Heart Disease and the Type-A Personality

Back in the early 1970s, two researchers, Friedman and Rosenman, found that more men had heart disease than women, and not because of any dietary or hormonal differences. They discovered that their personalities were quite different. More men had what they called Type-A personalities: They were excessively competitive and felt like they had to continually meet deadlines. Women, who were more likely to possess Type B personalities, were more relaxed, made time for leisure activities, and worked more for personal satisfaction than for money.

The Type-A personality is toxic — always striving for the external, the material; the Type-B personality takes better care of itself and is healing. In the two decades following this research on Type-A and Type-B personalities, women have achieved more in the workplace. And, as a result, there are now more women who have taken on the toxic Type-A personality — along with all the harmful effects it produces.

Climbing the corporate ladder, however, needn't result in toxic emotions. Many high-achieving women benefit health-wise from higher levels of personal satisfaction and self-esteem.

In addition, the feelings of frustration and powerlessness that are common among pink-collar workers, as well as many homemakers and mothers, are toxic and have been linked to higher rates of heart disease.

Heart disease is now as prevalent among women as men. In fact, it's the number-one killer of postmenopausal women. One reason for female heart disease is our natural decline in estrogen after menopause, a hormone that serves as a calcium channel blocker, preventing deposits of calcium in the arteries. But the increase in heart disease is probably due to increased cholesterol production in the liver because of stress. When we're under stress, our liver manufactures more cholesterol.

Taking a Look at Stress

Living in a state of toxic emotions is draining. It leads to chronic mental stress and illness. We all know what stress feels like, but just what is it? According to pioneer biologist Hans Selye, it is "the rate of wear and tear within the body." This means that worrying about your job or a relationship produces stress, and so does traveling around the world or going on a weekend ski vacation. All stress is not bad, it's just creating wear and tear (and, along with it, a need for more nutrients to help repair both your mind and your body).

Sometimes when we're experiencing overwhelming stress we make ourselves sick so we don't have to deal with it — like getting a headache. At other times, stress causes us to use up protective vitamins and minerals that support our immune system and we "catch a cold" or get some other sickness, like heart disease or cancer. Fear and mental stress are two toxic emotional components that can lead directly to high blood pressure (hypertension) and possibly stroke.

DHEA for Depression?

The hormone DHEA (dehydroepiandrosterone) is considered by many to be the "mother of all hormones." It's produced by the brain, the adrenal glands, the skin, and is the most abundant steroid hormone in the body. Its behavior is very unique and until the last decade or so, DHEA was probably the most misunderstood key hormone.

Studies to date have found that DHEA lowers cholesterol and prevents blood clots, improves memory, strengthens the immune system, prevents bone loss, fights fatigue and depression, enhances feelings of well-being, increases strength, reduces body fat, increases libido, and alleviates menopause symptoms. DHEA may also protect against diabetes and autoimmune diseases. And important research is currently underway into DHEA's ability to prevent cancer.

Perhaps DHEA is best-known, however, for its overall energizing effects. In a six-month study conducted at the University of San Diego, participants taking DHEA reported a "remarkable* increase in perceived physical and psychological well-being." They also reported sleeping better, feeling more relaxed, being less affected by stress, and experiencing relief from joint pain (among arthritis sufferers).

*In medical jargon, remarkable means significant.

But stress has great value for us in our lives. It can also be a pivotal point of our personal transformation. Psychotherapist Carl Jung observed that primitive people looked at illness as the strength coming from their unconscious minds that led them from one stage of life to another. Numerous people with cancer, AIDS, chronic fatigue, and other debilitating illnesses have found the quality of their lives increased greatly after facing their health issues. They adapted a different point of view and "detoxified" their emotions. They forgave people in their lives who had caused them emotional pain. They began expressing love to their friends, started doing what they wanted to do with their time, rather than what they thought they should do, and they started living life more fully. These were all benefits that came out of the stress of their illnesses.

Feeling Good With Endorphins

When you're under stress, your body uses more of certain vitamins and minerals. A lack of even some of these nutrients can alter your mood, creating irritability, mood swings, and negative thoughts. So which comes first, a diet lacking in sufficient nutrients to support your stress, or stresses in life that cause your body to be deficient in nutrients? It doesn't matter.

Endorphins are "feel good" chemicals released by the pituitary gland. Exercise helps release them. So does acupuncture. And so do certain nutrients like vitamin B_6, magnesium, and amino acids found in protein. Your thoughts do, too, through a powerful phenomenon known as the "placebo effect." Placebos are like sugar pills — worthless substances that won't change anyone's physical condition. Unless, of course, the patient believes they will. Time and again, studies have shown that when placebos were given along with the message that they would work — they did! Dr. Melvyn Werbach, author of the nutrition textbook *Nutritional Influences on Illness* has stated, "We don't need better medicines, we need better placebos."

Your mind can crank out chemicals that make you feel good emotionally and even take away pain, because endorphins are chemically similar to morphine. What's the difference between them? Endorphins are hundreds of times more potent, and you have the ability to create them with your healing thoughts. Endorphins are caused by positive emotions. Toxic emotions don't stimulate their production.

Gary Schwartz, PhD, professor of psychology at the University of Arizona, has been researching emotions and health for more than 20 years. He has found that the ACE Factor (our ability to attend, connect, and express) can affect our immune systems, blood sugar, and heart in a positive way. People who repressed their emotions, Schwartz found, made too many endorphins in an effort to block out their physical and emotional pain. These excessive endorphins had a toxic effect on the body by causing high blood sugar, which promoted an emotional roller coaster, creating more anxiety and mood swings. People who had the ACE personality, by contrast, had normal blood sugar and the right amount of endorphins.

Feeling Good With Serotonin

Serotonin is a chemical manufactured in the brain that gives a feeling of well-being. One particular amino acid (part of protein) is needed to help your brain make serotonin. That amino acid is tryptophan, and tryptophan needs vitamin B_6 and magnesium to work. When you're under stress, your body uses up more B_6 and magne-

---

Pass on These Energy Bars

Yohimbe Strength and Energy Formula bar by Mega Pro. Yohimbe is an herb that induces erections in men, and the advertising on this energy bar talks about a "rock hard physique." When asked about how much yohimbe was in the bar, and how it could be metabolized without citric acid (little did the sales rep know I am knowledgeable in the use of yohimbe), I was told there wasn't enough in it to do anything, so the lack of citric acid wasn't important.

This Yohimbe bar also contains Damiana (said to be an aphrodisiac) and Guarana (which contains a chemical almost identical to caffeine). The Guarana might give some energy, but the rest is placebo. The same company makes an Energy Max bar. Since there are much better products out there for your money, pass these two up!

sium. That leaves very little of these nutrients for the brain to make tryptophan and then serotonin.

Here we have a vitamin/mineral deficiency caused by the stress from toxic emotions that creates more toxic negative feelings, which cause more stress and negativity. It's a toxic emotional roller coaster ride without an end. The only way to stop it is to recognize what you're doing and just start thinking and acting differently.

Premenstrual depression is a familiar condition to many women that has a documented link to B_6, magnesium, and tryptophan deficiencies. During our monthly cycles, those of us who are affected become more depressed and negative. We create more toxicity. The best way to stop this cycle is to balance our bodies' biochemistry.

In the past, many doctors recommended tryptophan supplementation for PMS-associated depression. Now, due to the overreaction of the FDA to a tainted source of tryptophan that resulted in a handful of deaths (far fewer than those caused by aspirin or other over-the-counter drugs), tryptophan is unavailable except by prescription. Of course, monthly depression is not life-threatening. But it is threatening to your *quality* of life. And depression can be toxic because it often leads to lowered immunity, which can result in more serious illnesses

To increase your body's ability to utilize the tryptophan in your foods (turkey is one of the highest foods in tryptophan, but it is found in all complete protein — both animal and vegetable), begin by raising your quantities of vitamin B_6 and magnesium. Both of these nutrients are found in whole grains and beans. And there are also some women's vitamin/mineral formulas with extra B_6 and magnesium already in them.

It is not only premenstrual depression that affects your health, but depression, in general. This depression may be caused by blood-sugar fluctuations (alcohol and high sugar intake can contribute to this), food allergies, a biochemical imbalance, nutrient deficiency, or emotional upheavals like the loss of a loved one (either death, divorce, or separation). The first step is to identify the source of your depression, then to take action to break the cycle of toxicity and neutralize any toxic emotions.

Love and Fear — Our Primary Emotions

Joan Borysenko, PhD, is co-founder of the Mind/Body Clinic in New England. She is an instructor at Harvard Medical School and a teacher of yoga and meditation. In her book, *Minding the Body, Mending the Mind,* she says, "Emotions fall into two broad categories, fear and love." Fear is the toxic emotion; love the healer.

Other toxic emotions, like guilt and shame, come out of our fears that others will learn something about us that we want to keep hidden. Anger, another toxic emotion, can come from a fear of confronting someone rationally who does not behave rationally toward us. Whether we stuff these toxic emotions deep inside ourselves or spew them out at others, they are making us sick and wasting our precious time.

Numerous metaphysicians have said that fear is the absence

The Strong and Sexy Hormone, Testosterone

Although testosterone is considered a male hormone, women's bodies produce and use testosterone, too. Women who have had their ovaries removed are often testosterone deficient. And a deficiency can occur even when the ovaries are still intact. In the event of a true deficiency (documented through testing), natural (not methyl) testosterone supplements to correct the deficiency can help protect against heart disease and other problems associated with a lack of testosterone. The risk is believed to be minimal. Testosterone creams and gels are also available and some women and their doctors prefer these. For best results, also get total and HDL cholesterol levels checked regularly, since too much testosterone can adversely affect these levels.

In addition to boosting your libido, testosterone can also be used to treat depression, increase energy, and strengthen muscle and bone tissue, and even relieve menopause symptoms. While higher testosterone levels are traditionally associated with greater aggressiveness, this isn't necessarily bad: Women with higher testosterone levels tend to be higher achievers.

An interesting study by Dr. Barbara Sherwin of McGill University in Montreal found that premenopausal women who had undergone hysterectomies, fared better receiving a combination estrogen and testosterone supplements, than those supplemented only with estrogen. Other studies have found that the estrogen/testosterone combination is more effective than estrogen alone against osteoporosis.

of love. Now more physicians and health care professionals are say-ing the same thing. Fear and love are not only primary emotions, they are opposite emotions. They cannot occupy the same emotion-al space at the same time. If you are feeling love, you have no room in that moment for fear. Sometimes all we can do is push away our fear for a few minutes. Then the fear comes back. When you accom-pany love with other positive emotions, like helpfulness and under-standing, it stays longer.

With love comes joy, peace, and laughter. After a serious heart attack, writer Norman Cousins took charge of his life. He found, and documented his findings, that laughter has curative powers. It neutralizes toxic emotions, rendering them harmless. In *Anatomy of an Illness,* he writes: "Just as the negative emotions produce nega-tive chemical changes in the body, so the positive emotions are con-nected to positive chemical changes."

Cousins and other heart patients have reversed blockages in the arteries of their heart by manufacturing more of these healing chemicals through laughter and a positive outlook. And they're not alone. Every bookstore contains dozens of books written by people with deadly illnesses who went into remission — and stayed there — using a good diet, exercise, stress reduction ... and positive thoughts. Whether or not you rent comedy videos, read funny books, or engage in friendly banter with someone you love, laugh-ter produces healthy chemicals that neutralize the toxic ones.

Is a Hysterectomy in Your Future?

When Katie first visited her doctor, she suffered from heavy menstrual bleeding and several uterine fibroids (benign tumors), which were almost two inches in diameter. The bleeding was painful and caused her to become anemic.

After undergoing an ultrasound to diagnose the problem, her doctor strongly recommended she have a hysterectomy. But Katie was uneasy about having her uterus removed, so she decided to look into her problem on her own.

Katie's first step was to visit a holistic doctor who went through a thorough health survey and evaluation with her. What he found was quite different than anything she had heard before.

First, the doctor picked up on the fact that Katie didn't start menstruating until her mid-teens, which is late by most standards. Her mother, who had fibroids and a subsequent hysterectomy in her late 50s, also began menstruation late, indicating the problem ran in the family.

For some reason, women who begin menstruating late will almost always develop some type of reproductive problem at some point in their life. It's almost as if the woman's body never wanted to start menses in the first place and, so, it prevents the cycle from functioning properly.

But why had Katie's mother not had trouble until her late 50s and Katie was having problems in her early 40s? The issue troubled Katie's doctor until she told him that the problems started about the same time she and her husband began having serious marital difficulties. Month after month, the stress of the relationship took a toll on her. She was constantly worried that he might have an affair or leave her altogether.

Once the doctor understood the underlying cause of her problems, he was able to begin treating her medically without using any harmful drugs or surgeries. He encouraged Katie to get some counseling for her emotional state, as well as for her marriage.

She did, and within two months her fibroids had shrunk by half. The pain was completely gone and her periods returned to normal after three months.

Unbelievable? Maybe, but it's a true story. I changed a few of the details to protect those involved, but the essentials of the story are all there.

Are Hysterectomies Really Necessary?

The reality is that any ongoing stressful situation, whether it's a bad marriage (or any bad relationship for that matter), a tough job, or a prolonged physical illness can mess with a woman's hormones to the point that it causes problems with her reproductive organs.

Fortunately, most of the problems that develop are not life-threatening, though some can be.

Most gynecologists are quick to recommend a hysterectomy any time problems appear. But it's important to remember that while the hysterectomy Katie's original doctor wanted to perform would have solved the physical symptoms, it couldn't cure the underlying cause.

Hysterectomy in America is a $3 billion-a-year business, second only to Caesarean sections (another overused surgery on American women). In the U.S., one in three women will have a hysterectomy by the age of 60. Compare that to Italy, where the ratio is one in six. Or France, where it is only one in 18!

The two most common problems that lead to hysterectomy are persistent bleeding and fibroid tumors of the uterus. Other indicators include severe, long-term infections, severe endometriosis, cervical cancer, and ovarian cancer.

With persistent heavy bleeding, a hysterectomy may be necessary. But it should always be the last resort.

Interestingly, if you are 55 or older and suffer from heavy bleeding, chances are very good that the bleeding will stop spontaneously. Modern medicine doesn't know the reason for this, but it could have something to do with a reduction in the stress levels in your life. If this describes your situation, have your blood count checked every six weeks to be sure you're not getting anemic and try to deal with anything stressful that might be affecting your health.

Fibroid tumors of the uterus often cause no symptoms and many times are found during routine examinations. Fibroids can vary in size from microscopic to the dimensions of a cantaloupe — or even larger. If you have a fibroid tumor, and it's not causing any symptoms such as bleeding, problems with your sex life, or disfigurement, it's better to avoid major surgery and try some less invasive treatments, such as doctor-administered homeopathy or acupuncture.

Is Cancer a Good Enough Reason?

Possibly. But don't think that just because you're diagnosed with ovarian or cervical cancer, you must have a hysterectomy.

I read recently of a woman who was diagnosed with Stage III metastatic ovarian cancer and immediately scheduled a hysterectomy. In the interim, she met with a doctor who helped her deal with some of the stress in her life.

According to *Alternative Medicine* magazine, "Vera...had endured a highly abusive relationship with her husband, so abusive that at times she would lock herself in the bathroom to get away from him."

After dealing with the hurt and anger built up inside her, as well as some other related issues, Vera went in for surgery. In Vera's own words, here is what happened: "My surgeon said he found only a very small cyst-like mass, and the pathology report of neighboring tissues confirmed that no cancer cells were present."

So don't assume that a cancer diagnosis automatically means it's time to have your uterus removed.

More Reasons to Avoid Major Surgery

There are many reasons *not* to have a hysterectomy and few good reasons, other than uncontrollable bleeding or cancer, for having one. We've detailed a couple of reasons to avoid the surgery already, but one thing you must always remember is that no operation is completely safe. Here are a few more things to think about before submitting to a hysterectomy:

(1) A study done several years ago by researchers at UCLA and reported in the *Journal of Women's Health*, showed that many hysterectomies are done at the whim of the surgeon. The shocking report confirmed that doctors are having patients sign a pre-surgical permit that allows the surgeon to remove the uterus if he deems it necessary. Most of these operations are for ovarian cysts and have nothing to do with the health of the uterus. Patients are often told "this absolutely has to be done," says Dr. Joseph Gambone of UCLA.

The study compared 100 women who had only simple removal of the cysts with 100 who had hysterectomies as well. Those having a hysterectomy had five times the complications, lost twice as much blood, and stayed twice as long in the hospital.

(2) Although doctors claim that a hysterectomy will not affect a woman's sex life, it is not always true. They will point to many studies that "prove" a hysterectomy has no effect on a woman's sex life, except for those cases where it actually improves it. However, a study conducted in Japan goes completely contrary to what most American gynecologists are telling their patients. The study found that 27 percent of women who had undergone a hysterectomy experienced an emptiness due to the awareness of the uterus being gone. This decreased their sexual pleasure and 70 percent experienced difficulty reaching orgasm.

A Finnish study also found a "significant reduction" in the frequency of orgasm in patients one year after the operation.

(3) Many doctors will claim that the uterus serves no hormonal function, so why not take it out once its reproductive function is over? But, as with so many things in medicine, this has proven to be false reasoning.

We now know that the uterus is an active, hormone-secreting

Pregnenolone: Food for Thought

A second hormone that has recently appeared for purchase over-the-counter is pregnenolone. It is a key brain hormone, credited with memory enhancement and concentration improvement, as well as being a fighter of mental fatigue and reliever of arthritis. In the opinion of many experts, pregnenolone is the most potent memory enhancer available.

Human studies have confirmed pregnenolone's ability to improve mental functioning. Additional research also suggests that this is the result of increasing testosterone levels in men (who show improved ability to perform visual spatial tasks), and estrogen levels in women (who show improvement in verbal recall), rather than a simple across-the-board increase in pregnenolone. Instead, pregnenolone is broken down and used differently by men and women.

Another promising use of pregnenolone is to treat depression. A study from the National Institutes of Mental Health found that people with clinical depression have subnormal levels of pregnenolone. Hormone expert Dr. Regelson, is highly optimistic about pregnenolone's potential to treat age-related depression and advocates its use to treat mild cases, before higher-risk drugs such as Prozac are considered.

organ just like the thyroid and the ovaries. It is an integral part of the body's hormonal system that continues to perform essential functions even after menopause. It produces beta-endorphins, the body's internal painkillers, and prostacyclin, which inhibits blood clotting.

This could be why women who have had hysterectomies are more prone to cardiovascular problems, such as heart attacks and hypertension, though this has not been proven as yet.

This diminution in essential hormones can also explain some frequently reported symptoms of women following the operation, such as loss of energy and stamina, loss of not only sexual sensations, but physical ones, and diminished maternal feelings — in other words, feelings of being less of a woman.

Time to Take Action

As I said earlier, there are times when a hysterectomy is necessary. But if it has been suggested that you have a hysterectomy, it's time to take action and do some research.

First, find a gynecologist who does not do surgery and ask his opinion related to your particular complaint. In most cases, you'll find that the operation is completely unnecessary.

Next, buy a copy of the book *The No-Hysterectomy Option*, by Herbert A. Goldberg, MD, FACOG. It is a well-balanced and thorough book on hysterectomy and your options. It's worth the $15 and can be picked up or ordered at most major bookstores. It explains when a hysterectomy is absolutely necessary and what you need to know about your life after the operation.

And, finally, make sure you seek out a holistic doctor who can help you find the underlying cause of your uterine problems. He won't be able to counsel you through your relational problems, but he might help you figure out what stressors you have in your life. Once you've discovered the root cause(s), then you can begin to work through the real issues in your life.

Don't just assume that surgery is your only option. In fact, assume that it's not an option unless all else fails.

Six Ways to Be More Stress-Resistant

1. Get Plenty of Sleep. Since the invention of the light bulb, people have been sleeping less and less. But this hasn't been to our benefit. In 1988, sleepiness was the cause of 41.6 percent of all reported traffic accidents — costing $37.9 billion, 769,184 disabling injuries, and 17,689 deaths. Sleep researchers have discovered that plenty of sleep helps us function better at work and in relationships and increases our ability to enjoy life. It also helps us maintain stronger immune systems. A lack of sleep is a source of stress that is detrimental at best and deadly at worst.

How much sleep do you need? Dr. Thomas Wehr, a psychiatrist and researcher at the National Institutes of Mental Health, found that with no time cues and 14 hours of darkness (as in winter), people slept 10 to 12 hours for 21 days. After snoozing off their cumulative sleep debt (about 17.5 hours), the men settled at eight hours and 15 minutes, and the women settled at an average of 9 hours and 15 minutes per night. Older persons may need less sleep.

If you have trouble getting to sleep early, try initiating a TV-free bedtime ritual to help yourself wind down. It might include a warm bath, a good book, and a calming herbal tea such as chamomile. Also, men aren't the only ones inclined to fall asleep soon after orgasm. Women are, too. Find what works best for you.

If you have trouble falling asleep and staying asleep, most experts agree it's also safe for persons age 45 and older to take low doses of melatonin, the sleep hormone, 30 minutes before you want to fall asleep. Start off with .5 mg. and increase if necessary. Try to stay under 1.5 mg. and see if taking it every other night or less is sufficient to keep you well-rested. Melatonin is preferable to other sleeping pills. It is not addictive. And, unlike other sleeping pills, it helps reestablish normal sleep cycles — what a good night's sleep is all about.

2. Eat the Best Quality Diet Possible. You should know what this means by now.... A nutrient-dense diet comprised mainly of whole grains, legumes, lots of fresh fruits and vegetables, some raw nuts and seeds for essential fatty acids, and little if any dairy foods and flesh. Comparing a meal that fits these perimeters to a typical frozen, fast-food, or highly processed meal is like comparing jet fuel to low octane gasoline with water added. Our body's daily operation is fueled by the nutrients in our diets. A good, nutrient-dense diet boosts stress resistance. A poor diet is a source of stress in itself — so stressful that the Center for Science in the Public Interest estimates that poor nutrition (which includes eating habits that produce obesity) is the cause of most deaths. Be sure to drink plenty of pure water throughout the day as well — about four oz. per hour, more if you consume caffeinated beverages (which are dehydrating).

3. Take Nutritional Supplements. Start with a good, basic multivitamin/mineral. Avoid the one-a-day variety that provide only the RDA amounts. These are barely enough to prevent serious mal-

Remember to Sleep Enough

Sleep does much more than allow your body to rest and repair itself. It also helps your memory and your mood, according to Pierre Maquet from the Institute of Neurology at University College in London. Maquet was part of a team that compared brain activity in people who were learning a new task with brain activity during rapid eye movement (REM) sleep. Similar brain patterns were seen in both, suggesting to Maquet that when we sleep, we remember what we learned while we were awake.

This preliminary study is just the beginning of our understanding between memory and sleep. But don't worry. If you have insomnia or don't spend a lot of time in REM sleep, you won't forget what you know. The connection appears to be with learning new activities, not remembering old ones.

Until the final answers are in, you may want to address any insomnia with kava (for anxiety) or melatonin (a hormone that is reduced as we age and is linked to sleep). Both can be found in natural food stores and both appear to be safe, even when taken with medications. In fact, some medications suppress melatonin production. But melatonin only increases the effectiveness of benzodiazepines (like Xanas, Halcion, Valium, and Dalmane) and tamoxifen. Talk with your health-care practitioner about using small amounts of melatonin (1/2 to 1 mg one hour before bed) to help you sleep more deeply. When you sleep better, you feel better.

Larkin, Marilynn. "Sleep on it, say scientists," *The Lancet,* July 29, 2000.

Lininger, Schuyler, W., Jr., DC, editor, *A-Z Guide to Drug-Herb-Vitamin Interactions,* Prima Publishing, 1999.

nutrition diseases like scurvy. Instead, take the newer mega-dose multis in which the daily dose is six pills taken at three time intervals throughout the day (for maximum absorption). Remember to avoid a formula with too much calcium.

My favorites are Vitality, which can be ordered through customer service at 1-800-728-2288, and Optimox, which offers pre- and postmenopausal formulas and can be ordered by calling 1-800-722-9040. Your multi should provide a broad base of key nutrients. From there you can add more specialized supplements, determined by you or your health-care provider. Together, your multi and other supplements will provide you extra health protection and stress resistance. And always remember, they're called supplements because they're to be taken in addition to, not in place of, a good quality diet.

4. Try These Homeopathic Remedies for Stress and Anxiety:

Lycopodium: This remedy is used to soothe anxiety about a new situation, such as a new job, relocating to a new area, and even new relationships or prenuptial jitters.

Nux vomica: This is a remedy for workaholics. Often, however, their stress and anxiety is compounded by a lack of sleep, exercise, poor diet, and little or no personal life. Therefore, results are best if nux vomica is used for initial relief while positive lifestyle changes are being made.

Phosphoric acid: This remedy is for people who are normally lively, energetic, and affectionate, but have become exhausted and irritable as a result of stress.

Picric acid: This remedy is for the stress and tension that can arise from a simple case of too much work. For example, working moms who put in a full day at the office or other place of work only to leave at the end of the work day for a second work shift of shopping, cooking, cleaning, and parenting.

A few notes about using homeopathic remedies are in order. First, some prescription drugs such as birth control pills and antihistamines may interfere with the action of a homeopathic remedy. Aromatherapy and herbs can also interfere, as can coffee, alcohol, tobacco, and strong-smelling household and personal care products such as mint toothpaste. Do not use these items a half hour before or after taking a homeopathic remedy.

Many homeopathic solutions can be found at health food stores, and some conventional pharmacies are also beginning to stock them. Follow the instructions on the label and discontinue the solution when you notice your condition is improving. If a remedy has no effect, try another. Rather than spend more time and money trying to treat yourself, however, it might be wise to visit a homeopathic doctor who can recommend a remedy based on an in-depth evaluation.

Finally, as in the case of the remedy for workaholism I mentioned earlier, many homeopaths also encourage lifestyle changes as a complement to homeopathy. These might include more exercise, improved nutrition and posture, meditation, and professional counseling.

5. Avoid Substance Abuse. Smoking, excessive alcohol consumption, heavy coffee drinking (more than 16 oz./day), and prescription and over-the-counter medications with side effects, all

---

Stress and Surgery

The thought of surgery is stressful, and stress has a direct impact on our health. Now, a study is showing that when a woman hears stress-reducing messages when she's under anesthesia, her recovery time is shortened.

Nearly 40 women who had hysterectomies (a procedure we discourage since 90 percent are estimated to be unnecessary and actually more harmful than beneficial), were separated into two groups. One group listened to a blank tape during the operation; the other group heard a tape with nine minutes of suggestions that they would not feel pain afterward, would not be sick, and the more they relaxed the better they would feel. The women who heard these suggestions improved greatly over those who heard nothing.

If you're undergoing surgery, consider finding or making a tape with these kinds of suggestions on it. Or bring a tape of your favorite inspirational music to be played. Often, surgeons talk about sports, failed operations, and other negative things. You have a right to ask your surgeon and the attending nurses to keep the talk positive and encouraging. By doing so, you may even surprise them in your recovery.

Anderson, Robert A., MD. "Surgical recovery and intraoperative suggestion," *Townsend Letter,* June 1997.

place extra stress on our bodies (which, in turn, must work overtime to fight the adverse effects these substances have on our health).

6. Get Plenty of Exercise. I've said many times that exercise produces a dramatic reduction in breast-cancer risk, but the bottom-line results are even more impressive: A recent study of Swedish women ages 38 to 60 found that jobs that included moderate physical activity reduced the risk of dying by two-thirds. And moderate leisure activities reduced risk by nearly half. Exercise helps us overcome stress by keeping our bodies healthier and therefore, better able to rebound from the adverse effects of stress. Aim for a combination of aerobic and weight-resistance exercise, for at least four hours each week.

Techniques for Transforming Your Toxic Emotions

Live a healthy life. Eat a good diet high in whole grains and beans for the magnesium and vitamin B_6 your body needs to make chemicals that help you feel good both physically and emotionally. Limit your intake of fats, sugar, and caffeine. They use up these and other important nutrients that contribute to your emotional well-being. Don't eat foods that make you sick. If you have food allergies or sensitivities, stop eating these substances for a few weeks. See how you can easily transform your toxic emotions into ones that heal by simply avoiding foods that are toxic to your body.

Get some exercise regularly. Whenever you feel emotionally "stuck," move your body. Put on upbeat music and dance around the house. Clean a closet that you've been meaning to get to. Go for a walk or a run, or dust off your new and unused exercise equipment and start walking, rowing, or cycling. Do 10 minutes of exercise every day, then slowly build up to half an hour or more. When you go shopping, park your car farther away from the store, rather than as close as you can. Even that short walk will help.

Meditate for 10 minutes — every day you eat. That should be most days. Meditation, prayer, and relaxation exercises help center you and allow toxic emotions to melt away.

Larry Dossey, MD, author of *Healing Words,* has done research on the effects of prayer with large groups of people. He found that when people prayed for someone, even when that person didn't know they were being prayed for, their healing accelerated. Meditation and prayer are healing because they neutralize toxic emotions and allow the body's immune system to repair itself.

Tears are also cleansing and are part of healing emotions. They actually help you get better faster. William Fry, Jr., PhD was the first biochemist to suggest that emotional distress produces toxic chemicals in the body — and tears contain other chemicals that literally wash these toxins away. He is now studying the specific chemicals in emotionally caused tears to understand this biochemical activity.

In time, we should have a better understanding of the toxic

Depression and PMS

I have learned the most about premenstrual depression from a research gynecologist and endocrinologist, Dr. Guy E. Abraham, who has been conducting and publishing studies on nutrient deficiencies and PMS for more than 20 years. His studies show that you can correct premenstrual depression, anxiety, and mood swings with a diet high in magnesium and vitamin B_6, and lower in calcium. He suggests twice as much magnesium as calcium.

In 1993, a study on depression was published that showed a connection between the hypothalamus (in the brain), pituitary gland, and thyroid. All have an influence on the amount of magnesium we have in our bloodstream and brain. The doctors who conducted this study observed that magnesium seems to help regulate our moods. In fact, the study showed that the most depressed people had the lowest levels of magnesium.

A diet to reduce and eliminate PMS-related depression is high in whole grains and beans (which contain B_6 and magnesium), and low in dairy products (which are high in calcium). Nuts and seeds are also high in magnesium, and many women have eliminated them in an effort to keep their weight down. Small amounts added to your cereal or salads usually do more good than harm.

What you're eating may be contributing to your depression, and if you're depressed you may not be eating foods high in the nutrients you need, like B_6 and magnesium. If you are drinking more than 700 mg of caffeine a day (four to five cups of coffee or cola), or taking medications that contain a lot of caffeine, you may be contributing to your depression. Limit caffeinated beverages to one cup a day.

chemicals produced by stress and the neutralizing chemicals produced in tears. For now, think of your tears as cleansing, and allow yourself to cry when it's appropriate. Then adapt a positive attitude and get on with your life.

Letting Go

Transforming your health, transforming your life, is all about letting go. And let go we must. Someday you will let go of everything tangible — your possessions, your friends, your home, your pets, your life. Practice now by letting go of the negative. Use the remainder of your life feeling and expressing love. Your beliefs are powerful. If you believe you can change, you can. Begin by believing.

Forgiveness is a form of letting go. It allows you to let go of pain and negative emotions. It allows you to move on with your life. Along with forgiveness comes the ability to say, "I was wrong." We all are, at times. Admit it to yourself and others, and move on.

Be patient with yourself. Then you can be more patient with the people in your life. Recognize you're doing the best you can — and so are they — and let go of impatience.

Take Care of Yourself

Most of all, have fun. Every day, do something that's fun. Play with a child and become like that child for a few minutes. Remember what it felt like when you were playing happily with someone. Allow yourself to feel good for even a few minutes. Let that time expand.

Do something wonderful and unexpected for someone else. Get out of yourself. Find a group that needs your time and give them an hour a week; an hour a month. Get outside yourself and feel how good it feels to help someone else. You're helping them heal, and you're helping yourself as well. You're producing healing emotions and getting rid of some of the toxic ones that have been causing so much harm. Live each day, love each day, and enjoy every moment you can for the rest of your life.

My Favorite Way
to Calm Toxic Emotions

One great way to take care of yourself and lift your spirits is to use flower essences, a tincture made from the essence of particular herbs and flowers.

Physician Edward Bach discovered the first flower essences in the early 1900s. But what's the story behind them? What can a tincture infused with the energy of a single plant do for you if you're sick, unhappy, or can't stop your mind from running in the same unpleasant groove?

The sight and aroma of flowers calms us, puts us in a positive frame of mind, and helps us heal. Perhaps that's why they're given as gifts for both happy and sad occasions. But what would happen if instead of smelling a bouquet of flowers you took a tincture made from one of them? Could a plant tincture help you heal as well?

These were questions nature lover and English physician Edward Bach asked in the early 1900s as he saw patients in his private practice on London's Harley Street. Bach's specialty as a physician was in formulating vaccines made from various bacteria. The vaccines he developed have been used for nearly a decade to prevent smallpox, polio, diphtheria, and other illnesses. But approaching healing from this point of view did not satisfy Bach. Medicine only addressed the physical side of illness, and he saw that an individual's personality plays a determining role in his ability to get well.

Bach combined his study of bacterial vaccine therapy with that of homeopathy, where minute amounts of a substance corrected toxic amounts of the same substance. This homeopathic principle is called "Like cures like." For instance, someone who had arsenic poisoning would be given minute quantities of arsenic in a tincture, and their condition would improve. Sound ridiculous? It's the same principle as that used in vaccines.

But Edward Bach wanted to move away from using products of disease (the toxic bacterial vaccines) and substitute healthier substances. This search led him to the plant kingdom. His goal was to find a way to make plant substances as strong and effective as the bacterial vaccines he had been using. Bach studied the characteristics, moods, and habits of people and matched them with specific plant extracts. The results were encouraging, and he was on his way to developing a drugless system of 38 different plant tinctures that have a direct effect on a person's emotional state. "Disease is a kind of consolidation of a mental attitude," Bach wrote to a friend, "and it is only necessary to treat the mood of a patient and the disease will disappear."

Bach began by picking blossoms of various plants and putting them in a glass container filled with pure spring water. The container sat in the sun for several hours, as it became infused with the energy of the plant. These infusions were then added to alcohol, to stabilize them. Today, followers of the Bach Flower Remedy theory still make plant tinctures, according to Bach's methods. These can be found in health food stores. Other people have found additional benefits from different plants, so today there are the original Bach remedies and flower essences as well as other flower essences. You can try any of them, but you may want to begin with the original Bach remedies.

Begin With Rescue Remedy

You can also find numerous books and guides to the Bach flower remedies at most health food stores. Some have the history of Bach's path of discovery, and some concentrate on the specific plant essences and what type of person they're good for. By reading through the properties of each plant, you can put together individual mixtures. In addition, consider buying a small bottle of Bach's Rescue Remedy, a combination of five of the Bach remedies that was formulated for panic, anxiety, hysteria, extreme sadness, and other states of emotional emergency. It works on animals and it works on people — very effectively and very quickly.

Rescue Remedy contains **Star of Bethlehem**, for trauma and numbness; **Rock Rose** for panic; **Impatiens** for irritability and tension; **Cherry Plum** for fear of losing control; and **Clematis** for people who have a tendency to pass out.

Some Single Remedies

Here are a few of the single Bach flower remedies with some of the personality types who would benefit from them. Any book or

Depression and Amino Acids

Your brain contains chemicals called neurotransmitters that send various messages from one cell to another. Two particular neurotransmitters have been found to be low in people with depression: serotonin and norepinephrine. When you take large quantities of specific amino acids, you can stimulate the production of these brain chemicals. Many anti-depressant medications do this, but often with toxic side effects. Amino acid therapy can be a more natural and safer solution.

Serotonin is produced with the help of l-tryptophan, an amino acid used for more than 20 years without side effects. Several years ago, one contaminated batch of this nutrient purchased from a single Japanese manufacturer caused serious health problems and resulted in a few deaths. The FDA then took l-tryptophan off the market despite protestations from doctors, patients, and amino acid distributors that it was safe. Now, in a concessionary move, l-tryptophan has been made a prescription item much more expensive than ever — but available.

Tryptophan is the least abundant amino acid you can find in food; large quantities of food must be eaten to affect a chemical change. Tryptophan is relatively high in turkey and soy. Since high dietary soy intake is also associated with a lower incidence of breast cancer (as well as many other serious health threats), you may want to add soybeans to soups, tofu to stir-fried vegetables, and add veggie burgers made from soy (we think the Boca Burgers taste the best) to your diet.

L-phenylalanine and l-tyrosine are amino acids available through health food stores that increase the production of norepinephrine. Amino-acid treatments can be a bit complicated, so you may want to coordinate yours with a physician or health-care provider familiar with this approach. (To find one, you can call the American College for the Advancement of Medicine at 1-800-532-3688.)

If you'd like to go ahead on your own, consider the following protocol based on conversations with several doctors: l-tyrosine, from 500 to 3,500 mg in the morning as soon as you awake, and the same amount mid-afternoon without food. If you feel this program is not working as well for you as you'd like, substitute the afternoon dosage of l-tyrosine for 1,000 to 3,000 mg of l-phenylalanine or d-l-phenylalanine in the afternoon. Take this amino acid with food.

booklet on the remedies will give you more detailed information on each remedy and emotional state.

Agrimony is for people who don't like to be a burden to others, and who suffer in silence with a facade of cheerfulness. They don't like confrontations, and may use drugs or alcohol as an escape.

Aspen is for apprehensive people who have vague, unknown fears.

Beech is for critical people who tend to overreact.

Honeysuckle is for people who dwell on the past and the "good old days" when things were better.

Gorse is for feelings of hopelessness and futility.

Walnut is to help stabilize emotional transition times, including menopause, as well as moving into other new patterns, like a new job, relationship, or moving to a different location.

Sweet Chestnut is for people who feel they're at the end of their rope and have moments of deep despair.

Mimulus is for people who are afraid of known things, like heights, airplanes, or being alone.

You can buy individual essences and put together the combination that suits you best. Usually, two or three drops of a single tincture are put into distilled water and preserved with alcohol. Most combinations should be limited to three or four tinctures. Rosemary's Garden herb store will put together a formula with four flower essences for around $5.50 plus shipping. You can reach them at 800-493-5523. Or single tinctures sell for around $8-$9 for a one-ounce bottle. A bottle of Rescue Remedy is $9-$10. You can take the remedies frequently, a few drops (a typical homeopathic dosage) or a dropper full at a time. Experiment a little to see what works best for you.

If you use the Internet, try www.medicinegarden.com for more information.

Two Solutions to Depression

If your emotions or other toxins have put you into a constant state of depression, there are two supplements you need to consider. St. John's wort and 5-HTP (5-Hydroxytryptophan).

St. John's Wort: Why All the Fuss?

It's hot. It's the latest remedy for depression. You can find it anywhere from health food stores to mainstream drug stores. But is it safe for you to take if you're depressed? Maybe. It depends on many factors from why you're depressed to how depressed you are.

St. John's wort has never been an appropriate remedy for severe depression. Nor do I believe it should be used over a long period of time, especially since there are no long-term studies that would give us information about side effects with long-term use. Still, St. John's wort seems to be a safer answer for many people than current medications.

Remember that no food, vitamin, mineral, or herb works in the same way for everyone. Everything we ingest can cause some side effects, and our bodies vary tremendously in the quantity that is beneficial or harmful. So as good as it may be, St. John's wort is not for everyone. But then, neither is Prozac, one of several popular antidepressant medications that can have numerous side effects. A number of large, double-blind studies have shown that St. John's wort can be as effective as an antidepressant with very few side effects.

What Is It and What Makes It Work?

St. John's wort is an herb called *Hypericum perforatum,* a shrub with bright yellow flowers that grows in Northern California and Southern Oregon. It's also cultivated throughout the world, where it has been used for centuries. In Germany, for example, millions of people take St. John's wort every year.

This plant contains a number of chemicals that appear to help regulate your body, including hypericin, flavonoids, xanthones, phloroglucinol derivatives, essential oils, and carotenoids. Some of these ingredients are antiviral (against the herpes and hepatitis C viruses, Epstein-Barr virus, and influenza types A and B), some antibacterial (ointments can help heal burns more quickly), and others antifungal. St. John's wort has been used for numerous conditions in addition to depression.

It is thought that one action of St. John's wort is that it may inhibit your brain's uptake of serotonin in a similar way to Prozac, Paxil, and Zoloft, thus alleviating depression. The roots of the plant contain an anti-fungal agent, which has been shown to reduce Candida albicans.

Dr. Michael T. Murray, ND, has also found St. John's wort to be helpful for people with fibromyalgia — non-specific muscle pain — because he believes the central cause for this condition is low serotonin levels, which amplify the sensations of pain. The herb is one of a number of nutrients he uses for fibromyalgia. The others are magnesium and 5-HTP (5-hydroxytryptophan, a precursor to serotonin).

When to Consider Taking St. John's Wort

Researchers agree about when to use St. John's wort for depression. It is most appropriately used for mild to moderate depression, not when your depression is severe. But Dr. Murray cautions against using St. John's wort for a long time as a crutch. I agree with him. Diet, hormone levels, lifestyle, and attitude need to be evaluated and the appropriate changes need to be made. St. John's wort may be an excellent tool to use — but not instead of addressing any underlying problems.

Q: After reading your suggestions for increasing magnesium for bone strength, I find I'm no longer constipated. However, I read an article that says the magnesium and phosphates in many laxatives may cause fatigue, weakness, and pulse irregularities. Could my loss of energy be due to my taking magnesium? — *M.S., Joplin, MO*

A: No, magnesium is needed to give you energy. It also reduces or eliminates arrhythmias in many people, since magnesium relaxes all muscles, and the heart is a muscle. Magnesium deficiency appears to be common in this country. Stress, diet, and imbalanced supplements all contribute to a lack of magnesium. I would be surprised if it is causing your fatigue, but by all means, check with your doctor on this. It is more likely the phosphates (which pull calcium out of bones) or some other ingredient that is causing problems if, in fact, your fatigue is coming from your laxative. Remember that magnesium oxide is usually not very well absorbed. I recommend magnesium citrate, aspartate, or malate as better-utilized forms of this mineral.

Dr. Murray finds that only 25 percent of his depressed patients need to take the herb for more than six months. For people who may have a genetic tendency toward depression, long-term use may be appropriate. But not for most people.

What About Side Effects?

St. John's wort has fewer side effects than any antidepressant medication, but it has a few. The most common are gastrointestinal irritation, allergic reactions, fatigue, and restlessness. No toxicity has been reported in Germany, where more than three million prescriptions a year are given. However, if you suspect any reaction, stop taking the herb for three to five days and see if the symptom goes away.

What Should I Do About Continuing My Anti-Depressant?

First, talk with your doctor. Some people do best with a combination of medications and this herb, but they risk a phenomena called the "serotonin syndrome," a series of side effects including confusion, fever, shivering, sweating, diarrhea, and muscle spasms. If you continue taking any medications, be closely monitored by a health-care practitioner who can recognize if you're getting yourself in trouble.

Dr. Murray is both a naturopath and writer on herbs. He begins giving his patients St. John's wort extract while they're still taking their antidepressants. Then he reduces their antidepressants for two weeks, stopping them completely if all is going well.

Before You Begin

Don't fool around with your body and be your own doctor. If you're depressed, you need to do more than pop a few pills or take a tincture a few times a day. Your body needs specific nutrients. Either find a health practitioner to work with (doctor, naturopath, nutritionist) or run, don't walk, to your local health food store or book store and get a copy of *St. John's Wort: Nature's Blues Buster,* by Hyla Cass, MD.

I have personally known Dr. Cass for a dozen years. A psychiatrist who has used nutrition, herbs, natural hormone therapy, and lifestyle changes with her patients for decades, she is extremely knowledgeable about how and when to use St. John's wort, and what else you need to do. Her book, published by Avery Publishing (1998) is one of the best ones available.

A Solution You Might Have Missed: 5-HTP

One reason for depression is a lack of production of a particular neurotransmitter in the brain called serotonin. In fact, you could say that serotonin is one of your body's natural antidepressants.

Here's how it works: Neuro-transmitters carry messages to your brain cells. When the levels of neurotransmitters vary, this can cause a change in your mood. According to Dr. Cass, low serotonin production can cause a variety of symptoms including depression, obsessive thinking, anxiety, violent behavior, alcohol and drug abuse, premenstrual syndrome, and increased sensitivity to pain.

Medical doctors treat this form of depression with medications called SSRIs (selective serotonin re-uptake inhibitors), which increase the body's production of serotonin. Doctors who use complementary medicine and other health practitioners, are now suggesting 5-HTP, a safe form of tryptophan, as an alternative. Tryptophan is an amino acid that helps the body make serotonin. If your depression is not due to a lack of serotonin, 5-HTP may not be your answer. If it is, however, you may be on your way to a more natural, safer type of serotonin-producer.

Prozac is the first SSRI that came on the market in 1987. Today, more than six million people in this country alone use it regularly. In fact, Prozac was considered so effective as an antidepressant that other pharmaceutical companies came out with their own SSRI medications like Zoloft and Paxil. One problem with SSRIs is the side effects they may cause. These include headaches, nausea, anxiety (just what it's supposed to treat!), insomnia, drowsiness, diarrhea, and on and on. SSRIs also cause a lack of libido. This side effect alone is enough to make you depressed!

Tryptophan and 5-HTP

For decades, a single amino acid (part of protein) called tryptophan has been used safely and effectively to treat depression. Tryptophan exists naturally in many sources of protein and is especially high in turkey. But the problem with getting enough tryptophan from food is that other amino acids in protein foods compete with tryptophan in crossing the blood brain barrier (this means, getting from your bloodstream into your brain). So eating a lot of protein won't do very much to lift your mood.

Interestingly, a meal high in carbohydrates has the opposite effect. Carbohydrates cause your body to make insulin, and insulin acts on the other amino acids that compete with tryptophan. It lowers the amount of competing amino acids, but does not affect tryptophan. So you could feel more depressed or anxious before eating a high carbohydrate meal, and feel better afterward. Food can affect your depression, but most people need something more — a booster. Is tryptophan the answer?

Tryptophan is a nutrient that affects neurotransmitters, but before it can do this, it has to be converted in your body into 5-HTP. Then, 5-HTP converts into serotonin with the help of two of our favorite nutrients: vitamin B_6 and magnesium. When you take 5-HTP, you start out a step ahead on the process. It's a faster way of

Q: Does a high level of stress increase breast-cancer risk?

A: I know of no studies that have addressed this question, but believe it is certainly one of the most important of all. I do know that women with breast cancer who join support groups as part of their treatment have longer average survival rates than women who don't. One of the main functions of these support groups is stress reduction. Numerous studies have also established a significant link between high stress levels and numerous other diseases, including cancer in general and heart disease. This is because stress significantly weakens the immune system — which includes our body's ability to prevent cancer development. In view of these facts, there's an excel-lent possibility that women with lower stress levels also have lower breast cancer rates. More importantly, stress reduction is one of the most important steps you can take to prevent disease in general.

making serotonin than taking tryptophan.

Even if you want to take tryptophan, the cost is prohibitive for most people. And 5-HTP is one step closer to serotonin production than tryptophan. In addition, it's a naturally occurring substance found in some plants. Much of the 5-HTP found in health food stores is extracted from the seeds of a plant called *Griffonia simplicifolia*. While there can be contamination in any product, from SSRIs and other prescription drugs to processed foods, when bacteria are not present in large quantities, as is the case with 5-HTP, the risk is very, very low.

Last September, researchers at the Mayo Clinic implied that contamination in 5-HTP had, indeed occurred. Using a sophisticated laboratory test, the researchers found indications that all six samples of 5-HTP they tested had markers, they claimed, that were similar in chemical structure to two contaminants once found in a batch of tryptophan from the 1980s. None of the contaminants in the bad tryptophan, however, have ever been identified as the particular contaminant(s) that caused serious side effects.

The research from the esteemed Mayo Clinic was not from a study published in a peer-reviewed journal (this is what often separates good science from possibly bad science), but as a letter to the editor in *Nature Medicine* journal (September 1998). There is no indication at present that 5-HTP has any contaminants that can cause problems. The markers found in the tested samples of 5-HTP are not found in all products. If you decide to use 5-HTP, get it from the best source possible. Preferably, from a company known to you or your health-care provider.

5-HTP and Depression

More than a dozen studies using 5-HTP for depression have appeared since the early 1970s. These have included more than 500 people with various kinds of depression, including some seriously depressed patients. More than 50 percent of the patients were significantly improved after taking 5-HTP. In a Swiss study, 5-HTP was compared with SSRIs. Both groups improved, with slightly more people on 5-HTP improving over those on conventional antidepressants. In addition, there were fewer side effects with people taking 5-HTP (the most common side effects, mild nausea or slight gastrointestinal discomfort, usually disappear within a few days).

The dosage of 5-HTP for depression is usually 50 mg three times a day with meals. After a few weeks, if there is not sufficient response, it can be increased to 100 mg three times daily. 5-HTP should not be taken along with Prozac or other SSRIs. Check with your doctor before taking this supplement, especially if you're on any medication for depression. A month's supply of good quality 5-HTP will cost between $25-$30.

Added Benefits and a Caution...

In addition to producing serotonin, the "feel good" brain chemical, 5-HTP also helps make melatonin, a hormone that diminishes as we age. Melatonin helps us sleep, so you may find you sleep better when you take 5-HTP. This supplement has been found effective in numerous studies for fibromyalgia, migraine headaches, and obesity (by decreasing the craving for carbohydrates).

Using 5-HTP is really using a supplement like a medication. I urge you to talk with your health-care practitioner about all supplements you are taking or are contemplating taking. At the very least, we all lack objectivity when it comes to ourselves. Supplements like 5-HTP are generally very safe. Probably a lot safer than aspirin. Still, you want your health-care team to be aware of all you're taking. At some point, either they will educate you, or you will educate them, on the benefits, interactions, and side effects of various substances. Nutritional science is in its infancy, and it's tempting to take everything we hear about that may be beneficial. Be smart. Be in charge of your health, but don't attempt to be your own doctor.

Chapter 5

Are Hormones Making You Sick?

Currently, the National Institutes of Health (NIH) spends approximately $9.8 billion on research, yet virtually none of this is spent on researching one of the most intriguing topics in health today: natural hormones.

What most people don't realize is that an out-of-balance hormonal system can cause a multitude of illnesses, from cancer to chronic fatigue to heart disease. There are a number of things that can cause our hormones to cause problems, including environmental toxins, which I've already discussed, surgery or an accident that affects a hormone-secreting organ (e.g., hysterectomy), or improper hormone supplementation.

Scientists are now aware of hundreds of hormones that course through our bodies. And a small but growing number of researchers and doctors are now advocating full-spectrum hormone supplementation as a means to delay aging and ultimately increase longevity, as well as prevent disease and treat advanced disease.

Some of these hormones, including DHEA, melatonin, progesterone, and pregnenolone, are now available to consumers over-the-counter. But one important fact you need to keep in mind when considering any type of hormone supplementation is that, whether a prescription is needed or not, all hormones are powerful drugs.

Another key concern to keep in mind as you consider using hormones is that, in general, there are many unanswered questions regarding whether these supplements are safe for long-term, human use.

Only time and additional human studies will provide specific answers.

While there are a tremendous number of benefits hormone supplements can provide, there are also a variety of problems that can arise if your hormone levels are out of balance, you use the wrong hormones, or incorrectly use the right hormones. We'll discuss the positive uses of hormones throughout this book and in future issues of my newsletter, *Women's Health Letter*. But in this chapter, I intend to cover some of the problems you might encounter if your hormones are out of balance or if you use hormones inappropriately.

What Every Woman Must Know About Estrogen Replacement Therapy*

"Menopause is not a disease," says medical anthropologist Margaret Lock in a 1991 article in *The Lancet*, the esteemed weekly British medical journal, "but a life-cycle transition to which powerful symbolic meanings, individual and social, are attached."

That's not what most medical doctors believe, however. And their beliefs are making thousands of sane menopausal women crazy with confusion.

Chances are your doctor looks at menopause as an estrogen deficiency disease. This disease concept originated in 1966 in a book, *Feminine Forever,* written by Robert A. Wilson, MD His theory — and that's all it was — is now accepted as fact by many medical doctors. This is understandable, although unfortunate for women, because doctors are trained to treat diseases with drugs and hormones, not to look at natural life transitions and offer drug-free solutions to uncomfortable menopausal symptoms.

Since the majority of women live long enough to go through menopause, doctors have a ready market of hundreds of thousands of women every year who are potential patients. Pharmaceutical companies have lined up with hormones, antidepressants, and other medications to help solve your menopausal "problems," like hot flashes, osteoporosis, and heart attacks.

---

* Section reprinted from *The Giant Book of Women's Health Secrets.*

What if you didn't need these drugs and hormones? The majority of women, after all, report little if any menopausal discomfort. And what if most of the discomfort could be addressed through dietary and lifestyle changes? Well, you can be sure the drug companies wouldn't want you to find out. But, fortunately, you can.

This is a big relief for the many women who cannot or decide not to use estrogen replacement therapy (ERT). All medications have side effects, and some women are simply not candidates for this approach. We're not saying that ERT is bad for everyone. But we disagree with the medical model that says drug intervention is necessary to prevent unwanted health and beauty changes. And we are not satisfied that it's as safe as some people say.

Menopause and Society

Germaine Greer's book, *The Change,* mentions a study on the effect of estrogen replacement on a woman's personality. According to the study, estrogen keeps us less outwardly aggressive, but more inwardly hostile. This may be good for motherhood, but it stifles our outward creativity and our ability to be more assertive. Estrogen replacement therapy may be greatly responsible for the high-level female bonding among older women we're seeing in our society today, says Cheri Quincy, DO (Doctor of Osteopathy).

But those women who don't take ERT may be much more likely to use their *increased individual power* to get out in the world and accomplish things they had put off while raising families.

Dr. Quincy also notes that "Economic power in old age is one of the most important predictors of both longevity and health. The retirement plan, the golden parachute, the vested annuity; these are rewards for those who work outside the home." With the hormone shifts of menopause comes the opportunity for a woman to enter parts of society she may have avoided by necessity when higher estrogen levels and the circumstances they created gently nudged her into nesting with family and close friends.

Dr. Susan Love promotes the idea of menopause mirroring puberty: Like puberty, menopause is a transition into a new hormonal state.

Anthropologist Margaret Mead coined the term "post-menopausal zest" to describe the leading characteristic that provides us direction and meaning as we make the symbolic transition from mating-and-mothering mode to matriarch.

Forever Young

To avoid this transition and help keep us "feminine (as defined by our reproductive years) forever," there is a wide selection of estrogen replacement therapy (ERT) products available to us. They are taken to supplement and thus counteract the body's natural decline of estrogen and progesterone production that takes place at menopause. Let's take a good look at these estrogen supplements.

Traditional ERT (Estrogens and progestins — synthetic progesterone): Most hormones currently on the market are synthetic. In the case of Premarin, the most widely studied and prescribed estrogen supplement for women, it is made of horse estrogen, not human estrogen. One of the most important things every woman needs to know about these hormones is that they are not exactly identical to any form of estrogen or progesterone normally found in the human female body.

This also means that the term estrogen replacement therapy, (when applied to these hormones), is a misnomer. When these hormones are taken, your hormones are not being replaced. Instead, a more accurate way to describe ERT would be to call it similar estrogen supplementation. In essence, the synthetic hormones used in ERT mimic your hormones. But they don't always do a satisfactory job. And they certainly aren't the real thing.

If synthetic hormones were identical to naturally occurring hormones (those found in your body), their marketing potential would be too poor to interest drug manufacturers. Since the synthetic hormones are all slightly different than the real thing, however, they are patented. This gives the manufacturer exclusive rights to sell a particular synthetic hormone — at very impressive prices.

This makes synthetic estrogen pills a near-perfect product for pharmaceutical companies: You don't have to be sick to take them. Instead, every woman is a potential customer from the time her menopause begins. And you can take these pills for as long as you like! The longer you take them, the more money the manufacturer makes. And if you stop taking them, you have menopause symptoms. In short, millions of healthy women taking synthetic hormones every day adds up to one of the highest profit potentials of any drug ever approved for the U.S. market.

Drug companies are keenly aware of this and their marketing efforts reflect this fact. Consider *Seasons* magazine, which is published by Wyeth-Ayerst — America's largest estrogen supplement manufacturer. This magazine is not available by subscription. Instead, it is available only to women who have prescriptions to Premarin (Wyeth-Ayerst's estrogen supplements). All it takes is one quick examination of this magazine, however, and it's easy to see that this magazine is an expensive propaganda tool — designed to brainwash women into taking Premarin indefinitely.

Seasons magazine even misleads women about what exactly Premarin is made of. It states that Premarin is made of "natural substances." This is technically true. Premarin is horse estrogen from real horses. But, *Seasons* magazine and other promotional literature conveniently omit the fact that the main natural substances are extracted from the urine of pregnant mares. In fact, the name Premarin is derived from the phrase "PREgnant MARe urINe" and was probably approved for use by top marketing executives because it sounded pleasant. They knew that if they gave it a more truthful name, such as horse-pee-in-a-pill, they would quickly lose the interest of millions of potential lifetime customers.

If this weren't bad enough, there's more. To collect the urine, horses are impregnated, fitted with a rubber device, and made to stand for most of their pregnancies, so the urine can be collected. Places where this happens are called pee farms. As you can imagine, many animal lovers are very upset about the goings-on at these places.

Around here, though, I am more concerned about what these synthetic hormones do to women's bodies. Numerous studies have linked them to breast cancer. One large study that appeared in the *New England Journal of Medicine* (mid-June 1995) found that women aged 60 to 64 who had taken synthetic estrogen five years or more had a 71 percent higher breast-cancer risk than those who didn't take estrogen. Taking progestin boosted risk even higher.

Other health problems, for which studies suggest traditional ERT increases risk, include asthma, lupus, endometrial cancer, ovarian cancer, brain cancer, depression, rheumatoid arthritis, and heart disease. Some of these will be discussed more, later in this book.

Names of Synthetic Female Hormones

Synthetic Estrogens Pills: Estrace, estratab, Ogen, Estinly, Estrovis
Synthetic Estrogen Creams: Premain, Estrace, Ogen, Ortho
    Dienestrol
Synthetic Progestogens (man-made versions of progesterone):
    Provera, Curretab, Cyrin, Amen, Aygestin, Norlutate, Norlutin, Megace, Oveerette, Micronor, Nor-Q.D.
Note: New hormone products continue to be approved for marketing. To be absolutely sure about what an unlisted hormone is made of, ask your doctor or pharmacist.

Compounded Estrogens

Compound estrogens are forms of estrogen that are chemically identical to the real thing found in the body. They include:

Tri-estrogen — contains three forms of estrogen: estrone, estriol and estradiol.

Di-estrogen — contains two forms of estrogen that have not been linked to breast cancer — estriol and estradiol.

Like synthetic estrogens and progestogens, compounded estrogens are available by prescription only. Are they safe?

Myths About Postmenopausal Health

If you listen to the media and look at advertisements for calcium supplements, you may believe that you're destined to be a bent-over old woman with a wrinkled face and fragile bones unless you take a lot of calcium and hormones. This is not necessarily true. There are, in fact, a number of myths surrounding how you will look and feel after menopause with or without ERT. The first myth is one on which other myths are built. It contends that menopause is an estrogen-deficiency disease.

Anthropologist Margaret Lock disagrees. She points out that people have lived into old age for thousands of years. The idea that modern women are living longer lives and for that reason alone require estrogen replacement is simply invalid. She also says, "Most women do not seek help at menopause, and this part of the life cycle is not subject to medical attention to the same extent as childbirth."

Susan E. Brown of the National Women's Health Network supports Margaret Lock's position. She states that "blaming osteoporosis on an estrogen deficiency is just a little less absurd than blaming heart attacks on a deficiency of bypass surgery. Surgery might solve the problem for a while, but it is not a deficiency of the operation that caused the problem."

Calcium and Bone Loss

Another prevalent myth is that postmenopausal women need high amounts of calcium to prevent bone loss — about 1,500 mg/day. Yet a 1985 study by Gordan and Genant, which has been duplicated many times, showed that 1,500 mg of daily oral calcium supplement has no preventive effect on bone loss. We can think of several reasons why a lot of calcium doesn't prevent osteoporosis. One is that calcium is poorly absorbed unless you have sufficient acid in your stomach, and postmenopausal women often have lowered concentrations of hydrochloric acid.

Many people think that because vitamin C is made from an acid (ascorbic), it should help calcium be absorbed. But an alarming study published just last year in the *Journal of Epidemiology* showed that women who took large amounts of both calcium and vitamin C — what looks like a winning bone-strengthening combination — had a higher incidence of hip fracture than women who took only one of these supplements.

I've said it before and I'll say it until every woman who's interested hears it: Just because you take calcium or eat calcium-rich foods doesn't mean this mineral gets into your bones. This is a

myth perpetrated by vested interest groups who sell calcium supplements and dairy products.

Research gynecologist and endocrinologist Guy E. Abraham,
MD conducted a prospective study with Dr. Harinder Grewal that
was published in the *Journal of Reproductive Medicine* in 1990.
This small, double-blind study showed that postmenopausal women
who took more magnesium than calcium had an average increase in
bone density of 11 percent after just one year. These women took
only 500 mg of calcium and from 600 to 1,000 mg of magnesium.
A higher magnesium intake seems to be correlated with increased
bone density.

This isn't news. It was discussed in 1988 in an article in *Bone
Mineral* written by Rosalind Angus. She found that there was no
significant correlation between calcium intake and bone mass.
Instead, iron, zinc, and magnesium intake were indicators of
stronger bones. Add boron to that list, based on studies by Forrest
H. Nielsen, and you'll better understand why vegetarians have a
lower risk for osteoporosis than meat eaters. Boron, like magnesium, is high in plant material and low in animal products.

ERT and Heart Disease

Another myth surrounding menopause is that estrogen
replacement is necessary to prevent heart disease. It's true that heart
disease is the number one killer of postmenopausal women. But it's
also true that unabsorbed calcium — from high-calcium diets and
supplements — can collect in the arteries and become atherosclerosis (build-up in, and blockage of, the arteries). It's also true that
numerous dietary and exercise factors contribute to a higher or
lower risk for heart disease. If you don't want to take ERT, you need
to exercise regularly and eat well.

Most physicians believe that ERT reduces a woman's heart-
disease risk. Yet, to date, studies that support this idea have neg-
lected to take into account the fact that women who take estrogen
also tend to eat healthier foods, get more exercise, and, in general,
usually take better care of themselves than other women.

Preliminary results for the first three years of a more equitable study were published in the *Journal of the American Medical Association.* This study is comparing 875 healthy postmenopausal women who are taking either a placebo or one of four estrogen regimens.

The preliminary results are impressive:

1. The women receiving ERT had more favorable cholesterol ratios.

2. Five new cases of heart disease developed among the ERT groups, yet none developed among women in the placebo group.

3. Ten women in the ERT groups developed blood clots, yet none in the placebo group developed blood clots.

Overall, in spite of "better" cholesterol ratios, the ERT group didn't fare any better than their placebo-taking counterparts when it came to heart disease. Instead, the ERT group experienced significant turns for the worse with a combined total of 15 new cases of blood clots and heart disease — while not a single woman in the placebo group developed either problem.

ERT is neither good nor bad. It's one option. But you shouldn't be frightened into taking it. It should be your choice after looking at both sides. And this includes looking at its benefits.

The Benefits of ERT

Estrogen and progesterone replacement offers relief from temporary menopause symptoms, such as hot flashes and severe mood swings. Proponents also claim that, in the long run, it helps protect women against osteoporosis, heart disease, and strokes. Estrogen appears to lower the bad cholesterol (LDL) through its antioxidizing actions. Other antioxidants, however, are found naturally in foods. Vitamins A, C, and E, for instance, are found in abundance in fresh fruits, vegetables, and vegetable oils. This gives you a choice of where you get your protective antioxidants.

One more reason doctors suggest women take hormones is to protect brain function. But you may be being brainwashed about taking estrogen replacement therapy (ERT) to lower your risk for memory loss and Alzheimer's. Yes, studies are showing that ERT may protect your brain. But are these good studies? I think not. For one, vested interests can heavily influence results of scientific studies by omitting or adding data that throws off the results.

For example, one large study conducted by Annlia Paganini-Hill at Leisure World in Southern California linked ERT to a lower risk for dementia. The study was funded in part by Wyeth-Ayerst, the pharmaceutical company that makes Premarin. And Premarin is the most widely used form of estrogen at Leisure World, as well as in the United States. Also, the new nine-year Women's Health Initiative study on hormone therapy now in progress is being funded 100 percent by Wyeth-Ayerst. Don't be surprised if the results say ERT prevents dementia.

An article in the National Women's Health Network newsletter, *The Network News,* points out that "the failure to control for socio-economic status (SES) in the conduct of this research is its greatest shortcoming." It has been found that the less money a person has, the higher the incidences of Alzheimer's. I think this is because women with less money are less likely to use hormones due to their expense. So women who were most likely to get any form of dementia are least likely to use hormones. Women on a limited income are also more likely, I believe, to ignore information on the aluminum content of underarm deodorants and the absorption of aluminum from cooking utensils. And, if I were to search further, I would no doubt uncover other associations between possible dementia and low income.

But perhaps most important is for us to realize that Alzheimer's is not a woman's disease. There is no evidence to show that more women get Alzheimer's than men. And there is no conclusive evidence that ERT prevents this disorder. At present, there have not been any long-term studies that show ERT prevents dementia. And the nine-year study currently in progress is funded by a pharmaceutical firm.

The risks associated with synthetic ERT often greatly outweigh its benefits for many women. And few benefits exist with short-term use. If you take ERT for menopause symptoms, these will reappear as soon as hormones are stopped. And conventional treatment for osteoporosis and heart disease prevention requires decades of usage. If you plan to use ERT, plan to use it for many years.

ERT Side Effects

As long as you use ERT your estrogen levels will remain high, placing you at an increased risk for breast cancer. Studies on the relationship between ERT and breast cancer show this may be as much as a 30 percent overall increase in risk. The longer you have high estrogen levels, the greater your risk for breast cancer. We don't believe hormone therapy would be made available to men if it increased their risk for prostate cancer by 30 percent. Why is it safe for us?

Nearly 70,000 nurses over a period of 14 years showed an increased risk for lupus, an inflammatory disorder of the connective tissues that occurs mostly in young women. It can attack any organ of the body from the liver to the heart. People with lupus appear to have estrogen metabolism abnormalities. In this nurses' study, the increased risk for lupus coincided with an increased use of estrogen, primarily Premarin. Your risk for lupus may increase proportionally with the length of time you use synthetic hormones.

If you take hormones, you may continue to menstruate into your 70s and 80s. And you may increase your risk of blood clots and gallstones. Since blood clots can lead to strokes or heart attacks, you may not be helping your heart with ERT.

Painful uterine fibroid tumors and endometriosis will shrink when your estrogen levels decrease naturally at menopause. But they will continue to grow if you are on ERT. In some cases, this means they will need to be surgically removed.

Breast tenderness, depression, liver problems, blood-sugar imbalances, nausea, headaches, fluid retention and weight gain are all side effects of taking synthetic estrogen. In a study of over 36,000 postmenopausal women during a 10-year period, women who used estrogen had a higher incidence of asthma than those who never used it. In fact, side effects are so severe that the ERT compliance rate is quite poor: Approximately 50 percent of women who take it, end up discontinuing it because of unwanted side effects.

The Progesterone Controversy

There's a growing movement toward self-care, and I'm all for it as long as people don't hurt themselves. In fact, that's my job — to help you discover what really works — and what's safe.

This brings me to the subject of progesterone in its synthetic and natural forms. Progesterone is used by many women for PMS and as an alternative to, or in combination with, estrogen therapy. In theory, these uses make sense. Natural products are also generally perceived as being safe. And popular author and retired physician John R. Lee, MD keeps saying that natural progesterone is safe and effective, without negative side effects. However, doctors I've talked with disagree.

What I Found About Progesterone

I spent hours on the phone talking with pharmacists who compound natural progesterone for doctors to use with their patients, and with physicians who have extensive knowledge about progesterone therapy. Some of what I heard astonished me.

Let's first look at progesterone therapy for PMS. When you take a close look at this monthly condition, you find that many premenstrual symptoms occur one or two weeks before menstruation when progesterone levels drop and estrogen remains high. In some women, progesterone levels drop too low, which make them candidates for hormone therapy.

How It All Began

The use of progesterone for PMS began in the 1930s, when several doctors observed that progesterone levels in many women dropped the week or two before menstruation, coinciding with a number of uncomfortable emotional symptoms. At that time, synthetic products called progestins were being used. Originally, it was thought that while excessive estrogens may contribute to a woman's risk for breast cancer, progestins were thought to decrease the risk by having anti-estrogenic activity. Progestins, however, are not identical to the body's own progesterone, and they were found to cause undesirable side effects.

It wasn't until the 1950s, when a doctor's assistant, Katharina Dalton, began using natural progesterone with women with PMS in an English clinic. This natural progesterone had the same molecular structure as the progesterone made in your body. Katharina Dalton went on to become a physician, and studied PMS and progesterone for years, doing clinical studies on the subject with good results. In fact, you could say that Dr. Dalton is the "mother" of progesterone therapy.

And staying with the family analogy, retired physician John R. Lee is considered the "father" of natural progesterone creams. He took 20 years of observations of the women who came to his practice in a Northern California city, and drew conclusions as to the efficacy of a natural progesterone cream.

Progestins vs. Progesterone

Drs. Dalton and Lee are talking about natural progesterone, not progestins. Progestins are synthetically made hormones that have been found to be quite harmful.

A study, funded partly by the National Institutes of Health, was published in *Scientific American* in 1995. The authors of this study, published through the Johns Hopkins University School of Hygiene and Public Health, said that progestins can contribute to breast cancer. These professors of medicine, Darcy V. Spicer and Malcolm C. Pike, were not alone in their allegations. Another study, published in the *New England Journal of Medicine,* looked at over 120,000 nurses and found the women who took progestins alone had more of a risk for breast cancer than women on estrogen alone.

There are three types of progesterone: synthetic (called progestin), natural (compounded by specialized pharmacies and available by prescription), and over-the-counter creams (made from wild yam extract). All have different amounts of hormone activity from none to too much. Confused? Let's make sense of this.

Progestins are the synthetic form of progesterone. Uzzi Reiss, MD author of *Natural Hormone Balance for Women* (Simon &

Schuster, 2001) calls them "patented, chemicalized, progesterone substitutes." They are more powerful than the progesterone your body makes and all have side effects. Progestins, such as Provera, have been found to be carcinogenic, cause water retention, nausea, depression, and abnormal menstrual flow. In fact, progestins can actually cause some symptoms of PMS. An article published in the *Journal of Reproductive Medicine* (June 1987) by Zaven H. Chakmakjian, MD and Nannepaga Y. Zachariah, PhD, states that progestins may affect cholesterol, can cause facial hair, and even stimulate estrogen production. Most progesterone studies have been done on progestins, rather than natural progesterone.

Natural progesterone products, made in laboratories may be used as transdermal patches, injections, suppositories, or oral tablets. The natural progesterone creams found in natural health food stores often contain too little progesterone to raise hormone levels. Dr Reiss has not found them to be particularly effective.

Some naturally compounding pharmacies now make these various types of natural progesterone into products with sufficient quantities to raise progesterone levels in your blood, but they may be obtained only by prescription. These pharmacies work closely with doctors in helping to provide products designed for a woman's particular hormone needs. I personally know of two such pharmacies, both of which compound excellent quality hormones. You can call them for an information packet and ask them to send their technical information directly to your doctor. They are the Belmar Pharmacy (800-525-9473) and the Women's International Pharmacy (800-279-5708). The Belmar Pharmacy can also send your doctor copies of double-blind studies that were conducted using their particular natural progesterone products. No other natural progesterone has been studied in this manner.

And Then There's Progesterone Cream

The progesterone most popular among health-conscious women is the over-the-counter natural progesterone cream found in natural health stores and drugstores. These creams are often made from an extract of an inedible wild yam. They contain substances, called progesterone precursors that can theoretically turn into progesterone. Unfortunately, these creams, applied topically to your skin, don't convert into progesterone because your skin doesn't have the ability to turn these precursors into progesterone. It's important for you to understand that unless natural progesterone has been added to the wild yam extract, these creams contain no progesterone activity.

Wild yam extracts *cannot possibly affect your hormone levels* unless real natural progesterone hormone, made in a laboratory, has been added to them. Yet, some women insist that they feel better when they use these creams. And well they might. Some of the creams you pick up in natural food stores or pharmacies do have small quantities of the hormone added to them, even if it doesn't say so on the label. And they may contain other substances as well. You see, some natural progesterone creams don't say they have hormones added to them, but they do.

I heard of one doctor who took the wild yam cream his patient had been using to a laboratory for analysis. The cream did not say it had progesterone or anything else added to it. Not only did it contain some natural progesterone, but it also had some pregnenolone in it as well. Pregnenolone is a substance that is used by the body to make a variety of hormones: estrogen, testosterone, aldosterone, and progesterone. This means that a progesterone cream you pick up might cause facial hair or cause some of the problems you're using progesterone to correct. It is very possible that some of the side effects women are experiencing from natural progesterone creams are from these added ingredients. But there's no way to know.

Natural progesterone creams are not regulated. Because there are no regulations and specifications for progesterone creams, they vary considerably. Some have added hormones, some don't. Over-the-counter progesterone creams have not been studied in sound, scientific double-blind studies, nor is their labeling always accurate. While the manufacturers of these over-the-counter creams grow rich from the reported observations of various doctors, they have not funded independent studies to show their products are either effective or safe. When I contacted the heads of several natural hormone pharmacies, there was a lack of controlled scientific studies on natural progesterone creams.

But Is Natural Progesterone Safe?

If your body lacks sufficient progesterone and you give it just the amount it needs in the form of natural progesterone (not progestin), it's probably very safe. But what if your body needs a lot or just the tiniest amount? Then that's the amount you should take. No more. Although it appears that natural progesterone is safe, Guy E. Abraham, MD, a research gynecologist and endocrinologist, believes it is not just progestin that can cause problems. He told me in a long interview that taking large doses of either progestins or progesterone can lower your immunity. Interestingly, while natural progesterone has been used to reverse vaginal atrophy, Dr. Abraham told us that when you take progesterone without having sufficient estrogen, it can actually contribute to vaginal atrophy. He believes the only way women should take hormones is by determining exactly how much they need and taking that amount, no more.

What about Dr. John Lee's statement that natural progesterone cream doesn't cause any side effects? First, I have talked with dozens of women first-hand who have found it impossible to continue using these creams because of a variety of negative symptoms. I also have spoken with a number of doctors throughout the state who have had patients with symptoms from self-medicating with natural hormone creams. In addition, the heads of several natural compounding pharmacies related the same stories to me. They have heard from medical doctors that even natural progesterone can cause side effects if a woman doesn't take just the amount she needs in a form identical to her body's.

Dr. Lee was a pioneer in the observation of the possible uses of natural progesterone cream, but his research was not a carefully designed and controlled double-blind study. That's the next step we need after his excellent observations. Yet, even though Dr. Lee's study was done in the 1980s, no one has taken this research to the next level.

Since Dr. Lee's findings were published, numerous companies

have come out with natural progesterone creams. They vary considerably in quality and hormone activity, so Dr. Lee's observations and belief in their safety may or may not even apply to women using these newer products. Adriane Fugh-Bergman, who authored an article in the newsletter for the *National Women's Health Network* (Jan/Feb 1999), believes as I do that natural progesterone appears to be much more beneficial than progestins. But just because it's natural, she cautions, doesn't mean it's safe. Dr. Abraham would agree. The amount of a natural hormone is as important as its molecular structure. What's frightening is that there's no way for you to know what's in any particular product without taking it to an independent laboratory and having it tested at great expense.

When to Take Progesterone

Before you take any progesterone product, make sure you need it. Get your hormone levels tested.

There are three types of hormone tests: a blood test that your doctor's laboratory can do, a 24-hour urine test, and a saliva test. Which is best?

It appears that the common blood hormone tests, which give a snapshot view of your hormones at any one moment in time, are the ones you want. Remember that your progesterone level may be either higher or lower than the values given by any laboratory. So it's important for your doctor to assess your needs according to symptoms as well as lab levels. Some doctors do a blood test to determine a baseline, prescribe progesterone, and watch what happens. If your progesterone levels rise and symptoms decrease, you're taking the correct amount. You need a doctor skilled in hormone therapy, and natural hormone therapies if that's what you want, to help you achieve the results you're looking for. As limited as a blood test is, the medical doctors and pharmacists I talked with all agree that it is the best method we know of right now to measure hormone levels.

Saliva tests have become very popular with practitioners of complementary medicine. A sample of your saliva is sent to a laboratory where the progesterone level is measured. I talked about it with Guy E. Abraham, MD. He, as well as the heads of several pharmacies that compound natural hormones, say they are finding in actual practice that results don't seem to correlate as well with the symptoms of hormone deficiency women experience. Dr. Reiss agrees. He has not found it to be accurate, either.

Another hormone test that's becoming popular is the 24-hour urine test. A few specialized laboratories do this test. The theory behind it is that if you take a full day's amount of urine, and have a small amount of it analyzed, it can give a wider view of hormone activity than a blood test. But here's the problem: It can't accurately tell you about your progesterone level because progesterone is not excreted in urine. A metabolite, or part, of progesterone is, but this chemical is made in your liver. If your liver or kidney functions are not up to par, and if your water intake the day before you collect your urine is not the same amount as you usually drink, you may not get a correct picture of your hormones. Still, Dr. Reiss finds it useful when assessing total hormone levels in his patients. But he uses the 24-hour urine test along with blood tests. If you're getting one, get blood tests.

Raising Your Progesterone, Naturally

If your progesterone is low, you have other options for increasing your body's production of this hormone that are safe, natural, and often effective. You see, your body has built-in safety mechanisms that help regulate hormone activity. It just naturally makes various chemicals that either promote or inhibit the production of various hormones, including progesterone. While you won't be able to raise your progesterone levels very high, you may get some additional hormonal activity.

Dietary animal fats help make hormone-like substances called prostaglandins that inhibit, or block, progesterone production. Not all prostaglandins inhibit progesterone, but the ones made from animal fats do. One option is to greatly decrease your intake of animal fats. Another option is to block production of the inhibitor! This allows your ovaries to produce progesterone that can then be used. Magnesium and vitamin B_6 block the progesterone-producing prostaglandin. While you decrease animal fats, you can increase magnesium and vitamin B_6 by eating more whole grains and beans.

And taking supplemental B$_6$ and magnesium could be a good idea, too. Some PMS formulas already have higher amounts of magnesium and vitamin B$_6$, like Optivite. Look for these formulas at health food stores. Or adjust your current total nutritional supplement intake to include 300 mg of vitamin B$_6$ and at least 250 mg of magnesium.

Other treatment options we like for rebalancing hormones naturally include moderate exercise, Traditional Chinese Medicine, and Osteopathic treatment. It's worth investing some of your time and money with a skillful health-care provider who understands hormones in the greater context of your overall health. If hormone imbalance is a symptom of another condition, it should be treated first.

If You Need Supplemental Progesterone

If hormone imbalance persists, a doctor, who understands natural hormones and uses tests as well as his or her expertise in determining your specific needs, is essential. You want someone who will track your progress and adjust your hormones, and who will work with a good pharmacy to provide you with the product your body can use in the dose it needs. If you can't find such a physician near you, call the Belmar Pharmacy (800-525-9473) or the Women's International Pharmacy (800-279-5708) and ask them for the names of practitioners in your area who use their products.

It may be tempting to pick a cream off the shelf of a nearby store in the hopes that you'll get the same results as a friend, or a friend of a friend. But remember, these products are often very low in hormonal activity and you may not be getting the amounts your body needs. Hormone balance is critical for good health, and your hormones fluctuate during your menstrual cycle and as you approach menopause. Hormones affect your energy, your libido, your anxiety or calmness, and your water retention, to mention just a few. They are dependent upon a number of factors like nutrients and stress. Certain vitamins and minerals can help the body's production of hormones, and stress causes other hormones to be produced. You can be certain about one thing: Hormones are nothing to

fool around with. Still, thousands of women are doing just that —
naively using over-the-counter creams that can affect their hormone
levels without knowing first what they need or how much.

What's more, some of the more popular tests for hormones
may not give accurate information. It's time women learned the
truth about natural hormones and started to use them wisely, under
a knowledgeable doctor's supervision. This is one example of taking precautions to be safe now and in the future, rather than being
sorry later. Don't be a guinea pig. Be the wise woman you are. To
help your doctor help you with evaluating your hormone levels,
pick up a copy of Dr. Reiss's book and share it with him or her. It's
a guide to doctors and patients alike in the safe and effective ways
of replacing hormones…naturally.

Do You Need DHEA?

DHEA (dehydroepiandrosterone) is a steroid hormone made
from cholesterol by your adrenal glands. Your adrenal glands are
tiny workhorses that help you handle all the stresses in your life.
DHEA helps stimulate the immune system and acts as a buffer
against stress. DHEA both slows down bone loss and increases bone
formation, reducing your risk for osteoporosis.

Structurally, DHEA is similar to other steroid hormones like
estrogen, progesterone, and testosterone. In fact, DHEA can be converted into both estrogen and testosterone, boosting estrogen levels.
But DHEA is more than a reservoir for these hormones. It helps
regulate various hormones and enzymes. Animal studies indicate it
can help prevent diseases such as cancer, lupus, rheumatoid arthritis, Alzheimer's, heart disease, and chronic fatigue. It may even help
slow down aging and increase your libido. DHEA is abundant in
brain tissue and has been found to increase neurons in laboratory
tests with nerve-cell tissue cultures. This means that DHEA could,
conceivably, support brain function as we age. How this translates
into benefits for humans is yet to be seen.

Does this sound too good to be true? It may be. You see, when
you look at the many studies done with DHEA, it sometimes works

and it sometimes doesn't. According to Dr. Reiss, studies using DHEA have been too short and have used doses much too high. Many of his patients who take DHEA can take only five milligrams without experiencing side effects.

Is DHEA effective? While some women swear that they feel better after taking it, two studies published in the *Journal of Clinical Endocrinology Metabolism* found that DHEA did not increase any feelings of well-being in women. My suggestion, as with all hormone therapy, is to do some homework before deciding to take it. DHEA may do wonders for you. Or it may do nothing.

Author and physician Hyla Cass, MD, says, "It's a delicate balance, this hormonal dance." She points out that our bodies handle hormones like DHEA differently. In some women, it remains as DHEA; in others, it is converted to testosterone or estrogen. This is why it's so important to be monitored by a physician.

To determine whether or not you need this hormone, have your doctor do a DHEA-Sulfate blood test. Discuss a slow method of gradually increasing your levels. Taking too much too soon will give you undesirable side effects.

Buying and Taking DHEA

Elmer Cranton, MD, past president of the American Holistic Medical Association and co-author of *Resetting the Clock: 5 Anti-aging Hormones That Improve and Extend Life,* also advises that before taking DHEA you should test your blood levels of DHEA-Sulfate. Then have your blood re-tested again after taking it for a month or two. Dr. Reiss, who has given natural hormones to more than 20,000 women, agrees. So do I.

While I often lean toward "cutting edge" health solutions, my position on hormone therapy is more prudent and conservative. I believe you should first determine that you have a hormone deficiency with symptoms or risk factors that indicate hormones would be helpful in improving your life. Then work with your doctor to take the lowest amount of the best quality natural hormone you can get.

Dr. Cranton cautions against taking megadoses of hormones: "With hormones, more is almost never better. Too much DHEA can produce a testosterone-like effect with symptoms such as facial hair, acne, and irritability. DHEA is a hormone, not a vitamin." In his own practice at the Mount Rogers Clinic in Trout Dale, Va. (540-677-3631) he has found that 25-50 mg of DHEA a day works for many women, but you may need much less. Some studies indicate that as little as five to 10 mg daily is sufficient. The doctors, like Dr. Reiss, and the pharmacists I have talked with have all found that the lower amount is often enough and is quite effective.

Some DHEA is better quality than others. The head of a natural compounding pharmacy found that many DHEA products sold in natural food stores that claimed to be 25-50 mg contained only five to 10 mg of the hormone. "At least people aren't hurting themselves," he told me. Because of this, Dr. Reiss, who has had experience giving natural hormones to more women than any other doctor I know, prefers DHEA made by natural compounding pharmacies or some nutritional supplement companies that primarily sell to health-care practitioners. Some products in natural food stores have only a fraction of the DHEA listed on their labels.

What about precursors to DHEA like the Mexican yam or herbs? Dr. Cranton points out that your body's ability to convert precursors into DHEA diminishes with age, so these natural products are less likely to have an effect. Any increased feeling of well being, he says, most likely comes from a stimulant effect in these products. "The only proven method of raising your DHEA level is by taking DHEA itself," he says.

One study in the *Journal of the American Medical Association* found a correlation between high DHEA levels and ovarian cancer, while another study showed high DHEA levels in women with breast cancer. Yet, Dr. Reiss, who I know personally to be a very cautious doctor, found some studies that associate high levels of DHEA with lowered incidence of cancer. He admits there isn't enough research to know just how DHEA influences cancer. This is another reason why I think doctors should assess all hormone levels before you start taking them.

The benefits of DHEA that Dr. Reiss has seen include mental clarity, increased energy and stamina, and better moods. As good as it may be, he believes it should be just one of several hormones used in hormone replacement therapy.

Does the Fountain of Youth Flow With Human Growth Hormone?

Maybe!

When other hormone supplement regimens aren't enough, many enthusiasts claim it's time to try human growth hormone. It is by far the most controversial, perhaps the least understood, and definitely the most expensive — somewhere in the market of $9,000 to $12,000 a year — although this could soon change. It does boast capabilities that other key hormones don't, including the ability to revive a dying heart and stave off kidney failure. It also holds promise for persons experiencing wasting syndrome, which is often seen in elderly convalescent home populations and persons with AIDS. While much remains to be understood about growth hormone, scientists do know that growth hormone stimulates production of another hormone called insulin-like growth factor (IGF-1). This is what makes growth hormone a particularly promising therapy for life-threatening, late-stage diabetes.

Currently, substances called Growth Hormone Releasing Agents are in development and may soon be available to offer the benefits of growth hormone without the side effects. Drug-maker Merck is developing an agent for treating immune problems and the diseases that accompany them, such as cancer. Release of growth hormone can also be stimulated with vigorous exercise, and estrogen supplements for women and testosterone supplements for men.

As the name implies, human growth hormone is what makes children grow. It is produced by the pituitary gland throughout our lives, but like other hormones, the level declines with age. In adults, growth hormone has a rejuvenating effect. A 1990 study reported in the *New England Journal of Medicine* that men taking growth hormone just six months experienced the equivalent of reversing 10 to 20 years of aging, with significant increases in muscle and bone mass accompanied with a 15 percent reduction in body fat.

According to Dr. Edward Chein of the Palm Springs Life Extension Institute in California, "Only growth hormone can actually reverse biological aging. Lung capacity improves, body fat decreases, muscle mass increases, cardiac function improves, kidney function improves, bone density increases, fingernails and toenails grow faster, the skin is more resilient, the immune system improves — antibody production goes up, natural killer cell activity is restored."

Another MD, Dr. Sam Baxas, founder of the Swiss Rejuvenation Centre in Basel, Switzerland, and who also has extensive experience treating patients with growth hormone, says this:

Postmenopausal Hair Loss

Thinning hair is common in postmenopausal women, caused by changing hormone levels. Naturopath Tori Hudson, ND, points out that reduced androgen and testosterone production, and changes in the sensitivity of their receptors, can result in hair loss. So can elevated androstendione, a hormone secreted by the adrenal glands that has been linked to male pattern baldness. When hormones are the cause, hormone therapy may be your best solution. Estrogen with testosterone may be worth considering, since testosterone increases the utilization of androgen.

John R. Lee, MD, who has studied and written about the use of natural progesterone for postmenopausal women, finds that when progesterone levels are raised, hair growth returns to normal. Increased progesterone causes a decrease in androstenedione, resulting in hair growth. Many women self-administer DHEA, a hormone that can help the ovaries produce small amounts of estrogen after menopause. But this is one case where more is not better. Dr. Lee cautions about using too much DHEA since it can contribute to hair loss. Clearly, hormone therapy is not advised without partnering with a savvy MD or naturopath. Talk with your doctor about the risks and benefits for you of natural hormone therapy if your thinning hair is particularly worrisome.

Another approach would be to do everything you can to stimulate hair growth other than taking hormones. Diet, supplementation, scalp massage, and exercise can all provide a good foundation for healthy hair and maximum hair growth. Some women find they can live with thinner hair and either cannot take hormones because of a family history of breast cancer, or would rather avoid taking them.

"Growth hormone brings you back to a youthful state in which the organs are returned to ... the size they were at age 25 or 30. Nothing else can do this."

As glowing as these reports may sound, there are also reports of severe side effects — so much so that studies have fairly high dropout rates because many cannot tolerate growth hormone. Known adverse effects include carpal tunnel syndrome, diabetes, and severe fluid retention. Many doctors continue to defend growth hormone, though, explaining that these adverse effects are the result of improper dosage. There is probably some validity to this since studies usually give the same dose to everyone across the board. In hormone therapy, however, individualized dosage, based on test results, is of utmost importance. This is definitely an area where one size does not fit all.

Your Chronic Fatigue Could Be Due to Hypothyroidism

As I said at the outset, hormonal imbalance can cause all kinds of problems. One example of this is hypothyroidism, which can cause a number of problems including chronic fatigue. How big is this problem? We don't really know how many cases of chronic fatigue are caused by hypothyroidism, but we do know that "fatigue is one of the most oft-cited reasons for visiting the doctor, right behind the common cold," says internist Mark Moskowitz, of Boston University.

What Is Hypothyroidism?

Hypothyroidism, also known as an underactive thyroid, usually hits women who are around 50 years old and occurs when the thyroid gland (which is located just beneath the Adam's apple in your neck) produces an insufficient amount of thyroid hormone. This hormone is integrally involved in many body functions and is regulated by the hypothalamus, which is located in the brain just above the pituitary gland. The hypothalamus secretes a thyrotrophin-releasing hormone, which causes the pituitary to release a thyroid-stimulating hormone (TSH). When the blood level of thyroid hormone reaches a certain point, the pituitary will produce more or less thyroid-stimulating hormone, depending on the body's needs.

What Are the Symptoms?

If you have hypothyroidism, but haven't yet been diagnosed by a doctor, there are several symptoms you can look for before seeing a physician. In addition to the fatigue we mentioned earlier, symptoms would include: constipation, depression, dry skin, feeling cold, hair loss, high cholesterol, hoarseness, infertility, irregular periods, low sex drive, memory loss, sluggishness, tingling hands/feet, or weight gain that wasn't caused by your diet.

You might also suffer from some related conditions that might accompany hypothyroidism. These include: carpal tunnel syndrome, difficult menopause, fibromyalgia, Grave's disease, mitral valve prolapse, recurrent pregnancy loss, and resistant high cholesterol. (Untreated, the condition may progress to myxedema, an extreme and life-threatening form of hypothyroidism.)

If you suffer from any of these conditions or the previously listed symptoms, you'll want to conduct a simple test at home. The Basal Body Temperature test was developed by Broda Barnes, MD, and should be done as follows:

• Shake down an oral glass thermometer and leave it on your nightstand before going to bed.

• In the morning when you wake up, with as little movement as possible, place the thermometer firmly in your armpit or under your tongue. (Menstruating women should do this test only on the second and third days of their menstrual flow.)

• Leave the thermometer in place for 10 minutes.

• Do this for three consecutive days and record the readings.

A normal functioning thyroid should have a reading of 97.8 to 98.2. If you have a reading of 97.8 or lower all three days, you may have a low thyroid function, according to Dr. Barnes. You'll also want to see a doctor and have the necessary blood tests conducted.

How Can You Know If You Have It?

The tests you'll need to have done are the normal TSH (thyroid stimulating hormone) blood test, along with the T4, T3, Free T4, and Free T3 tests.

After you get the blood tests back from your doctor, you'll want to sit down with him or her and discuss the results. What follows is a little technical, but it will help you understand what your doctor is talking about.

The TSH test will tell your doctor if you've got primary hypothyroidism (in which the defect is in the gland itself), but it won't tell him if you've got secondary hypothyroidism (the defect is in the pituitary gland or the hypothalamus gland). The normal range is approximately 0.5 to 5.5. If the TSH level is at the higher end of the range, or above the range, you may be hypothyroid (underactive thyroid). If you have secondary hypothyroidism, the TSH test will show your levels to be normal or on the low end of normal.

The T4 test is to find out the level of total thyroxine. The normal range is approximately 4.5 to 12.5. If your reading is low, and you have a high TSH, you may have hypothyroidism.

The normal range for the T3 test is approximately 80 to 220. A result under 80 is indicative of hypothyroidism.

Many doctors are still not running the Free T4 and Free T3 tests, but their importance is not to be underestimated. Dr. John Dommisse, author of *Natural Medicine* newsletter and an expert on hypothyroidism, says, "There are many circumstances in which one can dispense with the TSH test, but never, in my opinion, with the Free-T4 and Free-T3 levels."

The Free T4 test is to find out your level of free thyroxine, and the normal range is approximately 0.7 to 2.0. If your result is less than 0.7, you may have hypothyroidism.

The normal range for the Free T3 test is approximately 2.3 to 4.2. Your thyroid would be considered underactive if your test result is less than 2.3.

If all of these test results come back "normal," but you're still suffering from the symptoms or risk factors for thyroid disease, consider going to a reputable holistic doctor or alternative physician to get another opinion. They can give you further interpretation of the tests and a diagnosis.

Five Steps to Prevention

For those who don't currently suffer from hypothyroidism, preventive steps are definitely in order. According to Mary Shomon, author of *Living Well With Hypothyroidism: What Your Doctor Doesn't Tell You ... That You Need to Know*, there are several things you can do to reduce your chance of having thyroid problems.

1. Don't overdo soy — This may come as a surprise for long-time readers of **Women's Health Letter** because I've always been a strong advocate of eating plenty of soy. I'm not changing my tune on soy, but many people overdo a lot of good things. Too much of anything can be a problem. Soy's effect on the thyroid has become a very controversial topic, as many people believe soy causes thyroid problems. They insist that ingesting too many isoflavones, which are found in many of our favorite soy products and supplements, may cause hypothyroidism.

There are many experts, though, who don't agree with this. One is Mark Messina, PhD, author of *The Simple Soybean and Your Health* (Avery Publishers, 1994). He says, "In iodine deficient diets, soy does cause thyroid enlargement in animals. But in diets abundant with iodine, this is not the case in animals or humans, as several recent studies have shown. Theoretically, soy could be a problem for people who consume marginally adequate iodine diets, although even in this case, I am not convinced. In any event, the advice should be to get more iodine, not to avoid soy." I agree (see #2 below).

While healthy women can eat soy without worrying about thyroid problems, there are those who are at particular risk. If you have a family history of thyroid problems, previously treated/ untreated problems (nodules, hyperthyroidism, goiter, hypothyroidism, thyroid cancer), previous thyroid surgery, or another autoimmune disease, you may want to cut down on the amount of soy you intake. For anyone who fits in this group, Larrian Gillespie, MD, author of *The Goddess Diet*, says "one serving of tofu a day is all you need to enjoy soy's benefits."

2. Check your iodine levels — Iodine is necessary for the thyroid to manufacture thyroxin, the thyroid hormone. So if you're not getting enough iodine, you could damage your thyroid and cause hypothyroidism. But excessive iodine intake — including ingesting kelp or bladderwrack (two herbs high in iodine) — can also affect the thyroid.

A test to see if you're getting enough iodine was reported by the Swiss physician, Jean Surbeck, MD. According to Dr. Surbeck, take a Q-tip and paint an area about the size of a silver dollar with two-percent tincture of iodine (available at the drugstore). You might want to do your painting on the thigh or stomach, as it will make a yellowish stain. If your iodine level is normal, the stain will disappear after 24 hours. If it disappears in less than 24 hours, it means your body is deficient in iodine and has thirstily sucked it up.

If the iodine keeps disappearing in less than 24 hours, keep applying it, every 24 hours, at different sites, until the stain lasts 24 hours. Once the stain lasts 24 hours, you're store of iodine is at a normal level and you can discontinue the test. Include iodine-containing foods, such as beef liver, turkey, kelp (the highest concentration of iodine of any known food), asparagus, white onions, and broccoli, every now and then. Take the iodine test every three to six months to make sure your levels are normal.

If you are already on thyroid medication and find that the painted spot is consistently disappearing before the 24-hour period is up, you'll want to talk to your doctor about reducing your thyroid medication after your iodine levels are normalized. Low iodine levels could prevent your current medications from working properly.

However, the most accurate way to test your thyroid is through blood tests. If you suspect thyroid deficiency, talk to with your doctor.

3. Drink bottled water — Fluoride in water, and a rocket fuel manufacturing by-product known as perchlorate, and other toxic chemicals are among the many substances in water that may trigger or worsen the risk of thyroid problems. Consider drinking purified or bottled water.

4. Stop smoking — Not only can smoking damage your thyroid, it can actually cause some existing thyroid conditions to worsen ... yet another reason to quit — or never start — smoking.

5. Reduce your stress — Reducing your stress levels is an important step to take in preventing some autoimmune problems like thyroid disease.

What to Do If You Have Hypothyroidism

For those who do have hypothyroidism, there are basically two ways you can go with treatment.

The first is with the conventional mode of treatment, which involves the oral replacement of deficient thyroid hormones using synthetic hormones. The most popular of these is Synthroid and Levothroid. While these can treat some forms of hypothyroidism, they consist of mostly T4, which has to be converted by the body into T3 and other metabolites. If the thyroid gland isn't working properly, this could be a problem and may be the reason many people who take these synthetics still don't feel quite right. (Some doctors who understand Synthroid's limitations will prescribe the synthetic Cytomel, which metabolizes the T3 form of the thyroid hormone.) Other problems with the synthetics include serious side effects if the dosage is too large, and they usually have to be taken for life.

The second mode of treatment involves nutritional supplements and natural glandular concentrates. To follow this treatment protocol, you'll need to work with a doctor who is willing to prescribe the natural glandular concentrates, which include Armour Desiccated Thyroid Hormone, Nathroid, and Westhroid. These medications are all derived from the thyroid gland of a pig because it contains both T4 and T3 and very closely resembles that of natural human thyroid hormone.

The critics of the natural glandulars say that because the hormones are made from animal hormones and not synthetic, they can't be pure and consistent from dose to dose. However, all of the glandulars listed above are held to very tight standards that are approved by the United States Pharmacopoeia (USP). And the USP requires that the potency of each dose be accurately tested and labeled. If you or your doctor would like more information about natural glandular concentrates, you can contact the Broda O. Barnes Foundation at P.O. Box 110098, Trumbull, CT 06611; 203-261-2101 (www.brodabarnes.org). The Foundation has an educational package that costs $15 and, if requested, will include a list of referral physicians in your state.

In addition to the natural glandulars, you need to be sure to you're taking a quality multivitamin. If you are deficient in vitamin A, vitamin B complex, B_{12}, C, E, CoQ10, magnesium, manganese, selenium, or zinc, your body may not be able to efficiently convert T4 to T3. You can get sufficient dosages of these nutrients in Vitality by Women's Preferred or from many other quality multivitamins.

So if you're struggling with fatigue, make sure you look a little deeper. It could be hypothyroidism that's got you down.

Guidelines for Using Hormone Supplements

Used cautiously, and under the supervision of a knowledgeable doctor, these hormone supplements may be highly beneficial. But used carelessly, they may wreak havoc with our health. To avoid the latter, follow these general guidelines:

1. If you are premenopausal, still have your ovaries and uterus, and have good hormonal balance, be especially cautious about taking hormone supplements. Since hormones work interdependently and are carefully balanced against each other, taking a hormone supplement when no imbalance exists can result in hormone imbalance, and actually create health problems. Using melatonin (the sleep hormone) occasionally, such as to overcome jet lag, may be harmless.

2. Use hormones only under a knowledgeable doctor's supervision.

3. Pursue non-drug, and non-hormonal therapies as a first line of action.

4. If these do not produce satisfactory results, work with your doctor to have your hormone levels tested. In addition to estrogen and progesterone levels, testing should also check the levels of testosterone, thyroid, pregnenolone, and DHEA. Any hormone sup-

plementation should then be based on the results of these tests. For increased longevity, the goal is to replenish key hormone levels back to more youthful levels.

5. If you start taking hormones, monitor yourself closely for any adverse reactions and report these to your doctor right away. Also, continue to have your hormone levels checked regularly — every six months or so. This is the most prudent way to track your progress. It will also help protect you against one of our foremost concerns regarding women taking hormone supplements: Even if you don't take estrogen supplements, other hormone supplements can increase your estrogen levels. And increased estrogen levels have been linked to an increased incidence of breast cancer. Therefore, always include estrogen in your hormone level tests.

6. Take the lowest dosages possible to achieve desired results. In the case of hormones, more is not always better. In fact, overly high dosages can be highly detrimental to your health.

Whether or not you wish to use hormones is a decision that should be made with great care and attention. Although much is known about hormones, much is also left to be learned. One way to minimize unnecessary adverse risks, however, is to maintain superior health. Then if and when you do decide to begin taking any natural hormones, keep dosages as low as possible to achieve the desired benefits.

Weigh the pros and cons of hormone therapy as well as other hormone therapies and make your own decision. Your doctors are your partners, not your parents. It's your body and your life. Take care of it.

Section 2

Treating and Preventing Common Health Problems

Chapter 6

Arthritis and Pain Management

Osteoarthritis (OA) and rheumatoid arthritis (RA) are two different diseases that favor women over men. In fact, women over the age of 45 are 10 times as likely to get osteoarthritis — a degenerative joint disease—as men. Seventy-five percent of adults in this country get osteoarthritis by the time they're 65 years old, and the Centers for Disease Control in Atlanta estimates that by the year 2020 this number will increase by 57 percent.

Osteoarthritis primarily affects the knees, hips, spine, and hands. Cartilage in these joints is slowly destroyed, and bone spurs form there causing deformity, pain, and restricted motion. The more these joints are used, the more painful they become. The key to understanding this problem is cartilage destruction. If you can stop cartilage from being destroyed, and actually rebuild it, you can control osteoarthritis more effectively than by simply taking medications for pain and inflammation.

Rheumatoid arthritis does not limit itself to the joints; it affects the whole body, although the hands, feet, wrists, ankles, and knees are most often affected. This is an autoimmune disease, which means that the body's immune system turns on itself and attacks its own tissues. Here again, women with RA outnumber men three to one.

Since many people with OA also develop rheumatoid arthritis, if you have OA you will want to look at the suggestions I have for rheumatoid arthritis. You may benefit from changes that address either or both forms of arthritis.

Let's Start With Osteoarthritis

The most common type of arthritis is osteoarthritis (OA). It begins with a slight stiffness, and then the joints become truly sore. Because weight-bearing joints like the hips and knees are often affected, the first step to take is to lose weight if you are overweight. This puts less pressure on your joints. Some people find their osteoarthritis symptoms disappear after they lose weight. Don't wait to try this simple first step. If you do, increased joint pain may limit your ability to exercise and lose those extra pounds in the future.

Western medicine treats osteoarthritis with aspirin and non-steroidal anti-inflammatory drugs (NSAIDs). They treat the symptoms. But this band-aid approach has its consequences. Aside from not addressing the cause, frequent use of aspirin often causes a small but persistent bleeding in the stomach. So numerous people with osteoarthritis have an arthritis-related anemia that comes from this steady loss of blood. Bleeding in the stomach can also lead to ulcers as the stomach's acid eats into damaged tissue.

NSAIDs are not much better. While they may reduce inflammation and pain, they cause a condition called gut permeability. This means the lining of the small intestines, through which we absorb nutrients, becomes more open — more permeable. Vitamins, minerals and amino acids are very small particles. They don't require large openings in order to get into our cells. In fact, the linings of our intestines are designed to let through those substances we need and keep out larger particles that could be damaging. Stomach acids are one of the first substances our bodies produce to help break down our foods into usable tiny nutrient particles.

As we age, our stomachs produce less acid, even though we need sufficient amounts to digest our food — especially proteins. So it's very likely that if you're over 50 and have osteoarthritis, the proteins you eat are not being digested completely. With gut permeability present, larger pieces of partially digested proteins can move across the lining of the small intestines often leading to autoimmune diseases (rheumatoid arthritis, lupus) and arteriosclerosis. NSAIDs may make you feel better temporarily, but they could cause more serious problems later on.

Instead of looking for a better band-aid, let's look at possible solutions. Begin by cleaning up your diet. Eliminate white sugar and decrease all refined foods like white flour products. Stop eating fried foods, luncheon meats, and margarine. Eat real foods, concentrating on whole grains, vegetables and fruits. Reduce red meat and increase fish, which contain naturally occurring anti-inflammatory oils. By making these dietary changes you will be increasing your body's supply of vitamins, minerals, essential fatty acids, and amino acids — the building blocks for good health.

Talk with a complementary medicine health care practitioner (some MDs, chiropractors, acupuncturists, naturopaths, nutritionists) about whether or not your stomach may be producing enough hydrochloric acid (HCl). Low amounts of HCl not only affect your ability to digest protein, it is also needed to utilize minerals like calcium and magnesium. You may benefit from taking one or two HCl tablets after meals, but never take this supplement if you have an active gastric or peptic ulcer. And check with a health professional first, especially if you are under 50 years of age.

Take a good quality multivitamin/mineral in addition to improving your diet. Many OA patients have nutrient deficiencies that a good supplement can help reduce. Diet may not be sufficient. Choose a supplement with moderate, but not extra-high, amounts of B vitamins (10-25 mg is better than 50-100 mg according to a number of studies) and with a full compliment of minerals. And remember to avoid supplements that are high in calcium and low in magnesium, which can contribute to arthritis. Look for multivitamin/mineral supplements such as Optimox's Gynevite (1-800-722-9040), which is high in magnesium and low in calcium. Or try Vitality by Women's Preferred (1-800-728-2288), which has 500 mg each of calcium and magnesium.

Keep your antioxidants high. They destroy free radicals, and free radicals destroy cartilage. Take plenty of vitamin E (400-800 IU) in a dry form (TwinLab is one good brand of dry, encapsulated vitamin E). Vitamin C with bioflavonoids is also needed for cartilage health and is another anti-inflammatory nutrient. One or two grams a day of vitamin C are often sufficient (1,000-2,000 mg) to bring noticeable results after several months.

Cartilage needs plenty of sulfur to regenerate. Sulfur is found in eggs, and is high in some amino acids like cysteine, taurine, and methionine. Because large amounts of these particular amino acids may be necessary, it would be best for you to work with a health professional who is familiar with using them in supplement form. You may need as much as two or three grams of each a day, but don't just rush out and buy a supply of amino acids. They require particular vitamins and minerals, like magnesium and vitamin B_6, to be absorbed and utilized. Amino acid therapy can be powerful, but it is most effective when an experienced practitioner is guiding you.

Chondroitin Sulfates—Number One for Osteoarthritis

Now I'm going to get a bit more technical, but try to stay with me, because it's important to understand the reasoning behind an exciting nutrient that can greatly benefit people with OA. Cartilage is a hard, gristly, smooth tissue made up in part from mucopolysaccharides. Chondroitin sulfates (CS), the primary type of mucopolysaccharide, helps cartilage become elastic. This elasticity allows cartilage to cushion our bones and absorb the pounding that occurs when we walk or put pressure on any of our joints.

Chondroitin sulfates are found in calf trachea and green-lipped mussels, and you can find supplements in health food stores made from these substances. But some nutrient manufacturers have purified the CS from these sources into a better-absorbed, standardized form. When a supplement is standardized, it means that each tablet or capsule contains the same amount of the active ingredient as the next. It is in this form that CS can repair both connective tissue and cartilage, as well as reduce the pain from osteoarthritis. CS is non-toxic, and from one to two grams daily has been shown to regenerate cartilage in some cases. You need this much because it is poorly absorbed.

Pain Relief: Glucosamine Sulfate

Glucosamine sulfate is another building block of cartilage. It is a natural anti-inflammatory agent, which stimulates cartilage repair. Like CS, it is non-toxic. The usual dosage is 500 mg three times daily. This supplement takes longer to work than NSAIDs (from 2-3 months). But people who persist in using it often find great relief from their pain.

Herbal Solutions:

Numerous herbs have been found to be helpful with OA, for relief of pain and inflammation including the following:

• **Boswellia serrata.** The resin from this Indian tree, guggul, is found in some nutritional supplements. The usual dosage is 400 mg three times daily. Studies have shown no adverse effects.

• **Bromelain.** This is actually a mixture of sulfur-containing enzymes found in pineapple stems (not the flesh of the fruit — so don't just eat a lot of pineapple). Typically, 125-450 mg of bromelain is taken three times daily on an empty stomach.

• **Capsaicin.** This is the active ingredient from cayenne peppers. Used in a topical ointment, capsaicin often blocks pain receptors and reduces inflammation as well. These ointments are available over-the-counter.

• **Devil's claw.** This African herb has a history of use in arthritis, but unfortunately numerous studies have not found it to be effective.

• **Ginger.** One study showed that powdered ginger root alleviated pain and swelling in 75 percent of the participants. The suggested dose was 500-1,000 mg a day, but the people who had the most relief took three to four times that amount. Ginger root powder is inexpensive and easy to find in many health food and herb stores. It can be added to food, made into a tea, or put into capsules.

Osteoarthritis is not an easy condition to treat, but it is worth pursuing this avenue. A healthy diet will only improve your overall health; a multivitamin/mineral is added health insurance; and one or two supplements can be tried for a period of two or three months until you find which works best for you. Remember, if you have osteoarthritis, you may also have some rheumatoid arthritis.

Outsmarting Rheumatoid Arthritis

No one really knows how or why rheumatoid arthritis (RA) begins, although there are numerous theories. This is a painful, chronic inflammatory condition that primarily affects the joints of the hands, feet, wrists, ankles, and knees. And it is more common in women than in men. Many people with osteoarthritis also have RA. For this reason, some nutritional information specific to rheumatoid arthritis could help someone with osteoarthritis. Nutritional changes, including supplementation, have fewer side effects than anti-inflammatory drugs — the treatment of choice among most medical doctors.

Earlier in this chapter, I discussed the gastrointestinal problems associated with using aspirin and nonsteroidal anti-inflammatory drugs (NSAIDs) to ease arthritis pain and inflammation. In an effort to head off gastrointestinal problems — especially ulcers — associated with heavy NSAID use, many arthritis sufferers also take antacids. Unfortunately this, too, causes problems. Namely, antacids neutralize hydrochloric acid in the stomach, which results in poor digestion. In turn, poor digestion can lead to nutritional deficiencies. This further compromises an already compromised immune system.

RA is considered to be an autoimmune disease, which means the body makes antibodies — substances that fight specific germs or viruses — that attack joint tissues as though they were harmful foreign invaders, not just tissue that belongs there. These antibodies cause inflammation and pain when they come into contact with tissues. In rheumatoid arthritis, even more than in osteoarthritis, nutrition has been found to play a major role in correcting this biochemical error. Avoiding regular NSAID and antacid use is an absolute necessity for beating RA with nutrition.

RA's Possible Origin

Many diseases begin in the intestines. Many people believe that rheumatoid arthritis, through a condition called Leaky Gut Syndrome (or intestinal permeability), may be one of them. Here's what happens. A high sugar diet or the overuse of antibiotics or steroids allows the friendly bacteria (good bugs) in your intestines to be overtaken by pathogenic bacteria (bad bugs). Your intestinal lining becomes inflamed in response to this bad bug overgrowth, and the spaces between the gut cells become enlarged. This allows large pieces of partially digested foods to pass through the lining of the intestines (or gut) and leak into the bloodstream. But your body doesn't know how to break these large particles down or use them.

Once in the blood stream, your body sees these food particles as unwanted substances. Your system then makes chemicals called antibodies to fight and destroy them as if they were bacteria, not merely pieces of food. This causes your body to have a food allergy response and worse. According to Sherry A. Rogers, MD, in her excellent book, *Wellness Against All Odds* (Prestige Publishing, 1994), "Arthritis is a common result when these antigen-antibody complexes form and attach to the synovium of the joint. Once

Using Acupuncture

Often, when we're looking for alternative treatments for health problems, we overlook acupuncture – the most well-known modality used by doctors of Oriental medicine (diet, herbs, and massage are others). Acupuncture sounds painful (it isn't) and strange (it is, until you've experienced it). But it's now become mainstream. Traditional medical doctors and dentists use it for pain control, and OMDs (Oriental medical doctors) use it for numerous health problems. Even the National Institutes of Health has given acupuncture a thumb's up.

In 1997, NIH found acupuncture reduces the nausea from chemotherapy and morning sickness. Pain from fibromyalgia, tennis elbow, menstrual cramps, low back pain, and carpal tunnel syndrome also responded to acupuncture. Ask any practitioner of acupuncture and he or she will tell you that it does much more than alleviate pain. Oriental medicine is based on achieving balance within the body and restoring vital energy (called Chi), not on treating specific illnesses. So as the body returns to balance, symptoms from a variety of conditions are reduced or disappear. In this way, acupuncture also boosts the immune system.

If you have a health problem that has not responded to Western medicine, you might want to try acupuncture. Low in side effects and much less expensive than surgery and expensive medications, it's worth giving it a three-month trial.

attached to the joint tissue, the antigen-antibody complexes cause the release of mediators that trigger inflammation, swelling, and pain."

Leaky gut syndrome is also associated with an overgrowth of Candida albicans (yeast overgrowth) and ulcerative colitis. An involved program for healing the enlarged cells in the intestines can be found in Dr. Rogers' book. Digestive enzymes, mucilaginous herbs, and an elimination diet are all a part of this first important step.

Do not fool yourself into thinking you can just take an herb or eliminate one or two foods and get relief from your pain and swelling. Rheumatoid arthritis is more complicated than that. If you truly want to use nutrition as a primary tool, you must first be sure that your gut lining is not impaired. Your health provider can order a test through the Great Smokies Diagnostic Laboratory (800-522-4762) that will ascertain whether or not you have intestinal permeability.

The Role of Food

Obviously, if you know you have allergies or sensitivities to particular foods, it is important to completely avoid them to eliminate the antibody response found in the Leaky Gut Syndrome. If you are unaware of any allergies, begin, as Dr. Rogers suggests, by removing all grains high in gluten (wheat, rye, barley, and oats). Eliminate all traces of these grains for two weeks and see if there's an improvement in your arthritis pain or inflammation. Then reintroduce them one at a time and look for a recurrence of symptoms. You may need to find substitutes for these grains (rice crackers, rice bread, corn tortillas, millet, wild rice, quinoa, etc.) in your daily diet.

Nightshade family: Let's begin at the beginning. Cholinesterase is an enzyme that helps muscles stay supple. Solanine stops the absorption of this "agility" enzyme. Solanine is found in a group of plants called the nightshade family, which includes: tomatoes, white potatoes, bell peppers (and hot peppers like cayenne or jalapenos), eggplant, and tobacco. Solanine is not destroyed through cooking. Some people with RA find a tremendous improvement when they eliminate all nightshades from their diet. This includes avoiding even the amount of cayenne found in salad dressings, a lit-

tle ketchup on a burger, or an occasional baked potato (sweet potatoes and yams are not members of the nightshade family and are
fine to eat). If you have RA and smoke, you need to stop, because
the tobacco is probably contributing to your problem.

Food allergies: An impressive study reported in the *British
Medical Journal* (June 20, 1981) tells of a woman with progressive
RA who had no known food intolerances, but her diet was high in
dairy products — primarily milk and cheese. She eliminated all
dairy and for three weeks felt fewer symptoms. Eventually, they
completely disappeared, only to reappear after she ate dairy one
day. After trying gluten and foods in the nightshade family, try eliminating dairy foods. They could be your nemesis, too.

Fats: In general, a low-fat diet is most beneficial for RA.
Those fats you do eat should come more from vegetable than animal sources. Some fats are anti-inflammatory; some aren't. The fats
that have been shown to reduce inflammation are those found in fish
(EPA), raw nuts and seeds, flax oil, and borage oil.

Your body makes hormone-like substances called prostaglandins from different kinds of fats. Anti-inflammatory
prostaglandins (PGE1) are made with the help of vegetable oils like
those mentioned above and fish oils. They can be taken either in
capsule form or added to the diet. Fish with the highest amounts of
beneficial EPA are mackerel, herring, salmon, and tuna. Fats that
increase PGE2 (inflammation-causing prostaglandins) are those
found in animal products like meat and dairy products. Reduce
your animal fats until they are only used occasionally as a condiment. Try this for a month. If you get results, keep your animal fats
very, very low.

Herbs

Curcumin: This is the active, anti-inflammatory ingredient
from the herb turmeric (*Curcuma longa*). It's also the chemical in
turmeric that makes it yellow. If you are taking curcumin, the
dosage found to be helpful in research studies is 400-600 mg three
times a day. If you'd prefer taking the herb turmeric, you will need
8,000 to 60,000 mg. That's a lot. Sprinkling turmeric in your food

just won't get you the results you want. I'd recommend finding cur-cumin, preferably in a standardized form (each capsule has the same amount of active ingredient).

Ginger: Gingerroot (*Zingiber officinale*) has been found effective in reducing the pain and swelling from rheumatoid arthri-tis. It may be taken in powdered form (500 to 4,000 mg/day), used fresh (5 grams/ day), or lightly cooked (50 grams/day). All have been found to be effective.

Boswellia serrata: This is an Ayurvedic herb from an Indian tree. The gummy resin from which Boswellia extracts are made shrinks inflamed tissues, brings more blood to the affected area, and helps repair blood vessels that have been damaged by inflammation.

Supplements

Multivitamin/mineral: It's not unusual for arthritis patients to be deficient in a variety of vitamins and minerals including mag-nesium, zinc, vitamin E, folic acid, iron, pantothenic acid, and vita-min B_6. If you have arthritis, you may want to take a good quality multivitamin/mineral supplement each day. And make sure it includes plenty of antioxidants. In the journal *Veris,* researchers reported that persons with the lowest blood levels of antioxidants were 8.3 times more likely to develop arthritis than those with the highest levels.

Magnesium: Most women are magnesium deficient. Increasing magnesium up to 400-600 mg daily — and lowering cal-cium intake to around 500-600 mg daily can improve joint health and reduce pain for both OA and RA sufferers.

Bromelain: This enzyme, made from the green stem of pineapple plants, keeps PGE2, the harmful prostaglandins, from being formed. Bromelain also allows the good prostaglandins (PGE1) to work and reduce inflammations. Bromelain should be taken in large quantities in between meals to be most effective, but not by anyone with an ulcer. Consult with your health practitioner for the amount that would be safe for you to take.

Copper: Before the turn of the century, there was very little reported rheumatoid arthritis in Europe. Many cooking pots and utensils were made from copper, and it is thought that people absorbed more of this mineral through their foods. Industrialization resulted in people coming into contact with substances that block copper absorption — zinc, lead, and cadmium.

Copper salicylate may be an even stronger anti-inflammatory substance than aspirin, according to several scientific studies. In fact, the more severe RA symptoms are, the lower the blood levels of copper appear to be. Copper salicylate should not be used for long periods of time. Talk with your doctor about using it under professional guidance. To be on the safe side, you may, instead, want to try wearing a copper bracelet. Studies have shown that small amounts of copper are absorbed through the skin and do frequently reduce arthritis symptoms.

Design a Program and Begin Today

The way out of a problem is the way through. In other words, taking substances that block symptoms is no substitute for eliminating the cause of the symptoms. Rheumatoid arthritis is a painful, difficult condition to reverse or improve. It takes dedication, time, and a lot of effort. From all the studies I've read, and patients I've talked to who took the long hard way through, I believe it's worth giving nutrition a chance. Write out a step-by-step program you think you can follow, and give yourself six months. Do the very best you can, then let me know about your results. I think you'll find the effort you take worthwhile.

Other Arthritis Therapies

I've talked with you in the past about using supplements like glucosamine sulfate and chondroitin sulfate for the pain of osteo-arthritis instead of taking traditional painkillers or anti-inflammatory drugs. But if you have arthritis, there are other therapies you can, and should, use as well — no matter which form of medication you take.

Since arthritis results in pain along with limited joint function, just taking something for the pain does nothing to help your joints move.

Two doctors from Gainesville, Florida, Shahid Zeb, MD, and

N. Lawrence Edwards, MD, have examined the area of non-drug therapies for people with osteoarthritis. They stress the importance of becoming more educated about your disease. The Arthritis Self-Management Program, given through the Arthritis Foundation, can provide you with a better understanding of various types of arthritis and treatment protocols. This national organization has 150 chapters throughout the country. You can find them online at www.arthritis.org, or look in your phone book for a local chapter.

Lose Some Weight

If you weigh more than 10 percent of your ideal weight, losing weight could decrease your risk of getting arthritis in the knee by as much as 50 percent. If you already have arthritis in your knee or hip, losing weight will reduce your pain substantially. But this is

COX-2 Inhibitors Can Cause Kidney Problems

There's a new classification of drugs on the market called COX-2 inhibitors that are used to reduce inflammation. COX-2 is an enzyme needed to produce the type of prostaglandins (hormone-like substances) that contribute to inflammation. And COX-2 inhibitors fall into a category of non-steroidal anti-inflammatory drugs (NSAIDs). In the past, NSAIDs inhibited another enzyme called COX-1, needed for the normal function of many organs and tissues. Their side effects included gastrointestinal bleeding and kidney failure.

Because COX-2 inhibitors don't affect COX-1 (or if they do, it's to a very small degree), they have been called safe. Now some studies are showing that COX-2 inhibitors can cause dangerous side effects affecting kidney function. A recent study published in the *Annals of Internal Medicine* (2000, 133) compared the effects of the older COX-1/COX-2 inhibitors with the newer COX-2 inhibitor. It found that both drugs slowed down the rate at which kidneys filter out unwanted debris through the urine. If your doctor took you off the older anti-inflammatory drugs, you may not be a candidate for the newer ones. Be sure to discuss this thoroughly before deciding whether or not the anti-inflammatory drug of choice for you is an NSAID or such supplements as MSM or glucosamine sulfate.

McCarthy, Michael. "COX-2 inhibitors found to impair renal function," *The Lancet,* vol 356, July 8, 2000.

easier said than done. Weight loss combined with exercise works best, and the pain and inflammation from arthritis often don't permit the type of exercise that would encourage weight loss. You may need to work with a nutritionist or dietician — or use some of the techniques I've talked about in the past — to successfully lose weight. One simple step is to eat smaller portions and chew them well. Then wait 15-20 minutes before asking yourself if you're still hungry. Often, you'll find you've had enough, and you can cut back on calories without feeling deprived. Emotional support helps tremendously, so team up with a friend who has similar goals and work on a program together.

Exercises That Help Range of Motion

Arthritis limits your range motion (ROM) and often leads to weak muscles that tire easily. It places restrictions on simple daily tasks like reaching for something in a cupboard or zipping up a dress. When you do regular exercises to increase ROM, you'll have more mobility along with less pain and fatigue. Depression lessens, too, since even small improvements are encouraging. Drs. Zeb and Edwards suggest the following regime for ROM exercises:

- Exercise during the part of the day when your pain and stiffness are least.
- Use heat for mild or chronic pain.
- Use cold packs for inflammation.
- Exercise in the evening to decrease your stiffness the next morning.
- Do gentle stretching to avoid increased pain.
- When you have an inflammation, do a little less — but do something if you can.

Strengthening Exercises

If your arthritis is moderate to severe, or if you're not used to exercising, begin with isometric exercises to strengthen muscles around your arthritic joints. Isometric exercises use a constant tension instead of movement. Strengthening exercises help your stability and guard against injuries from falls. The exercises outlined by

Robert Swezey, MD, a rheumatologist who developed the OsteoBall (see box below), are isometric. Not only do they help reverse osteoporosis and frailty, they strengthen your muscles as well.

Exercises that cause joints and muscles to contract and relax are called isotonic. These may be done with elastic bands, free weights, and even machines. Even aerobic exercises are appropriate for some people. If walking is too painful, try aquatic exercises. Often, the reduction in gravity from exercises done in a pool can increase your range of motion without causing flare-ups or damaging your hips or knees. Another benefit of aerobics is increased weight loss and a cardiovascular workout.

Check with your doctor first about the appropriate type of exercises for you to do. Then make sure a physical therapist or someone who understands your needs and limitations supervises any exercise program you go on. It's important to get this expert information since some exercises can have negative effects. For

New Exercise for Osteoporosis

Not everyone can do strenuous exercise, even to save or build bones. Now, doctors in Santa Monica, CA have found a simple and effective way to increase bone density. The scientific study to back this up appeared in the May 2000 issue of the *Journal of Rheumatology*. The study's lead researcher, Robert L. Swezey, MD, from the Osteoporosis Prevention and Treatment Center found that women who performed isometric exercises using a partially inflated large rubber ball with handles, began to form new bone within two months. The women either pushed or pulled at the rubber ball for five seconds at a time, doing specific exercises. The exercises, which are designed to protect the neck and back from injury, work both the arm and leg muscles, helping to build bone throughout the body.

Dr. Swezey points out that new bone is formed when the muscles attached to them contract. The complete set of exercises used by Dr. Swezey and his colleagues takes just 10 minutes a day. Muscles needed for balance, good posture, and prevention of fractures are included in the regimen that was originally developed for people with rheumatoid arthritis. If you have physical limitations that keep you from walking or lifting weights, this may be your answer. The ball used in Dr. Swezey's study is called the OsteoBall. It comes with a user's manual that contains detailed exercises, and is available by calling 800-728-2288.

instance, Drs. Zeb and Edwards caution against doing isometric exercises if you have hypertension.

Heat or Cold? Which Is Best?

Traditionally, cold packs are used for the first day or two after an injury, and heat is indicated when you have chronic pain and stiffness. But people are different. I know a woman in her 90s who swears by cold packs although she has had osteoarthritis for decades. If you're using hot packs, understand that the heat only penetrates a few millimeters, so you need to apply heat for about 20 minutes for the best results. Ask your doctor about deep heat treatments using a diathermy machine or ultrasound. Many rheumatologists have these machines in their offices.

What's New?

Another machine — one you can use at home — is called a TENS unit (transcuteneous electrical nerve stimulation). These machines block your low frequency chronic pain by emitting a high-frequency pain. So it works as a counter-irritant. It can relieve you of pain temporarily, but its effects are short-lived. Still, for someone in constant pain, even a short respite is welcome.

A giant step up from TENS units is a small device called the Alpha-Stim 100. Daniel L. Kirsch, PhD, developed it in the early 1980s and a colleague of mine, Fred Lerner, DC, PhD, used it in his chiropractic practice from its inception. Dr. Lerner and I worked in the same office, and I was treated successfully with this unit many times. I also saw that many of his patients were helped by it. The Alpha-Stim 100 combines microcurrent electrotherapy with a cranial stimulator. It actually treats pain in the brain, where it originates. In addition to stopping pain signals, this device treats stress, anxiety, depression, and insomnia.

You know that chronic pain affects your mood. Well, the Alpha-Stim 100 works on your mood as well as your pain — and the effects are much longer lasting than with a TENS unit. In a recent survey, Electromedical Products International, the company that makes this device, found that 94 percent of users found the Alpha-Stim 100 significantly improved their pain from arthritis, and 91.5 percent had significant improvements in their psychological outlook.

To get an Alpha-Stim 100, you need a diagnosis from your licensed health care practitioner (MD, chiropractor, osteopath, acupuncturist, etc.) and a prescription. If your prescription is from an MD you may be able to get reimbursed by your insurance company (it depends on your policy, says Dr Kirsch).

Different devices may work differently, and your doctor may already know of another one that he or she feels would be more appropriate for you. TENS units and the Alpha-Stim 100 can be expensive (the Alpha-Stim 100 is $735 — but it works beautifully), so call and ask for information on it first and discuss it with your doctor (Electromedical Products International, 800-367-7246 or www.alpha-stim.com).

Topical Creams

A number of topical creams containing capsaicin, which is an ingredient in cayenne pepper, are available in over-the-counter products you can find in drugstores. These creams do help many people and are safe to use. Double-blind studies have found them to be effective in reducing the pain of arthritis. The creams act by intercepting pain signals sent to your brain when joints are inflamed.

Pain interrupts our lives. It causes fatigue and shuts down our ability to think clearly. It leads to chronic depression, lowering the quality of our lives. Everything we do becomes more of an effort, so we tend to do less, which perpetuates the cycle. You may be caught in this downward spiral, doing little or nothing to change it because your past efforts have yielded few if any results. But if you have chronic pain from arthritis, you may be able to further reduce it with some of these techniques. You're worth the effort.

Shark Cartilage

Over 15 percent of the nation's population suffers from arthritis: eight million from rheumatoid arthritis and over 40 million from osteoarthritis. Unfortunately, nonsteroidal anti-inflammatory drugs

(NSAID), which are used to relieve arthritis pain, have been known to cause stomach ulcers, intestinal bleeding, abdominal pain, constipation, diarrhea, nausea, and skin rash. Furthermore, NSAIDs can also inhibit cartilage repair and even accelerate degeneration of cartilage — thus promoting the problem they are being used to treat.

Shark cartilage is fast becoming a widely accepted and safe alternative to help ease the pain of degenerative diseases such as arthritis. Because shark cartilage has the greatest amount of anti-angiogenesis agents of any substance known on earth, researchers have found it to be a powerful anti-inflammatory agent. As a result, shark cartilage, which has been proven to be nontoxic, has become the therapy of choice for thousands of people who suffer from osteo or rheumatoid arthritis.

The first studies regarding cartilage began in 1958 when Dr. John F. Prudden developed a bovine (calf) cartilage extract, which he made into a topical cream. Prudden discovered there was something in the tissue that resisted the formation of blood vessels. This

Q. I have arthritis stennosis, and my X-rays show a whitish swirling cloud-like mass around where both the nerves and blood vessels exit the spine to feed my arms and legs. Doctors say it is calcification cutting off blood flow and feeling to my arms and legs. I take calcium supplements, some skim milk, and soy products. Can you help? — *D.D.M., address withheld*

A. If the mass you describe is, indeed, calcification, you may be contributing to the problem by taking calcium supplements and using dairy products. Neither have sufficient magnesium to help get calcium into your bones. Unabsorbed calcium can cause various calcium deposits outside the bone, like the one you've described. By increasing your magnesium and decreasing calcium in both your diet and supplementation, you will give your body the ability to better absorb calcium. Sources of dietary calcium that also contain magnesium include whole grains and beans. These might be better for you than eating a lot of dairy products.

Also, both calcium and magnesium need some kind of acid in order to be absorbed. If your stomach is not making enough acid, you may not be absorbing these nutrients. One simple solution would be to have something acidic, like vinegar or lemon juice, with any foods that contain calcium and/or magnesium. This will help you use the minerals you're eating.

substance also had anti-inflammatory properties that were shown to decrease inflammation. Later, in 1983, it was discovered that sharks had the same ingredient in their cartilage as bovine, but it was more potent and there was more cartilage pound for pound.

In 1989, Jose Orcasita of the University of Miami School of Medicine gave six elderly patients suffering from "significant-to-unbearable" osteoarthritis doses of dry shark cartilage for a period of three weeks. In all cases, each patient reported that their pain was greatly reduced and their quality of life was vastly improved. People with arthritis can usually notice a difference within two to three weeks of taking the shark cartilage. If after 30 days there are no positive improvements, this therapy would probably not be beneficial to that person.

Traditional and holistic doctors as well as chiropractors and naturopaths who recommend shark cartilage agree that it is most effective when the daily dose is taken orally, three times a day, and in equal amounts about 15 to 30 minutes before meals. It's recommended that one gram of dry powdered shark cartilage be taken for every three to five pounds of body weight. Because it's nontoxic, you can't overdose on it. Shark cartilage powder is best blended with nonacidic fruit juice or water or taken in easy-to-swallow capsules. The only reported side effect is a sometimes mildly upset stomach while your system adjusts.

Due to the antiangiogenetic effect of shark cartilage, it is advised that children, pregnant women, and people who have experienced a recent heart attack should not take shark cartilage. Shark cartilage should also not be used three weeks before or after any major surgical procedure.

If you're looking for an alternative to your arthritic pain medication and want to try something natural and nontoxic, you should give shark cartilage a try. You have nothing to lose but your pain.

Walking in High Heels Leads to Osteoarthritis

If you're a fashion plate and wear high-heeled shoes, you may be at twice the risk for getting osteoarthritis in your knees than if you don't. Women have twice as much osteoarthritis in their knees as men. Your chiropractor or osteopath could probably have told you this, if you have one.

What's the association? There's nearly a 25 percent greater compressive force on your knees when you walk on high-heels than when your shoes are flat. Obviously, the higher the heels, the greater the force, so a two-inch heel might increase knee compression some, but not as much as four-inch heels. And the length of time you wear them could contribute to a possible problem as well. So would walking up stairs or up hills, where more force naturally occurs around the knee joint.

You've heard that "the knee bone's connected to the thigh bone" ... etc. This compression is accompanied by a twisting, or torque, to the ankles and hips, adversely affecting all of these joints. As your body tries to stabilize itself, the pressure centers on the knee. I'm suggesting that if you have ankle, knee, or hip pain, you may want to step out of your high heels for a while. Then, if your pain doesn't lessen or go away, seek the help of a chiropractor or osteopath, preferably one who can fit you with orthotics — inserts in your shoes that help re-balance your stance.

The combination of adjustments and orthotics will often resolve these problems. And frequently numerous others, from headaches to backaches, and more.

Pain Is Too Common

A recent Gallup poll of more than 2,000 adults over 18 found that nearly half the women (46 percent) have daily pain. The most common type was joint pain. Backaches, sore feet, muscle pain, and arthritis were the next most common. There are numerous remedies for pain including over-the-counter medications to nutritional supplements and herbs. In a national survey on pain recently conducted by the Angus Reid Group, orthopedic surgeon Samuel J. Snyder, MD, from Westwood, NJ, said he had found the combination of glucosamine sulfate with chondroitan sulfate brought relief to many of his patients. Since the molecular size of chondroitan sulfate is too large to be well absorbed (only 5 percent of this nutrient actually gets into your cells), I suggest you first try glucosamine sulfate.

Many people believe that stress, tension, and just growing older are major causes of pain. I'd like to suggest another — immobility. And an important approach to pain reduction is movement.

Pain keeps many people from exercising, but deep breathing and relaxation exercises will relax tense muscles and allow increased circulation. You may not be able to do what is considered "exercise," but everyone can benefit from the relaxing effects that come from deep breathing and simple yoga exercises. Check with an osteopath or chiropractor to make sure your spine is in alignment. This can take pressure off pinched nerves that cause additional pain. Do simple shoulder shrugs and arm stretches. Take a brief walk. Pretend you're six years old again and very slowly move your hips as though you had a hula-hoop in motion. Move your way out of some of your pain.

Q. I am 74 years old and last year had knee surgery. My doctor prescribed Caltrate, which I have taken faithfully. But I noticed a big change — there is a stiffness and a tightness that I hadn't experienced. Should I stop taking the Caltrate? — *M.A.P.*

A. First, you should talk with your doctor to see if the stiffness can be due to the healing process. You may simply need to do some stretching exercises. Also, have him or her evaluate your knee for any inflammation. A knee weakened by surgery in an older person might become inflamed after bumping, twisting, or over-using it.

If these are not your problems, you might consider this: Calcium causes muscles to contract, while magnesium causes muscles to relax. I don't know how much calcium or magnesium is in your diet, but you may be taking in more calcium than you're able to use. Switching from calcium to magnesium for a few months might give you this information. Be sure to take your magnesium with a little lemon water. Calcium and magnesium both need acid in order to be utilized, and your stomach may be making less hydrochloric acid than it once did, simply as part of the aging process (that's why some foods don't "agree" with us as we get older!).

If you have an inflammation, glucosamine sulfate (without any other substances added to it) is a safe, natural anti-inflammatory agent that has no side effects. Most studies show that 500 mg taken three times a day is sufficient. It takes about three months to work, but is excellent for chronic inflammations. You can find it at any health food store.

Exercise Without Pain

One reason many women don't exercise is because they're in pain. Some of the pain is from arthritis and other illnesses, some is from repetitive stress injuries (RSI) like carpal tunnel syndrome, tendonitis, and chronic neck or back pain. If RSI is keeping you from exercising, I have good news for you. I found a medical doctor, Gail Dubinsky, MD, whose life work is devoted to healing soft tissue injuries through yoga. A yoga teacher in Northern California for more than 10 years, Dr. Dubinsky has produced a set of four videotapes designed for people with RSI. Not only will they allow you to practice yoga without pain, they can help your condition get better.

I appreciate seeing people on these tapes who don't have perfect bodies. Most of us don't. I also appreciate the expertise Dr. Dubinsky brings to this subject. While these tapes may be ordered individually (at $14.95 each), I prefer the entire set of four, which is only $49.95 plus shipping ($5.50). Californians add $3.75 tax. For more information, check Dr. Dubinsky's Web site at www.rxyoga.com. Or call for a brochure (707-829-7596) and leave your name and address if it's outside business hours.

Glucosamine for Osteoarthritis

Numerous double-blind studies have shown glucosamine sulfate to produce comparable (and sometimes even better) results to medical drugs in relieving pain and inflammation due to osteoarthritis. In addition, glucosamine goes one step further by helping to repair damaged joints. Studies show these results are achieved safely with little or no side effects. Glucosamine sulfate, a natural substance found in the joints, helps the body make collagen, which keeps connective tissue flexible. It can be purchased at your local health food store. The amounts used in studies range from 500 to 1,500 mg a day and were given for six to 12 weeks. Check with your doctor about what amount is best for you.

When You're in Pain

A recent case of shingles reminded me of some of the horrible consequences of pain. Fortunately, the pain I was feeling day and night was transient, and I knew that within a few weeks I would be back to normal.

But some people are in constant pain, like my 90-year-old mother who has had arthritis for most of her life.

After doing some research for my own benefit, I came up with some ideas about what you can do for pain, whether yours is chronic or acute. Most importantly, I discovered that no matter what was going on, there was still something I could do, and by taking action I was not at the mercy of my pain. We all have some power, although at times it doesn't feel like we have much. We can take some kind of action, even if that action means resting, stretching, or just moving into a different position. Because pain can be so debilitating, and you don't want to do too many things all at once, it's best to have a partner in your doctor or other health practitioner to make sure you're not doing anything that will cause more pain.

Heat or Cold?

Some pain responds to heat and some to cold. Find out which is best for you. When you strain a muscle, heat is often helpful. If your condition is one of any type of inflammation, like a sprain, broken bone, or arthritis, cold is often most helpful. I discovered that the pain from my shingles went away when I was in my hot tub. Friends told me it wasn't a good idea, but my chiropractor said it was. And when I went to my osteopath, she not only concurred, she explained why.

Heat causes the body to produce histamines, which deaden the pain. The consequence of this is that the condition may accelerate and become more acute before it gets better. But it can shorten the life of the condition. My osteopath told me about a patient of hers who would occasionally get poison oak. To treat it, he would take a hot shower and furiously scrub himself until he was raw. His poison oak hurt terribly, but left quickly. While she didn't suggest I do that, her information did give me the rationale behind soaking in a hot tub for relief of my pain.

If you have pain from an inflammation, cold packs are best. They cause tissues to contract, thus reducing inflammation-related swelling. Apply an ice pack, or use a package of frozen peas or other vegetables if you don't have an ice pack. Keep the area iced for 15-20 minutes, then remove the ice for 10 minutes. Repeat as needed. If you must use any heat for any reason, such as a bath or shower, ice the area immediately after.

But there's even more you can do for pain. But before using the following suggestions, check with your doctor. You don't want to create another problem on top of your pain by taking something, even an herb or vitamin that is not appropriate. The suggestions given here are all based on sound scientific studies, but the most important aspect is to find the most appropriate answer for your specific condition.

Natural Painkillers

Not all painkillers are pharmaceuticals. For instance, *glucosamine sulfate* is a natural product that reduces inflammation in chronic cases. Because it can take two or three months to work, it isn't the answer for an acute, temporary condition. However, many people are finding relief from tendonitis and arthritis with glucosamine sulfate (500 mg, three times a day).

Some glucosamine sulfate products contain chondroitan sulfate. There's a problem with this formula, because while glucosamine sulfate is more than 90 percent absorbable, chondroitan sulfate is only three to five percent absorbed when taken orally. Glucosamine sulfate alone is my suggestion.

Arnica montana is a homeopathic remedy that often stops pain. You can find it in an ointment, like Traumed (Heel, Inc., 800-621-7644) in health food stores and some drugstores, or in tablet form. Injested homeopathics should be taken away from food and beverages. The dose of homeopathics varies greatly. The higher the number (e.g., 6x or 30x), the lower the potency. Hypericum is another homeopathic remedy that reduces pain, but it's specific for cuts, stabs, and deep wounds.

Capsaicin is found in cayenne pepper and is used topically for arthritis and neuralgia in an ointment form and is available in drug and health food stores. Capsaicin stimulates and blocks small-diameter pain fibers. Some people find capsaicin burns, while other people have no problem with it. If you get results with capsaicin but find the burning afterward is uncomfortable, try applying five percent lidocaine ointment before using the capsaicin ointment. Capsaicin also stops bleeding from cuts almost instantly, according to Michael Blate, author and director of a natural health educational organization in Columbus, North Carolina.

Feverfew is an herb that works for some people with migraine headaches by inhibiting the production of substances that cause inflammation. From 50-100 mg of the dried encapsulated herb has been found to reduce migraines, but one to two grams may be needed for an acute migraine attack. Feverfew has been found to have similar properties as non-steroidal anti-inflammatory drugs (NSAIDS), and is a safe substance. NSAIDS, like ibuprofen, for instance, can cause side effects such as bleeding ulcers.

Vitamin C with bioflavonoids and vitamin E can be helpful for the shooting pains of neuralgia. This pain is common in shingles, otherwise known as herpes zoster. I took the dose suggested for postherpatic neuralgia (the pain that comes with and after the herpes lesions) and found the unbearable pain left overnight. Both vitamin C and vitamin E have anti-inflammatory actions. Vitamin C with bioflavonoids: 1,000 mg three to five times a day. Vitamin E: 400 IU three times a day. During the time you take high doses of vitamin E, avoid white flour, vitamin-enriched cereals, vitamins with inorganic iron, or conjugated estrogens, which inactivate vitamin E.

Magnesium can put a quick end to muscle spasms, muscle cramps, muscle tension, plus pain from weak bones, and even some types of back pain. Aim to take around 1,000 mg daily, more or less, depending on your bowel tolerance. In other words, take as much as you can without inducing diarrhea on yourself.

Because magnesium relaxes all muscles, it's an important mineral to increase during times of pain. Many people find they can tolerate more magnesium without having loose stools when they're in pain. All pain is stressful to your body, and stress causes you to use up important nutrients or to excrete them in greater amounts than usual. Magnesium is one of them. When you're under stress, your adrenal glands produce hormones that block the uptake of magnesium. At the same time, you excrete more magnesium. Both magnesium and vitamin B$_6$ are needed to produce serotonin and melatonin, brain hormones that give a feeling of well-being and allow you to sleep well. This is why some people in pain are depressed or sleep poorly.

Drugs and Doctors

When all else fails, take a *pharmaceutical* painkiller, either prescription or over-the-counter, prescribed by your doctor. It's important for you to be out of pain and to be able to sleep and rest. But don't self-medicate or look for a friend who can give you their prescription drugs. Some drugs have side effects or could be contraindicated for you. Others may not be appropriate for your particular type of pain. Take them for as long as your doctor suggests. Often it is easier to control pain by taking painkillers throughout the day than it is to play "catch up" and take them only before bed. Discuss this with your doctor.

Acupuncture is an effective form of pain management. In fact, pain control may be the area in which acupuncture is most frequently used in this country. Some medical doctors and dentists take short courses in acupuncture just to be able to free their patients from pain. Often, results are immediate and dramatic. In cases of chronic pain, it may take numerous visits.

Chiropractic or osteopathic adjustments may align your body so you're in less pain. Most chiropractors and osteopaths can give you exercises that can help correct your pain-causing imbalances. These techniques for reducing or eliminating pain are extraordinary, especially if you find a talented practitioner. Ask friends or people who work in health-related occupations, like the sales staff at a health food store, for recommendations. If you've gone to a chiropractor or osteopath without results, you may need someone with a different approach. Chiropractors and osteopaths are like other doctors: There are a few excellent ones. Seek one out.

Electrical Therapies

One of the most exciting areas of pain control is that of various types of electrical therapies. From electric acupuncture, where tiny electrodes are attached to thin acupuncture needles and stimulate specific acupuncture points, to TENS units (Transcutaneous Electro Neuro Stimulators) and biofeedback, the problem of chronic and acute pain may be greatly reduced through electricity.

A *TENS unit* is a small machine that's connected to your body by way of small electrode pads. These are placed at particular sites that will vary depending on the source of a person's pain. Years of studies have found this small hand-held machine to be one of the most effective ways of stopping pain. Many medical doctors who specialize in pain management are familiar with TENS units.

The Cadillac of TENS units is probably the Alpha Stim 100, made by Electromedical Products International. I have tried the Alpha Stim and worked with one of its developers, so I've experienced and seen its effectiveness with pain patients. You, or your doctor, can call 1-800-FOR PAIN for additional information. All TENS units are not alike.

Biofeedback utilizes an instrument that assists you in learning to recognize, monitor, and control muscle tension and chronic pain. A trained and certified practitioner hooks you up to an electronic machine that gives you visual or audible feedback so you can become aware of what tension and lack of tension feels like. Look in the Yellow Pages for a practitioner.

Pain Relief That Works!

As discussed previously, aspirin and NSAIDs often trade arthritis pain for other problems. Here are some alternatives that may work just as well, or better, without the side effects. The key to success is to experiment as much as possible in order to discover the treatment or combination of treatments that work best for you.

Acupuncture has proven to be an effective pain reliever in about 60 percent of arthritis patients. And in general, studies have shown acupuncture to be 55 to 85 percent effective in relieving all types of pain, according to acupuncture researcher George A. Ulett, MD, PhD and clinical professor of psychiatry at the University of Missouri School of Medicine. Acupuncture is also well known to be especially effective in treating a wide range of painful conditions.

Acupuncture and Chinese herbs are often used together. Chinese warming herbs that are sometimes helpful in the early stages of osteoarthritis include pubescent angelica root, ledebouriellua root, timospora stem, and cinnamon. Chinese herbs that are recommended for their anti-inflammatory power are bupleurum root, licorice, and Chinese skullcap.

Acupressure. This is acupuncture's cousin, which stimulates acupuncture points with touch instead of needles. This makes acupressure a good candidate for do-it-yourself treatment, even though acupuncture is considered more powerful and effective. To locate a particular point, probe the area with your fingertip until you pinpoint a specific spot that produces tenderness, tingling, soreness, or slight discomfort. Then press the point firmly for about 60 seconds, stop for a few seconds and repeat. Do this for five to 20 minutes while also breathing deeply. Work the points that produce the best results on an as-needed basis. Here are some acupressure points that are used specifically for relief of arthritis pain:

Point #1: Located in the tissue between the thumb and index finger. (This point may also stimulate uterine contractions so pregnant women should not use it unless they are trying to bring on labor.)

Point #2: Located 2 1/2 finger-widths above the wrist crease, between the two bones in the forearm, with palm facing down.

Point #3: Located four finger-widths below kneecap on the outer side of the lower leg.

Point #4: Located on the outer crease of the elbow.

Point #5: Located at the base of the back of the skull, in the hollow area above the two large vertical neck muscles.

Point #6: Located below the base of the skull, approximately two inches outward from the center point of the back of the neck.

Aromatherapy. Judith Jackson, aromatherapist and author of *Scentual Touch: A Personal Guide to Aromatherapy* recommends a special arthritis blend of six drops each of rosemary and chamomile essential oils in four ounces of a carrier oil, such as sesame oil (we sometimes use olive oil because it's always handy in the kitchen). This blend can be added to a warm bath or massaged into sore areas. Elliot Green, past president of the American Massage Therapy Association suggests that it is most effective to massage around sore joints, making small, gentle circles with your fingertips.

Flower remedies frequently combine Holly and Vine and can be found in some health food stores.

Ayurveda uses numerous therapies such as a warm oil massage of the affected areas, heat therapy, and herbs mentioned elsewhere in this book. Ayurvedic treatment, however, is very customized to the individual, so I recommend working with an Ayurvedic doctor if you are interested in pursuing such treatments further.

Dehumidifier. Simple changes in humidity can be the cause of your pain flare-ups. Therefore, a dehumidifier can help maintain a more stable level of humidity in your home and thus help calm weather-induced pain, says Joseph Hollander, MD, professor emeritus of medicine at the University of Pennsylvania Hospital in Philadelphia.

Exercise. Many arthritis sufferers find that exercising joints and muscles in painful areas helps relieve pain. In addition, exercise provides natural pain relief because it releases endorphins, the body's natural painkillers.

In one study conducted by the Cornell Multipurpose Arthritis Center in New York City, a regular walking program resulted in a 27 percent decrease in pain, less medication use, and the ability to walk greater distances without pain. For a more in-depth discussion of walking for arthritis pain relief, write the Arthritis Foundation, 1314 Spring St., N.W., Atlanta, Georgia 30309.

Another study by Ronenn Roubenoff, M.D., and assistant professor of medicine at Tufts University in Boston found that strength (weight) training reduced pain because it resulted in better muscle support for affected joints.

Many sufferers report less pain when they swim or exercise in warm water.

Finally, yoga is emerging as an especially appropriate form of exercise for arthritis pain relief because it promotes flexibility and strength. Many arthritis sufferers report that yoga results in overall improvement of their conditions, including reduced pain.

Fitness. "You'll find that the better your physical condition, the less arthritis pain you'll have," says Halsted R. Holman, MD, director and professor of medicine at the Stanford University Arthritis Center in California. This means making general fitness improvements wherever possible, including weight loss, better nutrition, a regular exercise program, reducing stress, strengthening your immune system, and getting any other health problems under better control.

Homeopathy. Common homeopathic remedies include the following:

Rhus toxicodendron is used for painful joints and stiffness in the neck and small of the back that become worse in cold weather.

Bryonia is used for stiff, painful joints that are swollen, and feel hot and worse in motion.

Cimicifuga is used for achy muscles that worsen with cold and in the morning.

Laughter. One of the most famous case studies of laughter as powerful medicine is that of Norman Cousins, former editor of the *Saturday Review*. In 1964, he was diagnosed with a serious form of arthritis (ankylosing spondylitis) with a one in 500 chance of recovery. He had read about mind-body healing and proceeded to treat himself with laughter by asking friends to bring him humorous books. His condition improved, and he checked out of the hospital and into a luxury hotel where he set up a movie projector and screen so he could begin watching Marx Brothers, Three Stooges, and Candid Camera films and laugh even more. Within a few months he returned to work. Eventually, the only symptom that remained was sluggishness in his fingers, but not severe enough to prevent him from typing.

This is an example of the powerful healing ability of intensive laugh therapy. Laughter is known to lower blood pressure, release endorphins, and boost immune-system strength.

Other approaches for improving mental well-being have also been proven effective in relieving arthritis pain. In 1978, Stanford University researchers discovered that mind-body relaxation exercises decreased arthritis pain by an average of 20 percent over the course of a four-year study. Guided imagery — visualizing the pain leaving the body and disappearing — is also highly effective, according to Dennis Gersten, San Diego MD and psychiatrist.

Rest. Sometimes brief periods of rest can relieve pain. These might include 15 to 30 minutes of lying down. Also, pacing yourself and resting periodically when doing painful activities such as household chores.

Sex. One study found that 70 percent of the participants experienced up to six hours of arthritic pain relief following sexual intercourse. Warren A. Katz, MD and chief of the Division of Rheumatology at Presbyterian Medical Center in Philadelphia, believes that this pain relief is brought on by a surge of cortisone that is triggered by sexual intercourse. Beta-endorphins are also released by the brain during orgasm and are natural painkillers. He also suggests that a warm bath or shower before intercourse can help relieve initial stiffness. Sex has also been found to boost the immune system. Although there are no specific studies, this could theoretically help offset arthritis-related autoimmune activity and, in turn, relieve pain.

Temperature Therapy, When it comes to treating arthritis, there is controversy over whether heat or cold therapy is most effective. Some swear by heat, others find cold therapy works best for them, and others embrace a combination of the two. Experimentation is the only way to discover which works best for you. Any convenient source will suffice such as hot baths, cold baths, heat pads, ice packs, etc.

A Final Word

Don't accept that you will always be in pain, even if you can't imagine there's an answer. For many unsolved health problems that exist today, solutions will be found tomorrow. Consider that there may be forms of therapy, both nutritional and physical, that can reduce or eliminate your pain. Keep looking for answers and explore one method at a time. Take it one step at a time, rather than trying three or four methods at once. Ultimately, this will enable you to find the combination of pain control therapies — adding one at a time — that works best for you. Know that there are options you have not explored, and move toward your solution rather than feeling stuck in your pain.

Chapter 7

Female Heart Disease, Part 1: Are You At Risk?*

What do we know about women and heart disease? An easier question to answer might be: What do we *not* know? Because the answer is: *a lot.*

We know much more about men and heart disease because most medical studies have been done with men rather than women. When it comes to some conditions — and heart disease is one of them — what works for men does not always work for women. The General Accounting Office, an investigative arm of Congress, published a booklet in 1990 that showed a bias against women in medical studies. The GAO stated that studies showing that healthy men could reduce their risk of heart attacks by taking an aspirin every other day simply don't apply to women because women were not included in the studies. Hundreds of studies on mice, rats, rabbits, and men have been conducted, but only a fraction of that amount have focused on women.

There has definitely been discrimination against women in the area of medical research until very recently. In fact, in 1993, three years after an investigation in the House of Representatives, Congress passed the National Institutes of Health (NIH) Revitalization Act. This act of Congress made it mandatory for researchers who are federally funded to include women in their clinical research trials.

In another 10 or 20 years, we should know more about women and AIDS, arthritis, irritable bowel ... and heart disease. The wheels of change move very slowly. Yet many of us don't have the time to

---

*Portions reprinted from *The Giant Book of Women's Health Secret.*

sit around and wait for more definitive answers. We need to understand some of the reasons so many women die annually from heart disease so we don't join their numbers and become another statistic. And we need to begin today to change our lives with the information that's available now.

Fortunately, as limited as medical research is in the area of women and heart disease, there's enough out there for us to change our cardiovascular picture and improve the quality and length of our lives.

Doctors Will Eventually Learn More

The 13,000-member American Medical Women's Association (AMWA) decided in 1994 to produce a three-year program to educate doctors on women and heart disease. The program focused on a mere 100 doctors in the first year and increased the number of doctors it would reach in subsequent years. AMWA's target is our primary care doctor who may not even be aware that there are differences between men and women in relation to cardiac disease.

Heart Attacks and Gender

As a woman, you're likely to receive less aggressive treatment for heart disease and less diagnostic testing than you would if you were a man. A two-year study with more than 650 patients who had experienced heart attacks showed that women's health deteriorated more than men's following their incident, and that they received less care than men. Interestingly, there was little difference in recurrence of heart attacks or mortality between men and women. Even when it came to using small doses of aspirin, only 55 percent of women compared with 70 percent of men were given this inexpensive blood thinner.

Perhaps with managed care, only the end results are of importance. With mortality rates similar, only the quality of life would differ. So if you have a heart condition, speak up loudly to your cardiologist, and demand that your case be taken every bit as seriously as a man's.

Arch Intern Med 1997;157:1545-51.
The Lancet, August 2, 1997.

Because more women in this country die from heart disease than from all cancers combined, the AMWA believes this program is imperative for our protection and health. Still, the educational process is slow. Don't expect this small group of information advocates to get to your personal doctor quickly. Become better educated yourself so you can encourage your doctor to learn more about this subject.

If doctors don't know much about women and heart disease, what do any of us know? We know that statistics from the National Center for Health, released some years ago by the American Heart Association, state that nearly 30,000 more women die each year of stroke and coronary heart disease (CHD) than men. In fact, heart disease is the number one killer of all women past menopause. Every year, about 2.5 million women of all ages are hospitalized in this country with some form of cardiovascular illness, and over 500,000 of them die of it.

We have been educated to look at our cholesterol levels to make sure they're not too high. High cholesterol is considered to be a risk for heart disease and for that reason has gotten a bad rap. *Cholesterol itself is not bad.* It is a necessary fat made up of several components, including HDL and LDL. HDL is the healthy, or "good," cholesterol that keeps cholesterol molecules from sticking to the sides of the arteries. LDL is the lousy or "bad" cholesterol that has sticky properties and can eventually slow down the flow of blood to the heart or block it entirely, causing heart attacks and death. (Here's how to remember the difference: HDL=healthy; LDL=lousy.)

Several large studies have shown that high levels of HDL in women put them at a greatly reduced level for heart disease. And low levels of the protective HDL increased their cardiovascular risk to a much greater degree than in men. In fact, these two studies indicated that low HDL is more harmful in women than high levels of sticky LDL. Low-fat diets decrease HDL in women, so it is important to include some fats, like monounsaturated olive oil, and essential fatty acids found in raw nuts and seeds (plus fatty fish if you eat flesh), and not be on a totally fat-free diet.

In summary, you want relatively higher levels of HDL; for women, over 45 is considered good and over 55 is excellent. A healthy LDL level is approximately 130 or lower. These ranges will vary somewhat among women with high cholesterol.

Women with coronary heart disease have been observed to have a worse prognosis than men with CHD. More women die after having an initial heart attack than men. Women are more likely to develop heart disease as they grow older, while in men it often starts at a younger age.

There is a reduction in our levels of many hormones, including DHEA, progesterone, and estrogen at menopause. Many in the medical community believe that a reduction in estrogen, explains in part, why so many women get heart disease, but estrogen is only one of many components. It also seems that more women fear getting breast cancer from taking estrogen replacement therapy than getting heart disease — so many women don't take estrogen.

Other women can't take estrogen. They have a family or personal history of estrogen-related cancers, like breast cancer, and would run too high a risk for getting another serious illness to feel comfortable taking hormone therapy. Other women prefer not taking it. After all, it is a medication and taking hormones requires being monitored regularly by our doctors. If menopause is not a disease, and it's not, why would all of us need to be treated? For all of us, there are many options — even with the little we know.

And we shouldn't discount the power of prevention, especially when it comes to female heart disease. Women are more likely to go untreated for heart disease, even after it develops, because doctors frequently fail to diagnose it in women. And when it is diagnosed, surgery is less likely, and effective, for women. One study from Cedars-Sinai Medical Center in Los Angeles found that the bypass-surgery death rate was 2.8 percent for men and 4.6 percent for women. Other studies confirm this discrepancy and attribute it to the fact that women have smaller arteries, which are more dangerous to operate on. Smaller-sized men have higher perioperative (during or soon after surgery) bypass death rates as well. Other studies show higher failure rates of bypass surgery in women, plus higher rates of repeat surgery.

Angioplasty surgery, bypass surgery's less expensive cousin, is also high risk, and has a similarly dismal track record when women are considered. We are 10 times more likely to die from angioplasty than men, according to a study by the National Heart, Lung, and Blood Institute. The fact that female heart disease patients are older, on average, may account for some of these deaths. Still, many are due to the fact that the surgical equipment used, such as the catheters for angioplasty, were originally developed for use on men's larger-size arteries.

Fewer bypasses and angioplasties for women may be a blessing in disguise. This sentiment is shared even by the American Heart Association, which has stated: "Women may want to think twice before asking for 'equal treatment' from their heart doctors."

It should also be noted here that many experts, including renown former cardiac surgeons Julian Whitaker and Robert Willix, MDs, question the current widespread use of heart surgery. Instead, they advocate less radical treatment first, including lifestyle modification (diet, exercise, and meditation), and in many cases, chelation therapy. This advice is especially appropriate for women in view of their poorer survival rates with conventional treatment.

What Is Heart Disease?

Coronary heart disease is a category that includes many different illnesses from atherosclerosis to stroke, cardiac arrhythmia, cerebrovascular and peripheral vascular diseases, and congestive heart failure. Since women are less likely than men to be diagnosed — for example chest pains in women are commonly written off as indigestion — women should be especially self-vigilant of any symptoms they experience.

Angina Pain

When arteries are sufficiently blocked by cholesterol, and/or calcium deposits, arterial circulation can be impaired, resulting in the pain of angina. Classic angina pain is best described as a dull pain deep within or across the chest. This pain may radiate to the left arm and/or shoulder, neck, jaw, and even teeth. Right side pain has also been reported. Sometimes angina pain runs down the back, accompanied by nausea, sweating, and shortness of breath (some women have described this as a sensation of inhaling cold air). Angina pain is often described as a sensation of tightness, heaviness, or squeezing. In women, more often than men, it can also present itself as a sharp stabbing pain.

Early-stage angina is usually fleeting and accompanied by physical exertion or emotional stress, stopping when you return to a more relaxed state. Advanced or unstable angina also occurs during relaxation.

Heart Attack

Untreated angina can result in blockage and/or a blood clot severe enough to produce a heart attack. Classic heart attack symptoms include crushing chest pain, which may radiate to the arm, neck, jaw, teeth, and back. This may be accompanied by difficulty breathing, palpitations, nausea and/or vomiting, cold sweats, turning pale and/or feeling weak, lethargic, and/or anxious.

If this happens to you or someone you are with, get to an emergency room *as soon as possible* and demand a magnesium IV. One Orange County study of 103 heart-attack patients found that of the 50 who received a magnesium IV in the emergency room, only one died. Of the 53 who didn't receive a magnesium IV, nine died! You can even demand a magnesium IV in an ambulance on your way to the emergency room. This is one of the most valuable life-saving tips you will ever read. Share it with your family members, friends, and doctor!

Silent Heart Disease

Thirty-five percent of all heart attacks in women are called "silent." In the Framingham study, half of these heart attacks occurred with no symptoms, while the other half were mistaken for indigestion, ulcers, arthritis, anxiety, apprehension, nervousness, and other conditions. Some patients even suspect they are having heart trouble, and share this information with their doctor, only to be told that it is something else. If this happens to you, or someone you know, you can demand definitive tests to rule out heart trouble. And remember, this is no time to let a doctor intimidate or talk you out of your desire for further investigation. If testing is negative, you will have greater peace of mind. If it is positive, you will have taken the first step toward saving your own life.

Finally, silent heart disease can also come in the form of denial of symptoms — causing women to delay seeking treatment. This is akin to playing Russian roulette: Doing so results in nearly 50 percent more female than male heart-attack victims dying before they leave the hospital. Long-term survival rates also decline with delays.

Women's Mixed Signals

As you can see, symptoms of heart trouble are not always clear-cut. And being female can confuse the issue even further.

Women frequently experience harmless chest pains and rhythm disturbances. This may be a case of your heart suddenly "jumping into your throat," skipping, or beating rapidly. Then just as quickly, your normal heart rhythm returns. Sharp twinges and burning or aching in the chest are also fairly common.

Sometimes sensations are the result of overexertion caused by carrying a heavy purse, baby, child, or even heavy breasts. Exercising without warming up can also produce chest pain in women.

Another painful condition, Tietze's syndrome, is an inflammation of the cartilage between the breastbone and ribs, and can last for weeks.

Anxiety can also produce chest pain that may wax and wane for hours. If accompanied by hyperventilation, it can produce a tingling or slight numbness of the fingertips, mouth, tongue, and even legs.

Other health problems can also produce pain similar to that experienced with heart trouble. These include hiatal hernias, gallbladder disease, and other less serious conditions.

With so many different possibilities of heart trouble presenting itself in women, a safe policy is to have any unusual sensations checked by a doctor. The good news is that, unlike men, women rarely are stricken with a heart attack without warning. If we are more informed and more vigilant over what our bodies are experiencing, we have the opportunity to identify and address heart trouble earlier rather than later. This is a case of "just do it."

Ultimately, treatment delays result in bleaker prognoses. In addition, heart attacks sometimes occur silently — without symptoms significant enough for the victim to seek treatment. If you suspect you have had a silent heart attack, your doctor can run some tests and confirm whether it happened. It is important to do this so you can know your status and receive necessary treatment.

Heart Disease Risk Factors

Lower Levels of Estrogen

As we said earlier, the primary risk factor for heart disease in women seems to be related to our production of estrogen. When estrogen production drops off, heart disease increases. Estrogen seems to have protective effects on the heart. This is why more women have heart disease after menopause than before. One reason for this may be found in a study published in *The Lancet* that indicates estrogen has antioxidizing actions, which may lower the bad cholesterol (LDL) and thus reduce heart attacks.

Of course, if you want the antioxidant protection of estrogen without the risks that come with taking hormones, you can add more antioxidants to your diet and supplements. This could very well give you similar beneficial results without increasing your risk for cancer, causing bleeding into your 70s, and requiring daily medication and constant medical supervision.

Another reason for estrogen's possible usefulness in preventing heart disease is that it appears to not only reduce the harmful cholesterol (LDL), but increase the helpful cholesterol (HDL) as well. And remember, low HDL is more of a risk for women than high LDL. The Framingham study, for example, found that a 10 mg/dl reduction in HDL increases a woman's risk of heart disease by 50 percent, while women with elevated LDL were only slightly more likely to develop heart disease than those with normal levels. A change in diet (low fat, high fiber) and regular aerobic exercise can improve your HDL levels without the risk of cancer that's associated with estrogen supplements.

An interesting hypothesis about how estrogen works, published in the *The Lancet* in 1993, suggests that it has a long-term effect of blocking calcium. Calcium causes muscles to contract, and your heart is a muscle. Too much calcium will cause excessive contracting, and yet, we are being told we need very high amounts of calcium (especially after menopause). The problem with this is that not all calcium gets absorbed. Some unabsorbed calcium from a high-calcium diet or supplements is often stored in joints (where it contributes to arthritis) or arteries (where it contributes to atherosclerosis). *WHL* has been informing women of the danger of taking more calcium than we are able to absorb for many years.

But it is not only estrogen that blocks the absorption of the excessive amounts of calcium we're constantly being told to take. Magnesium does the same thing by helping you absorb the appropriate amount of calcium — without the risks of arthritis or atherosclerosis. And magnesium causes muscles, including the heart, to relax. Would you rather have a heart that goes into spasm (heart attack) or relaxes?

How Protective Is Estrogen, Really?

It is very important for you to understand that there is a lack of research to back up the notion that estrogen supplements prevent heart disease in women. An article published in 1994 in the *The Lancet* says that "not one large-scale randomized study evaluating the benefits and risks of long-term unopposed estrogen treatment or long-term combined estrogen/progestogen treatment has ever been published." This includes the protective effects of estrogen against heart disease. Spokeswoman Cynthia Pearson of the National Women's Health Network agrees. She believes an increase in the number of women taking synthetic estrogen could result in more uterine cancer (studies show that estrogen greatly increases this risk) and breast cancer. A study from the June 1995 issue of the *New England Journal of Medicine,* and based on 65,000 women, found that those age 60 to 65 who had taken synthetic estrogen five years or longer had a 71 percent rate of breast cancer.

What we do know about estrogen and reducing heart disease in women is that the studies showing hormone replacement therapy is effective are based on observational studies. That means that a large group of women is selected, and over a period of time, is observed to have less heart disease when taking estrogen than women who didn't take it. However, there are many factors that are not being considered in these types of studies — like the type of diet

Heart Disease After Menopause May Be a Myth

I was surprised to find an article in the *The Lancet* (May 9, 1998) saying that women are *not* at greater risk for heart disease after menopause. It's all a myth, the authors say, perpetuated by doctors who prescribe hormone replacement therapy (HRT) and pharmaceutical companies that make huge profits by scaring postmenopausal women into taking their pricey prescription drugs on a long-term basis. The myth is that women are at a lower risk for heart disease before menopause and, at that point, their risk increases until it surpasses the risk for heart disease in men. Not so, says Dr. Hugh Tunstall-Pedoe, professor of cardiovascular epidemiology in Scotland.

Studies that have shown more heart disease in postmenopausal women were conducted with women who had an early surgical or natural menopause, high cholesterol, or other cardiovascular risk factors. Studies on women who go through menopause in their mid-50s, without increased risk factors for heart disease, have not shown sex-biased results. Dr. Tunstall-Pedoe's research into the available studies shows "there is no rebound acceleration in risk in women at or after age 50 years, there is no closing of the gap between the sexes, which continues to widen, and no age at which risk in the two sexes is the same." He has also found no protection in British women who have taken HRT.

But we know that unabsorbed calcium, if it is deposited in arteries, can lead to atherosclerosis and contribute to heart disease. So we're still seeing just part of a large picture — perhaps a part we haven't looked at in this way before. As part of the media, we stand corrected, if, in fact, this article is as accurate as it appears to be.

Turnstall-Pedoe, Hugh. "Myth and paradox of coronary risk and the menopause," *The Lancet,* vol 351, May 9, 1998.

and the exercise programs of the women who are being watched. Women who spend the time, energy, and money to get on hormone therapy and be checked periodically by their doctors are more likely to be eating less fats and more fresh fruits and vegetables than women who are not taking any preventive measures. They are also more likely to be exercising. It may just be that women on synthetic estrogen therapy are healthier in general than the women in these inconclusive studies who were not on hormone replacement.

If you look at the eight-year long Framingham study on estrogen and heart disease, where over 1,200 postmenopausal women were observed, the results were startling. They showed that women who used synthetic estrogen actually had over a 50 percent increase in deaths from heart disease, and twice as much risk for cerebrovascular disease, than women who did not take estrogen. So right now, the picture is cloudier than you may have been lead to believe.

It is possible that we are interpreting estrogen replacement therapy correctly as one answer to reducing heart disease, or we may be missing the forest for the trees. Whatever protection synthetic estrogen offers, it can be duplicated by other substances that offer no risks to your health (or changes in lifestyle), which could have only positive effects. Only time — and good randomized placebo-controlled studies — will tell, and more studies using natural hormones. In the meantime, you have to decide how to protect yourself against heart disease. You may want to begin by taking a look at known risks for heart disease in women.

Cholesterol — Not What We Thought

As shocking as it might seem, women have been brainwashed about cholesterol. Most of the studies linking heart disease to high cholesterol have been done with men only. And we know women and men have more physiological differences than appearance alone discloses. It's true that numerous studies have shown that men who die of heart disease frequently have high cholesterol. But men with high cholesterol don't always get heart disease. Cholesterol is only one of many risk factors.

So, what about women and cholesterol? We know very little, since few studies, until recently, have been conducted on women. However, a recent survey (Buchwald, et al. *Annals of Surgery*, 1996;224(4):486-500) compiled seven large studies on cholesterol and heart disease and looked at the facts and figures, separating them by gender. The findings indicated that high cholesterol was most definitely a significant risk factor for men ... but not for women.

In spite of these findings, a large number of women with high cholesterol are being given cholesterol-lowering drugs they might not need. As a result, many women suffer serious side effects from these drugs — which shouldn't have been prescribed in the first place. Doctors are just not looking at the recent body of scientific literature. They're still treating us as if we were living in men's bodies with larger breasts and hidden genitalia!

What Is Cholesterol and What Does It Do?

Cholesterol is a fat, manufactured from the raw materials found in the animal fats, sugars, and protein we eat. It has many important functions, like keeping cell membranes from breaking (too much cholesterol) or getting too fluid and falling apart (too little cholesterol). Your liver makes most of the cholesterol in your blood, cranking it out when your diet is high in saturated fats (from animals) and sugars.

Cholesterol also is an important building block of sex hormones — like estrogen, progesterone, and testosterone — as well as adrenal hormones which help regulate our fluids, help us handle stress, and suppress inflammation. Without sufficient cholesterol, a younger woman couldn't conceive or even have enough of a libido to want to.

Bile, which helps break down and use fats, is another substance made from cholesterol. And bile carries excess cholesterol out of our bodies.

Women and High Cholesterol

This doesn't give women permission to eat a lot of fats and

sugars or to ignore high cholesterol completely. After all, new information is constantly being brought to our attention, and we may find in the future that high cholesterol in women brings with it a risk factor for other deteriorating health conditions. We do know that a high-fat diet is implicated in cancers of the breast and colon.

If your doctor strongly suggests you take cholesterol-lowering medication, refer him or her to the aforementioned study before taking it. All medications have side effects, and if you don't have to take one, don't. Some cholesterol-lowering drugs suppress hormone activity, including the production of sex hormones and adrenal hormones. The adrenal glands help us handle stress. And stress contributes to high cholesterol, as well. So cholesterol-lowering drugs may lower your cholesterol, but at a high cost — especially in light of these new findings about women and cholesterol!

In addition, most drugs are approved by the FDA based on very limited testing. Afterward, when a drug is being used on a broader basis by the general public, more extensive studies are conducted. Also pre- and post-approval testing frequently focuses mainly on men, with women accounting for smaller percentages of study populations. Plus, drugs are often approved and prescribed based on an effect, such as lowering cholesterol (this is called a surrogate endpoint), not the ultimate outcome, such as lowering the number of deaths among persons with high cholesterol. One doesn't necessarily lead to the other!

Before taking a cholesterol-lowering (or other) drug, ask about specific study findings for women in your age bracket with a similar health profile to confirm whether there is a good likelihood that the drug will have the effect you're looking for. If so, weigh this benefit against the known risks. To find out about risks, request a patient-package insert from your doctor or pharmacist.

Sometimes cholesterol levels run high in a family, and no matter how you eat they stay high. Is that reason to ignore your diet? Not at all. A healthy diet is the foundation on which all other therapies sit. Whether or not you are on any medications for any condition, your diet needs to be a solid, healthful foundation.

Can Cholesterol Be Too Low?

Studies have shown a correlation between low cholesterol and depression. At times, this depression has led to suicide. One study of 20 women indicated a strong connection between low cholesterol following the birth of a child and postpartum depression. This small sample is an indication of a possible association that needs to be studied further. A larger study — of more than 6,000 men — showed that when cholesterol levels dropped significantly, suicide rates increased.

What about suicide and women? When studies are completed with women, perhaps we'll know more. But the postpartum depression findings at least give us an indication of an association between low cholesterol and mood changes.

Depression has been linked to low cholesterol by lowering serotonin levels. Serotonin is a "feel good" chemical produced in the brain. Low cholesterol appears to decrease the number of sero-

---

Phytoestrogens: A Safe Alternative to Estrogen

In view of the lack of clear-cut answers about estrogen's ability to reduce heart-disease risk, a safer alternative might be to increase your consumption of foods containing phytoestrogens. These are plant estrogens, found in foods, that act similarly to estrogen in your body. There are no studies on the specific effect of phytoestrogens and heart disease. But other studies suggest that phytoestrogens do have beneficial health effects — especially on women.

According to Dr. Hermal Adlercreutz, a leading phytoestrogen researcher, phytoestrogens may reduce hot flashes and other menopausal symptoms. In other words, phytoestrogens have an effect similar to hormone replacement therapy — without the risks. Soy is the only known source of genistein, a phytoestrogen that has been shown in test tube and animal experiments to block the growth of prostate and breast cancer cells, so eating soy foods regularly may protect you against breast cancer.

In addition, Japanese men who consume lots of phytoestrogen-containing foods (like soy) have the lowest rates of heart disease in the world. The heart-disease rate of Japanese women, who also consume lots of phytoestrogens, is also exceptionally low — much lower than that of American women. Phytoestrogens are found in whole grains and legumes. Soy foods such as soy milk, tofu, and miso, are also rich source of phytoestrogens.

tonin receptors in brain cells, meaning there's no place for serotonin to attach and allow us to feel good.

Other adverse effects of low cholesterol include an increased risk of lung cancer in older women. There have been numerous studies linking low cholesterol with increased death from various cancers. A study published in *Preventive Medicine 24* was one of the few to examine low cholesterol in women. Both men and women in this study had increased deaths from lung cancer during an 18-year period. It's possible that low cholesterol was just one marker of a suppressed immune system and was not directly responsible for these deaths. Still, it indicates that cholesterol can be too low.

How low is too low? A level lower than 140 (130 for vegetarians) may indicate a suppressed immune system and should be investigated. Once a cause of immune suppression is identified and treated, cholesterol levels should rise.

Watch Your Cholesterol

It's important to periodically check your cholesterol levels. Very high and very low cholesterol appear to be predictive of various health conditions from heart disease to depression and immune suppression. But have doctors made too much fuss over cholesterol? When it comes to women, I think so. High cholesterol may not be a problem for some people, especially when those people are women. Since most studies in the past have been conducted with men, we're not surprised there's been so much noise about lowering cholesterol at any cost, using medications with side effects.

The Fibrinogen Factor

Yet another major factor for female heart disease that is often overlooked is our fibrinogen level. A number of medical studies indicate that high fibrinogen leads to heart disease. In fact, the Northwick Park heart study from Britain reported in 1994 that elevated fibrinogen levels were more strongly linked to cardiovascular deaths than elevated cholesterol levels. Other epidemiological studies have come to the same conclusion.

Fibrinogen is a protein that is part of our blood's clotting system and viscosity (its stickiness and thickness). It also stimulates the growth and movement of some of our muscle cells into the walls of the arteries, causing these arteries to become clogged. During the blood-clotting process, fibrinogen becomes a substance called fibrin. Simply put, the more fibrin or fibrinogen you have, the thicker and stickier your blood and the insides of your arteries are likely to become. And the higher your risk for heart disease.

Between 200 and 400 mg/dL of fibrinogen is considered normal. Smoking, high blood pressure, and diabetes can cause elevated fibrinogen levels. Back in 1968, however, Framingham researchers noticed that women with fibrinogen levels as low as 334 mg/dL were still more susceptible to heart failure, heart attacks, and clot-related diseases. Higher fibrinogen can also contribute to problem varicose veins, and women comprise the large majority that suffers these. Clearly, it's better to be near the midpoint or on the low end of the current normal fibrinogen range scale for females.

In some people with varicose veins, their bodies just aren't able to break down fibrin, and their arteries get lumpy with fat and fibrin. Blood moves more slowly and pools and clots more easily. But it's not just the cosmetic condition of varicose veins that concerns us, or the pain they cause. Varicose vein complications claim over 100,000 lives annually. Veins clogged with fibrin can lead to heart attacks, stroke, and deadly pulmonary embolisms.

So if you have varicose veins or simply might want to know whether you might be more susceptible to heart disease because of higher fibrinogen, have your doctor check your fibrin levels through a blood test and keep in mind the following fibrin-lowering solutions.

The Trouble With Aspirin

Most doctors recommend taking aspirin each day to thin the blood. We don't like this idea because it has side effects and because there are more natural solutions to this problem that don't have side effects.

Aspirin has been shown to reduce the blood's ability to clot. So many doctors prescribe low doses of aspirin (325 mg/day) to reduce future heart attacks in people who have already had one episode. But according to Dr. Michael T. Murray, ND, "People who have experienced a heart-attack and live through it are very likely to experience another." And a number of studies looking at nearly 15,000 heart-attack survivors using aspirin for up to five years back up Dr. Murray's statement. I was very surprised to discover that these studies have not shown that aspirin lowers the death rate from heart attacks.

How can this be? Looking closely at the results of the studies, I found that while no single study showed that aspirin was effective, when all of the studies were lumped together there were fewer deaths in the people who took aspirin than those who didn't. However, all the deaths were not from heart disease! Today some doctors are beginning to suggest their patients take even lower doses of aspirin (sometimes baby aspirin) as a preventive measure, but there have been no good studies to show that lower amounts are effective, either.

What is the harm in taking aspirin, just in case? It can have serious side effects, like internal bleeding and peptic ulcers. A study published in the *British Medical Journal* showing the effects of various doses of aspirin — from 75 mg to 300 mg/day stated, "No conventionally used prophylactic aspirin regimen seems free of the risk of peptic ulcer complications." In other words, aspirin may give you a bleeding stomach ulcer! Some people cannot tolerate aspirin because it causes stomach pain. This pain often comes from small amounts of bleeding due to the irritating effects of aspirin.

Even if you accept the idea that aspirin reduces heart attacks, or are not willing to risk giving up trying aspirin, there's more to the story: U.S. studies on aspirin and heart disease have always used buffered aspirin. A British study used plain, unbuffered aspirin and could not replicate the findings of the U.S. studies — in which magnesium was included in the buffering agent. Knowing what I know about the medical industry, I wouldn't be a bit surprised to learn down the road that it is the magnesium in buffered aspirin, and not the aspirin itself, that reduces the blood's ability to clot. So if you still choose to use aspirin as a blood thinner, at least make sure you're getting a generous daily dose of magnesium (600 to 1,000 mg/day) along with it. In addition to helping thin blood, magnesium helps control high blood pressure and irregular heartbeats (arrythmia).

Other Natural Solutions to High Fibrinogen

Garlic, fish oils, and red wine also help break down fibrin (in a process which is called fibrinolysis) and in this way thin the blood.

Garlic is so potent that this breakdown occurs within six hours of ingestion and continues for half a day. If you add quantities of garlic to your diet or better yet, take garlic capsules which have higher amounts of the substances that cause this fibrinolysis, you can thin your blood and protect your heart in other ways as well. You see, garlic also lowers blood pressure and prevents the harmful cholesterol (LDL) from oxidizing. When oils oxidize, they are spoiled and create substances called free radicals that are associated with various cancers. So taking garlic protects against both heart disease and cancer.

How much garlic should you take? If it's the fresh herb, one or two cloves a day should be sufficient. If it's in capsule or tablet form, look for one that has about 4,000 mcg of allicin, one of its more protective chemicals.

Omega-3 fatty acids found in cold-water fish oils and flaxseed oil keep platelets in the blood from joining together and becoming thick. Adding several helpings of fish (salmon and herring are highest in fatty acids) to your diet each week is safer than taking large quantities of fish oils. The reason for this is that when you ingest a lot of any oil you need to also add more antioxidants to keep the oils from spoiling (oxidizing) in your body.

If you would rather not eat more fish, or if you are a vegetarian, you can add flax seed capsules, flax seed oil, or grind the seeds and add flax seed meal to your cereal or breakfast drink. The latter is an inexpensive way to increase your daily intake of omega-3 fatty acids. If you're looking for something quick and easy to take, flax seed oil capsules can be found in health food stores.

Red wine has been in the news over the past few years as a beneficial substance in reducing heart disease. Many people choose not to drink alcohol. Drinking alcoholic beverages daily puts additional stress on the liver, the organ that is responsible for excreting the ethanol found in all alcoholic beverages. Still, if you can drink alcoholic beverages in moderation and if you enjoy it occasionally, you should know that it may be the alcohol, and not the grapes, that lowers fibrinogen levels. So other alcoholic drinks could lower fibrinogen as well.

One recent Italian study showed that three glasses of red wine or three glasses of alcohol diluted in fruit juice, both produced lower fibrinogen levels. I do not recommend three glasses of wine a day for anyone, especially for women. In fact, I am not in favor of drinking alcohol daily. More than two glasses of alcohol a day has been implicated in other diseases like breast cancer, birth defects, and low blood sugar. It may have some positive qualities, but a number of cautions as well. Still I want you to know what this study found and how much alcohol was used to get these results.

There is a nutritional supplement that has been used to break down fibrin in people with varicose veins. It's an enzyme from pineapples called bromelain. The amount of bromelain used in stud-

When Cholesterol Is Too Low

If you're a woman who smokes heavily and is 60 or older, don't feel good if your cholesterol is low. It may mean you won't get heart disease, but a study published in *Preventive Medicine 24* last year indicates you're likely to die of lung cancer. This, of course, is a risk for all heavy smokers, but it is one of the first studies on cholesterol that has included women.

The authors of the article caution us in misreading the information. They are not suggesting that low cholesterol causes deaths from lung cancer. We have seen numerous studies indicating that low cholesterol is, most likely, a sign of a suppressed immune system. Women smokers with low cholesterol may already be sick, say the authors, with lower levels of antioxidants that could be protective against all cancers.

If you're older, smoke, and have very low cholesterol (less than 140, for instance), we suggest you speak with your doctor about what this could mean, and follow through until you have a clear understanding of any possible underlying problem.

Chang, A.K., et al. "Low plasma cholesterol predicts an increased risk of lung cancer in elderly women," *Prev Med* 24, 557-562 (1995) (*Int'l Clin Nutr Rev*, July 1996).

ies has been 500 to 750 mg taken three times a day between meals. If you have high levels of fibrinogen you may want to discuss using bromelain with your doctor.

A combined program may be your best approach in reducing fibrinogen. This could consist of using high quantities of garlic or garlic extract, increasing your intake of cold-water fish or adding flax seed oil to your diet each day, and having an occasional glass of red wine. Bromelain may also be a useful nutrient to take sup-plementally, especially if you have varicose veins. Whatever you do, know that there are more answers — and safe ones — to the var-ious aspects of heart disease than you may realize.

Other Risk Factors for Women

Active and Passive Smoking

When we go back to the Framingham study of 1,200 women over an eight-year period, we find that women who used synthetic estrogen and smoked had more heart attacks than women who did not smoke. While there were no more deaths in the smoking group, there was more cardiovascular disease. In the Harvard nurses study, women who only smoked between one and four cigarettes a day had nearly two and a half times the heart-disease rate of non-smoking females. That's a big price to pay for a few cigarettes. In a Mayo Clinic study, smoking was found to be the single cause of two of every three cases of severe coronary heart disease among women between the ages of 40 and 59.

This makes a lot of sense. Cigarettes contain substances that contribute to atherosclerosis and can cause you to have less oxygen in your bloodstream and more carbon monoxide, making conditions ideal for heart problems. It also raises LDL cholesterol, injures the lining of the arteries, and encourages the blood to clot (a primary factor in coronary heart disease) by raising levels of fibrinogen, the blood clotting factor. In addition, cigarettes contain high amounts of the toxic mineral cadmium, which causes adverse changes in the heart tissue.

Partially because of the cadmium content in smoke and partially because other substances in it are harmful, passive smoke is also a risk factor for heart attacks and strokes. Although the studies available are not gender-specific relating to women, I mention this because if you are a mother who smokes you are not only placing yourself at an increased risk for heart disease, you are risking your child's health as well. Their small, tender bodies are more susceptible to environmental and other toxins than are adults. Their livers and lungs are less able to move these poisons out of their bodies.

In addition, all non-smokers, children and adults alike, seem to be more sensitive to smoke and have more serious effects from exposure to it than smokers. More than 35,000 deaths from heart disease have been attributed to second-hand smoke. If your partner smokes, ask that there be no smoking inside your home or car or near your children — ever. If you smoke, especially if you have children, find a doctor, acupuncturist, or naturopath who can help you stop.

Different studies give conflicting information on the subject of smoking and heart disease. We need more controlled studies with a focus on women to see what effect smoking has on incidents of heart disease and death from heart-related problems. There are, of course, no benefits from smoking. Weight can be controlled in other ways, and less harmful energy surges can be obtained with a cup of green tea with resulting benefits to weight, tumor reduction, and energy.

Caffeine and Your Heart

Caffeine is a stimulant. When you drink it, it excites your central nervous system and can cause restlessness, nervousness, anxiety, and insomnia. As little as two or three cups of coffee can increase your blood pressure and pulse rate. Coffee contains a chemical called theophylline, which can cause your heart to race (tachycardia). And although, once again, most studies on heart disease and caffeine have been conducted with men, caffeine intake has been associated with increased heart disease in women.

In a study recently published in the *American Journal of Epidemiology,* 850 women between the ages of 45 and 69 who drank coffee and had non-fatal heart attacks were compared with 850 non-coffee drinking women. Those who drank five or more cups of coffee a day had more heart attacks than women who drank less coffee or none at all.

High triglycerides, fats manufactured in the liver usually from a high-sugar diet, also increase heart disease. Other substances can trigger your liver's production of triglycerides, as well. A recent study published in *Nutrition Research* reports that more than 200 mg of caffeine a day also increases triglycerides in women.

How much coffee or colas does that mean? Three five-ounce cups of percolated coffee (240 mg), five cokes (228 mg), or two coffees and two cokes (251). So try to limit your coffee to one or two cups a day and make them half decaf whenever possible. And switch to caffeine-free soft drinks (or avoid them altogether).

Although many people with heart disease have high-cholesterol levels, not everyone with high cholesterol gets heart disease. Still, cholesterol may be one predictive factor. In a large study of coffee drinkers, both men and women, each cup of caffeinated coffee caused cholesterol levels to increase by two mg/dl. That means that if your cholesterol was 200, considered by medical doctors to be on the borderline of safe vs. unsafe (I think it's a bit too high for good health), and you drink five cups of coffee, black tea, and colas a day and reduce them to one, your cholesterol could drop to 192 by making that simple change. Decaffeinated coffee does not change cholesterol levels and, so far as heart disease is concerned, is preferable and safe.

Don't Be a Couch Potato!

You don't have to train for a marathon and do heavy workouts every day to guard against heart disease. You can do housework and benefit your cardiovascular system! According to the U.S. National Institutes of Health (NIH), any activity that causes you to breathe a little harder and perspire a bit will help your heart. Try doing some physical housework like sweeping the driveway or scrubbing the floors, vacuuming or carrying unused things to the garage and storing them. If you can exercise at this level for at least 10 minutes at a time, 30 minutes or more a day, every day — you're protecting your heart. This means that doing some kinds of housework will work as well as a brisk walk. On the days when you don't do housework that meets this physical criteria, find a friend and go for a walk. Or get a yoga or aerobics video tape and give yourself a small workout each day.

If you have a sedentary job like sitting most of the day at a desk, consider a 10-15 minute walk at lunch time as part of your moderate activity. Then, when you get home, you only have 15 or 20 minutes to go. You may get away by doing this small amount of exercise each day, but staying a couch potato increases your risk of heart disease.

Increased Weight

We have known for many years that extreme obesity increases the risk of heart problems, but now we're finding that just moderate increases in weight contribute to heart disease in middle-aged women. More than 100,000 women aged 30-55 were followed for 14 years. At the end of the study, it was found that 37 percent of the incidence of coronary heart disease was related to being overweight. As little as a four-pound increase in weight was associated with an increase in heart disease. Estrogen-replacement therapy, lack of exercise, a diet high in sugars and fats, and overeating, all contribute to weight gain and an increased risk for heart problems.

The Pregnancy High-Risk Factor

Pregnancies can decrease your risk of breast cancer by giving your body a rest from producing estrogen (the longer you have estrogen in you body, the greater your risk). But pregnancies can also increase your risk for heart disease — if you have enough of them. Two studies, including the Framingham Heart Study, indicated that women who had six or more pregnancies were at a slightly higher risk for coronary heart disease and cardiovascular disease. At this time, we don't know why. With so many women working and being moms, the number of women in this category is not particularly high. Still, with so few studies on women, we wanted to include this information.

Fats and Oils Can Help or Hurt You

Not all fats and oils contribute to heart disease, but some do, like the trans-fatty acids found in vegetable oils that have been hardened through a process called hydrogenation (forcing air molecules into the fat and causing it to become solid). You wouldn't think a little air thrown into a vegetable oil would make it a harmful food, but it does. What happens during the process of hydrogenation is that the naturally occurring curved molecules get straightened out. These straight molecules resemble saturated-fat molecules, which are a known risk factor for heart disease in both men and women. Saturated fats are primarily those found in animal protein — red meat, chicken, pork, lamb, etc.

When you take a look at the Nurses' Health Study, which I've referred to in the past, you see that the trans-fatty acids in margarine, Crisco, and any other solid vegetable shortenings — and foods that contain them — increase LDL cholesterol (the bad kind) and decrease HDL cholesterol (healthy cholesterol). And they seem to be strongly associated with increased heart disease. Here's what the study said: "Women who ate four or more teaspoons of margarine per day were at higher risk of CHD than women who ate margarine less than once per month ... consumption of cookies and white bread was significantly associated with higher risk of CHD." Perhaps this is because many baked goods contain tropical oils (which also contain trans-fatty acids) or margarine, and the diets of women who ate these foods may have contained a higher total amount of trans-fatty acids. Tropical oils are also often used to replace lard by many fast-food restaurants that make deep fried foods.

When buying baked goods, read the labels. What you don't want to buy are those which have the word hydrogenated on the ingredient list. Many cookies and cakes are now being made with liquid vegetable oils like safflower, canola, sunflower, and corn. These do not contain trans-fatty acids and are safer to eat.

Are You at Risk for Heart Disease?

How susceptible to heart disease are you? Knowing can save your life.

To help you assess your personal vulnerability, researchers at the Arizona Heart Institute have compiled the following test. It was designed specifically for women based on our unique disease development patterns and physiology. The test covers all those risk factors that have been proven time and again to influence women's risk in a predictable way.

Take the test, total your score, and find out your risk level at the end of the test.

Heart Test for Women

Age

❑ 50 and over..5

❑ 35 to 50 2

❑ 34 and under..0

Family History

If you have parents, brothers, or sisters who have had a heart attack, stroke, or heart bypass surgery at:

❑ Age 55 or before 5

❑ Age 56 or after..3

❑ None or don't know 0

Personal History

Have you had:

❑ A heart attack 20

❑ Angina, heart bypass surgery, angioplasty,
    stroke, or blood vessel surgery 10

❑ None of the above 0

Smoking

Current smoker: how many cigarettes per day?

    ❑ 5 or more 20

    ❑ 4 or fewer..10

If you are a smoker currently taking oral contraceptives and are:

    ❑ 35 years old and over....................................5

    ❑ Under 35 years old..2

If you are a previous smoker who quit less than two years ago: How many cigarettes did you smoke?

    ❑ 5 or more 10

    ❑ 4 or fewer..5

Blood Pressure

If you have had your blood pressure taken in the last year, was it:

    ❑ Elevated or high (either or both
       readings above 160/95 mmHg) 6

    ❑ Borderline
       (between 140/90 and 160/95 mmHg) 3

    ❑ Normal
       (below 140/90 mmHg) or don't know 0

Hormone Status

If you have undergone natural menopause, your age at its start:

    ❑ 40 or younger...2

    ❑ 41 or older 1

If you have had a total hysterectomy, your age when it was done:

    ❑ 40 or younger...3

    ❑ 41 or older 1

❑ If you are still menstruating ....-1

❑ If you take an oral estrogen supplement .....-2

Exercise

Do you engage in any aerobic activity, such as brisk walking, jogging, bicycling, or swimming for more than 20 minutes:

❑ Less than once a week 6

❑ One or two times a week 3

❑ Three or more times a week 0

Blood Fats

If you have had your cholesterol and blood fat levels checked in the last year, score your risk here:

❑ Over 240 mg/dL...6

❑ 200 to 240 mg/dL...3

❑ If your HDLs are lower than 45 1

❑ Cholesterol under 200 mg/dL 0

Or if you do not know your cholesterol and blood fat levels, use this section to score your risk: Which of the following best describes your eating pattern:

❑ **High fat:** red meat, fast foods, and/or fried foods daily; more than seven eggs per week; regular consumption of butter, whole milk, and cheese......................6

❑ **Moderate fat:** red meat, fast foods, and/or fried foods four to six times per week; four to seven eggs weekly; regular use of margarine, vegetable oils, and/or low-fat dairy products..3

❑ **Low fat:** poultry, fish, and little or no red meat, fast foods, fried foods, or saturated fats; fewer than three eggs per week; minimal margarine and vegetable oils; primarily non-fat dairy products 0

Diabetes

If you have diabetes (blood sugar level above 140 mg/dL), your age when you found out:

    ❑ 40 or before 6

    ❑ 41 or older 4

    ❑ Do not have diabetes 0

Body Mass

Calculate your body mass index with the following formula:

    Weight (lbs.): _____ x 0.45= _____ (W)

    Height (inches):_____x 0.025= _____ (H)

    W/(HxH)=your Body Mass Index (BMI)

    ❑ If your BMI is 27 or greater 2

    ❑ If your BMI is below 27 0

Now measure your waist and hips and divide your waist measurement by your hip girth to calculate your hip to waist ratio:

    (waist)_____/(hips)_____=_____

    ❑ If your waist to hip ratio is
       0.8 or greater 1

    ❑ If your ratio is 0.79 or less............................0

Stress

Are you easily angered and frustrated:

    ❑ Most of the time...6

    ❑ Some of the time 3

    ❑ Rarely..0

What Your Score Means

15 points or below: Low Risk

Congratulations! Maintain your heart healthy status by watching your weight, blood pressure, and blood fat (cholesterol and HDL) levels; get regular check-ups and don't smoke. Retake this test every year to monitor your heart-health risk profile.

16 to 32 points: Medium Risk

My experience indicates that your medium risk level warrants attention. Personal factors or lifestyle habits may be increasing your vulnerability to heart disease. I strongly recommend you schedule an appointment with your doctor for an evaluation, and take this test with you to get advice on how you can improve your heart-health status.

33 points or above: High Risk

Your potential for experiencing a heart attack or stroke is significant. You must take action NOW. If you are not already being treated for heart disease, I urgently advise that you see your doctor immediately and take this test with you. Please seek ways to reduce your risk!

Chapter 8

Female Heart Disease, Part 2: Protecting Your Heart

Following are a number of ways to prevent and reverse heart disease. Keep in mind that many prevention techniques — such as improved diet, supplementation, exercise, and lowering stress — can also help reverse heart disease.

Antioxidants in Diet and Supplementation

Before you can understand antioxidants, you need to understand what it is they destroy. That would be molecules that circulate within your body called free radicals. Free radicals damage whatever is around them — enzymes, proteins inside cells, and the fat membrane around cells that keep our DNA coding (a code that tells the cell what to do, what to become, and how to behave) intact. Free radicals are constantly bombarding our cells. In fact, it is thought that each cell in our body gets attacked by free radicals 10,000 times each second! Obviously, your body has ways of protecting you against free radicals.

One of its protective devices is the use of antioxidants. They seek out and destroy free radicals. But once an antioxidant has destroyed a free radical it becomes inactive. So we need lots more antioxidants than free radicals.

Free radicals are produced in a number of ways. All cells in our body use oxygen, and when they do, they create free radicals. These damaging molecules are also created by cells involved in the process of detoxification. When your immune system is called upon to destroy viruses, bacteria, and parasites, it makes more white blood cells, which, in turn, manufacture free radicals to kill the foreign invaders. Finally, free radicals enter your body through environmental pollutants, medications, a poor diet, and even ultraviolet light. So the idea is to cut down on your production of free radicals by improving your diet (fresh fruits and vegetables naturally contain antioxidants, for example), eating as much organic food as possible, and breathing clean air (or at least not driving when traffic is heaviest on hot, smoggy days!).

We are at a disadvantage once again in the area of antioxidants since most studies have been done on men or do not differentiate between responses in each gender. So while we have seen many scientific studies that link antioxidants to protection against heart disease, I'd like to focus on those that specifically mention their effectiveness with women. You might still want to take other antioxidants that have not been studied as much.

Women, Heart Disease, and Antioxidants

There was one interesting 14-year-long study published in the *American Journal of Epidemiology* that indicated that women did benefit from high intakes of vitamin E, vitamin C, and carotenoids (the best known one of these is beta carotene, but the family of carotenoids includes others, as well). What is of great interest to all women is that all of these antioxidants were not only beneficial in reducing the risk of death from heart disease in men and women, but women had almost twice the protection as men. Perhaps this study infers that antioxidants in diet and supplementation is especially important for women. Fruits and vegetables contain the highest amount of these nutrients and may also contain additional protective factors (such as phytochemicals) that were not studied. The whole food, I believe, is always better than any pill, although a combined approach may be worth considering.

Looking back again on the Nurses' Health Study, I find that the women who took high amounts of vitamin E (100 IU or more) and multivitamin supplements had less major coronary heart disease than women who had a low intake of this vitamin. Long-term use of vitamin E seems to have a protective effect on atherosclerosis by reducing the LDL cholesterol (the sticky kind). The multivitamins also contained other antioxidants like vitamins A and C. If you are going to add vitamin E to your diet, I suggest you use a dry form of d-alpha tocopherol. Dry or water-soluble vitamin E is better absorbed than the oil-based variety, and d-alpha is better utilized than less-expensive mixed tocopherols or the synthetic dl-alpha tocopherol.

The Magic of Magnesium

Your doctor may be telling you to take more calcium, but studies indicate that the mineral to take more of is magnesium. Without enough magnesium, the calcium you take will not be absorbed. This doesn't mean it's harmless, either. Unabsorbed calcium that is not excreted (and most isn't) gets into the joints where it becomes arthritis or in arteries where it becomes atherosclerosis. According to a review of magnesium done back in the 1970s, taking more magnesium can prevent your blood vessels from calcifying and developing into atherosclerosis.

But it's not just hardening of the arteries that magnesium (through its natural chelating action) helps prevent. A deficiency of this mineral is also associated with a higher risk for heart attacks, cardiac arrhythmias (rapid heartbeat), hypertension, and unexpected cardiac death.

According to Dr. Alan Gaby, most of the people he sees in his practice have low levels of magnesium. A government survey shows the average American diet provides about 40 percent of the magnesium we need each day — based on the low RDA levels. Approximately 75 percent of U.S. females are magnesium deficient. And most doctors still don't check magnesium levels in sick or dying patients in hospitals who are showing signs of magnesium deficiency (cardiac arrhythmia, muscle spasms, depression, and hypertension). Dr. Jean Durlach, president of the International Society for the Development of Magnesium Research, found that throughout the world, higher amounts of magnesium in drinking water correlated with lower death rates from heart disease.

It's not easy to know if you are low in magnesium. Most blood tests are inaccurate. Red-blood-cell magnesium levels are better to check than the regular serum magnesium, according to Dr. Guy Abraham, a pioneer in the area of magnesium, PMS, and osteoporosis-reversal. If you prefer, you can just begin taking extra magnesium — up to 1,000 mg/day. Side effects from taking too much are loose stools. You can take the amount that will cause your stools to be loose without being runny. And you may be protecting yourself against heart disease as well as osteoporosis, stress, and other conditions.

That's magnesium in general. What about magnesium, women, and heart disease? As usual, few studies are on women only, but in a study of about 100 menopausal women with mild or moderate hypertension, none of whom were taking medication, the blood pressures of those who took oral magnesium for six months dropped significantly over those who did not take magnesium. High blood pressure leads to stroke. Other studies are not gender-specific, but indicate the broad necessity of including magnesium into the dietary and supplemental programs of all people at risk for heart disease.

Mildred Seelig, MD, a professor of nutrition at the University of North Carolina, is considered by many to be the world's authority on magnesium. She strongly suggests that magnesium be given intravenously as soon as a person has a heart attack. In the ambulance, if possible. The bottom line is don't wait until you're magnesium-deficient. Begin by increasing magnesium in your diet (whole grains and beans of all kinds are high in this mineral) and make sure any vitamin supplement you take has at least as much magnesium as calcium — and more magnesium if your bowels can take a bit more.

Green Tea and Heart Disease

Apparently, all caffeine isn't terrible for you. Green tea, which contains antioxidants that have been shown to protect us against some forms of cancer, also helps decrease total cholesterol, the harmful LDL cholesterol, and triglycerides. It also appears to increase the beneficial HDL (or healthy) cholesterol. If you like it, you might want to incorporate two or three cups of green tea into your daily program. Because of all the current research on the benefits of green tea, this beverage is now available in supermarkets, health food stores, and Asian markets.

Heart-Disease-Fighting Herbs

Herbal remedies for high blood pressure, a risk factor for heart disease, include garlic, hawthorn, Coleus forskohlii, and khella.

For angina, Michael T. Murry, ND and author of *The Healing Power of Herbs,* recommends hawthorn in the doses listed below for the various forms, taken three times daily:

✔ hawthorn berries or flowers (dried): 3 to 5 grams or as an infusion

✔ hawthorn tincture (1:5): 4 to 5 milliliters (alcohol may elicit pressor response in some individuals)

✔ hawthorn fluid extract (1:1): 1 to 2 milliliters

✔ hawthorn freeze-dried berries: 1 to 1.5 grams

✔ hawthorn flower extract (standardized to contain 1.8 percent vitexin-4'-rhamnoside or 20 percent procyanidins): 100 to 250 mg

For angina, Dr. Murray also recommends:

✔ carnitine: 300 mg, three times daily

✔ coenzyme Q10: 150 mg, one or two times daily

✔ magnesium (citrate, aspartate, or Krebs cycle chelate): 250 to 400 mg, three times daily

When treating a condition as serious as angina or heart disease with alternative and/or complimentary medicine, it's always a good idea to work closely with a naturopathic doctor or other health care professional who is knowledgeable about alternative treatments and can track your progress with the appropriate tests.

The Protect-Your-Heart Diet

Your best diet for preventing heart disease is one low in saturated fats found in animal protein. Monounsaturated and polyunsaturated fatty acids, found in vegetable oils, reduce your risk for heart disease. Still, all your fats should be low. Keep them below 30 percent, ideally around 20 percent, even if current fad diets tell you to eat more fats. More than 30 percent will not help prevent heart disease. But don't eat a very low-fat diet or a fat-free diet, because while they will lower you harmful LDLs, they'll also lower your helpful HDLs. And low HDL levels put women at a higher risk for heart disease. In addition:

✔ High fiber is a necessity, and you can get enough if you eat plenty of whole grains, beans, and vegetables. Constipation is frequently a sign you do not. Aim to eat enough fiber to have one bowel movement daily. (This will also significantly lower your risk of colon cancer.)

✔ Vegetable protein is more protective than animal protein. Tofu, lentils, and beans of all kinds turn into a complete protein when you eat them the same day as grains. You need not eat both at the same meal.

✔ The best animal protein for heart protection is cold-water fish that have high amounts of omega-3 fatty acids, which help your fat metabolism. However, cold-water fish, like salmon, which are farmed and not fed their usual diet of sea vegetation, are not high in these protective fatty acids. Make sure the fish you eat come from the ocean. When in doubt, ask.

✔ Keep your refined-sugar consumption low. In some people, it promotes atherosclerosis. In others, it raises cholesterol while lowering HDL. If you limit refined sugar to 10 percent of your caloric intake, you can still enjoy an occasional dessert, cookie, or muffin and have a healthy heart.

✔ Include raw nuts or seeds in your diet as well. One study of Seventh Day Adventists found that those who ate a handful of nuts a few times a week had significantly less heart disease. Nuts contain omega-6 fatty acids, and walnuts are one of the richest sources. Omega-6 and omega-3 are called essential fatty acids. Your body must have them for optimum performance. Yet it can't manufacture them — they must come from an outside source.

✔ Keep caffeine low and drink green tea instead of coffee when you can.

✔ If you can handle just a little alcohol and want to include it in your diet, limit yourself to one glass of red wine a day. If you have any liver disease, past or present, don't drink daily. Carefully weigh the data and make your choice a wise one. You can reduce stress by meditating, exercising, and getting antioxidants into your body in other ways. Daily alcohol may prove in time to not be as safe as it appears to be today. Caution is advised here.

Protective Supplements

Numerous vitamins, minerals, and fatty acids appear to be helpful in preventing heart disease, so take a good multivitamin/ mineral with equal amounts of calcium to magnesium, or a greater amount of magnesium. Folic acid is now in the news in relation to heart disease, but deficiencies of vitamin B_6 and B_{12}, chromium, copper, selenium, and others are also linked to heart disease. Don't wait for new studies to be published. A good multi is good, inexpensive insurance.

Do not be misled by the one-a-day type vitamins that provide 100 percent of various Recommended Daily Allowances. This is barely enough to prevent serious nutritional deficiency diseases such as scurvy. Your best bet is the newer mega multivitamin/mineral formulas that have a daily dose of six capsules, taken at three intervals throughout the day for best absorption. One brand I like is Vitality by Women's Preferred, which can be ordered by calling 1-800-728-2288.

Add magnesium to bowel tolerance. After you have modified your diet to include more whole grains and beans, after you have taken a good multivitamin/mineral for a month or so, increase your magnesium to an amount that gives you comfortable bowel movements. As you protect yourself from heart disease with magnesium you will be eliminating constipation and the resulting illnesses it often brings.

De-Stress

In the '60s and '70s, researchers expected heart-disease rates to climb among women as they began climbing corporate ladders. That didn't happen. The explanation for this surprise is that the increased personal satisfaction and higher levels of self-esteem that come with professional success appear to mitigate female stress.

Feelings of frustration and powerlessness among pink-collar workers, on the other hand, has been identified as a cause of higher heart-disease rates. In fact, female pink-collar workers suffer three times the heart disease rate of female white-collar workers. A study of the Cynomolgus Macaque monkey provided a biological explanation for this phenomenon. Researchers found that lower social status suppressed estrogen among this species, robbing them of the hormonal protection against heart disease that was enjoyed by the higher-status dominant female monkeys. Just last year the *Journal of the American Medical Association* published the results of a Duke University five-year study that concluded mental stress is more dangerous to the heart than physical stress.

If you find yourself frequently feeling frustrated, anxious, tense, edgy, restless, overwhelmed, or powerless, these feelings of stress may be increasing your heart-disease risk. You may be able to lower heart-disease risk, however, with stress reduction techniques. The ultimate stress-reduction technique may be meditation. In 1978, researcher and physiologist R. Keith Wallace of the University of California at Los Angeles discovered that a group of meditation practitioners experienced 80 percent less heart disease (and over 50 percent less cancer) than those in a control group.

The simplest way to meditate is to find a quiet place to sit comfortably, close your eyes, and direct your attention to your breathing. Repeat one word, such as "calm" slowly and continually. As thoughts come into your mind, let them go. Do this 15 minutes or longer. The goal is to be still, physically and mentally, until you feel extremely relaxed and peaceful. After stopping, try to keep the relaxed feeling with you. Some people find it helpful initially to receive more formal meditation instruction. Numerous meditation groups across the country offer this. Or pick up a copy of *How To*

Meditate by Lawrence Leshan. All forms of meditation work, even when you aren't sure initially whether it's working.

Five More Ways to Overcome Mental Stress

The following list of ways to reduce mental stress is not comprehensive. You may have some lesser-known favorites of your own, such as listening to music, relaxation tapes, or just getting away by yourself for a while. For best results, use the combination of techniques that works best for you:

Laughter. Have you ever laughed so hard you nearly fell out of your chair? And what about the ultra-relaxed feeling you had afterward? Whether we realize it or not, laughter is a powerful stress-relief tool. This probably explains in large part why prime-time TV is dominated by sit-coms — they help us unwind and de-stress. Other tools for regular laughter include funny movies, books, and taking a humorous approach whenever possible. Medical research has confirmed the healing power of laughter and includes many reports of persons actually healing themselves with intensive laughter therapy.

Fun and Games. A Swedish study found that persons who regularly attended cultural activities — movies, concerts, plays, artistic events, and even sporting events — were half as likely to die as persons in a control group who didn't. The lead researcher of this 12,000-person study even speculated that such activities have a stronger influence on longevity than income, physical activity, and even smoking by eliciting strong positive and healing emotions that, like simple laughter, boost the immune system's ability to fight stress.

Togetherness. Sexual arousal and orgasm, and just being with others also boost stress resistance. Numerous studies show that persons with the strongest ties to family, friends, church, and other community groups enjoy significantly greater longevity. Strained, unpleasant, and abusive relations with others, however, create stress.

A Positive, Proactive Approach. If you're prone to negativity, a little mindfulness can go a long way in helping you overcome it, and the dysfunctionality and illness it breeds. The reward? Your stress resistance, effectiveness as an individual, and enjoyment of life will soar. If your friends and family aren't enough, get professional help to overcome excessive negativity or fatalism.

Change Your Life

Protecting yourself against illness always changes your life. If you haven't already, be sure to include regular exercise — aerobic, five times a week when possible — and stress-reduction techniques into your life. If you don't have time for exercise or 10 minutes of relaxation exercises or meditation a day, how will you find time to recover from heart disease? Do you have time to spend sitting in doctors' offices waiting for appointments, tests, and prescriptions for medication?

Begin slowly. Start today by exercising for 10 minutes. Tomorrow, meditate or play a tape with a guided meditation or relaxation technique on it. Do this for 10 minutes. Each day, do one or the other for 10 minutes. At the end of a week or two, increase to 15 minutes. When you are up to 20 minutes a day, do 10 minutes of exercise and 10 of meditation. Eventually, get your exercise up to 20-30 minutes five times a week. Walks with friends count. So does housework and gardening. Get active. Make your heart work a little harder at times. And open it up more with meditation, relaxation exercises, and prayer.

To Drink or Not to Drink? That Is the Question

People who want to drink argue that the French, who drink wine daily, have a low incidence of heart disease. This is true. They also have a high mortality from alcohol-related liver disease. The amount of alcohol consumed seems to be the most predictive factor for prevention of heart disease vs. other harmful effects. Japanese men, however, are proof that red wine consumption is not a must for heart disease prevention. They have a lower incidence of heart disease than French men, yet drink little, if any wine. (They do drink lots of green tea, and eat a lot of fish and tofu, as recommended earlier.)

If you drink wine, look at other toxic substances you're ingesting in addition to alcohol. It takes the liver about three days to remove the ethanol from a glass of wine. A primary function of your liver is to remove harmful substances. If alcohol is one of many, drinking daily may cause you more problems than it solves. If your diet is clean (without a lot of additives, preservatives, pesticides, etc.) one or two glasses of wine a day could help you guard against heart disease.

What kind of wine is best? Again, we're not completely certain, but preliminary data suggests that red wine is more protective than white wine. Red wine seems to contain more flavonoids, naturally occurring antioxidants that protect against LDL cholesterol. Some studies have indicated that red wine contains antioxidants, while white wine contains pro-oxidants. But a very recent study indicates that if white wine comes in contact with grape skins while it's being made, it contains more antioxidants. To be safe, stick with one glass of red wine a day.

Or take vitamin C! One gram (1,000 mg) of vitamin C has a 22 percent antioxidant status at the end of one hour and 29 percent at the end of two hours. Red wine contains 18 percent and 11 percent, respectively; while white wine has only four percent and 11 percent of an antioxidant action.

In the area of alcohol and its protective effects on heart disease, we must remember that many people cannot drink just one or two glasses of alcohol. People with a genetic predisposition to alcoholism, or people who cannot control their intake for emotional or other reasons, should not even consider drinking a glass of wine as a preventive measure.

Not surprisingly, there is little data on women, alcohol, and heart disease. Most studies have been conducted on men. It is thought that the protective effect of alcohol appears to be that it raises levels of the protective HDL cholesterol (and women tend to have higher levels of HDL than men). In addition, women's livers are more sensitive to the effects of alcohol than are men's.

One study of over 120,000 nurses, conducted over a 10-year period of time, gives us at least a beginning look at this subject. It showed that women over the age of 50 who have one glass of wine or beer a day have fewer heart attacks and less heart disease than non-drinkers. They did, however, seem to have a higher risk for brain hemorrhages, which might be associated with both drinking alcohol and smoking. We just don't know at this point.

Still, the idea of having one glass of wine a day is appealing to some women. It may be causing beneficial results for two reasons: the antioxidants in the wine and the relaxation that having a drink at the end of a stressful day may produce. In both cases, options other than alcohol exists for women who do not drink alcohol.

Homocysteine and Your Heart: The Missing Link

At one time, not so long ago, we heard about the connection between high cholesterol levels and heart disease. Then cholesterol was broken down for us into HDL (healthy) and LDL (lousy). The ratio of the healthy, slick cholesterol to the unhealthy, sticky stuff was, we were told, a predictor of heart disease.

Next came the role of hormone replacement therapy (HRT), which kept calcium deposits on arterial walls at bay. Nutritional studies later showed, however, that this calcium build-up was due to unabsorbed calcium, and that magnesium, the mineral that helps with calcium absorption was an effective blocker of these deposits and also helped keep the heart muscle relaxed.

Then we heard about fibrinogen, a protein that is part of our blood's clotting system and viscosity (its stickiness and thickness). It stimulates the growth and movement of some of our muscle cells into the walls of the arteries, causing these arteries to become clogged. During blood-clotting, fibrinogen turns into fibrin. The more fibrin or fibrinogen you have, the thicker and stickier the insides of your arteries are likely to become. And the higher your risk for heart disease.

It seemed that we had to watch our cholesterol and boost the HDL with a low-fat diet and regular exercise, and either take HRT after menopause or increase our magnesium intake in diet and supplements. Then add a few nutrients like omega-3 fatty acids and a glass or two of red wine to lower fibrinogen levels. Now we hear there's more: homocysteine levels need to be factored into the equation. With all the aspects that need to be addressed to keep our heart healthy, no wonder there's so much heart disease!

As much as you may not want to hear one more thing to take into consideration concerning your heart, heart disease is still the biggest killer of postmenopausal women. And until the numbers drop, we must look at all aspects of preventing this deadly disease. Besides, we have more information, so let's use it to our advantage and put all the parts of the puzzle together.

Homocysteine: What Is It?

Homocysteine is one of the sulfur-containing amino acids, a chemical component of protein. It is closely related, chemically, to methionine, another sulfur amino acid known for its antioxidant properties. With the help of other nutrients, homocysteine is made from the breakdown of methionine, which is found in meats, legumes, soy, fish and eggs, as well as garlic, onions, corn, rice, and other grains. With the help of such nutrients as betaine, vitamins B_6 and B_{12}, and folic acid, homocysteine is then converted into other chemicals and then either turned back into methionine or excreted.

High amounts of homocysteine damage cell membranes, make collagen unstable, and lead to the formation of atherosclerotic plaques. End result: heart disease. Methionine helps prevent cholesterol deposits in the arteries.

One of the earliest researchers in the link between high homocysteine levels and heart disease is Kilmer S. McCully, MD, author of *The Homocysteine Revolution* (Keats Publishing, 1997). His book offers an extensive explanation of this formerly obscure amino acid and its effects on heart disease, aging, and hormone levels in both men and women. If you're looking for a more thorough explanation, you'll want to read this book.

How Do We Get Too Much Homocysteine?

Dr. McCully explains that aging is a factor in high homocysteine levels. For one, as we age our diets contain less of the vitamins

B_6, B_{12}, and folic acid needed to convert harmful homocysteine into helpful methionine. Studies have shown that elderly people in the Framingham (Mass.) Heart Study had lowered consumption and blood levels of these nutrients. I'm not surprised. Try going to New England and finding lots of vegetables in restaurants. They're not there. Green leafy vegetables are the primary source of folic acid (the name comes from "folate," or leaves). What would a study of elderly people in Southern California show? Or a study of vegetarians who eat plenty of fresh produce?

Folic acid has been found in some studies to be the nutrient deficiency most associated with high homocysteine levels. In a European study, normally healthy people with elevated homocysteine who took one mg/day of folic acid responded with lowered homocysteine during the first five days of treatment.

Vitamin B_{12} is often low in older people, because it needs a substance called "intrinsic factor," which comes from gastric juices, to be absorbed. Intrinsic factor is made in the large intestines. Intestinal bacteria also affect the amount of intrinsic factor. If you have digestive problems or not enough friendly bacteria like acidophilus and bifido, you may not be producing enough intrinsic factor to have sufficient vitamin B_{12}.

Other Risk Factors

While men usually have higher levels of homocysteine than women, as we age, our homocysteine levels rise. This means that postmenopausal women usually have more homocysteine than premenopausal women.

Genetic factors can cause high homocysteine in people of any age. Barring this inborn genetic error, smoking cigarettes combined with drinking eight cups of coffee or more a day, raises your levels. So will just drinking this amount of coffee without smoking. What about tea? Remember, folate is an important nutrient in lowering homocysteine, and folate comes from leaves. So does tea. Authors of a Norwegian study found that all caffeinated coffee contributed to elevated homocysteine, while caffeinated tea did not.

Helpful Foods

As complex as all this may seem, it's really not. I've been telling you for years to drink a couple of cups of green tea daily, increase your intake of soy (high in methionine), and to eat plenty of fresh green leafy vegetables. I've been telling you that smoking is more harmful than just affecting your lungs, and that too much coffee is not good for you. I've also stressed the importance of having enough friendly bacteria in your intestines. This is what it takes to lower homocysteine levels.

How to Test for Homocysteine

Many laboratories are now performing blood tests that show whether or not your homocysteine level is high. This test must be done after you have fasted for about 12 hours (nothing but water from 9:00 p.m. until you have your blood drawn in the morning). If you have a clear-cut high homocysteine level, this test will be accurate. If you don't, and many people do not, a more reliable test is called a methionine-loading test. You take 100 mg/kg of methionine and have your blood drawn six hours later to test for homocysteine levels. Speak with your doctor about either of these tests.

More on Homocysteine

In the past five years, more than 1,000 articles on homocysteine have been published in scientific journals. Elevated homocysteine has been implicated in neural tube defects, rheumatoid arthritis, diabetes, and is suspected to be connected to osteoporosis. Later, I'll explore these connections and give you some specific foods to add to your diet that are especially high in folic acid — thought to be the key nutrient needed to regulate homocysteine.

Why Women Need Low Homocysteine Levels

You've now seen that when the amino acid homocysteine is high, cell damage occurs and plaque builds up in the arteries of the heart, leading to atherosclerosis. But there are more reasons for wanting your homocysteine levels to be low, especially since you're a woman. High levels have been implicated in neural tube defects, osteoporosis, diabetes, and rheumatoid arthritis — conditions which, when added together, affect just about all women.

Homocysteine and pregnancy: Folic acid supplementation is now being touted as the nutrient that will prevent both neural tube defects and miscarriages. Research currently in progress in the Netherlands suggests that a defect in the metabolism of methionine and homocysteine may be both the cause of these problems and the reason folic acid corrects them.

Homocysteine and bone loss: The connection between high homocysteine and osteoporosis is less well-defined. A number of authors of scientific studies have suggested that because children with genetically high homocysteine commonly have osteoporosis, the same pathway that causes this condition in children may well contribute to bone loss in adults. At present it is only a theory, but one based on sound scientific principles. Until there are further studies we won't know for certain. But this connection may explain the reason for more osteoporosis in women whose homocysteine levels rise after menopause. Until we have more information, the wise approach would be to keep your homocysteine levels low, especially after menopause.

Homocysteine and diabetes: In the case of diabetes, homocysteine metabolism seems to be impaired in people with non-insulin-dependent diabetes mellitus (NIDDM) — as opposed to those with type I diabetes. This can lead to diabetic retinopathy, since elevated homocysteine is also a risk factor for this eye condition. Remember, high homocysteine causes cell damage, and injured cells within small vessels like the eyes appear to lead to retinopathy, as well as heart disease.

Homocysteine and arthritis: Rheumatoid arthritis patients also tend to have high homocysteine levels. When a number of them were given an arthritis medication that assists the conversion of homocysteine to methionine, their homocysteine levels dropped and their pain was reduced. Again, it's too early to do more than postulate, but for those of us who don't have the time to wait for research on these diseases, it is clear that there are numerous benefits in lowering homocysteine levels, especially as we grow older.

Nutrients You Need to Lower Homocysteine

Folic acid may be the most important nutrient to keep your homocysteine levels lower. Folic acid is most abundant in legumes (beans) and green leafy vegetables, and few people eat them daily. A salad plus a serving of broccoli, spinach, or chard is an easy way to get plenty of greens. The way you cook vegetables can also either reduce or retain folic acid. When you stir fry, you seal in a number of nutrients and retain more folic acid. Aim for a total folic acid intake of 400 to 800 mcg/day. For information on the amount of folic acid and other nutrients in various foods, look up the foods you eat in the *Nutrition Almanac* (John D. Kirschman, McGraw-Hill), an excellent reference book found in most bookstores and many health food stores.

While your diet could contain sufficient folic acid, some drugs block its absorption. These drugs include oral contraceptives, alcohol, nicotine, anticonvulsants, antibacterials, and some chemotherapy agents. If you are on medications, check with your doctor, pharmacist, or the *Physician's Desk Reference* to see if the medication you are taking or have taken blocks folic acid metabolism.

Alcoholics tend to have twice as much homocysteine as nondrinkers. And what you drink seems to influence your levels, as well. People who drink wine and hard liquor tend to have higher homocysteine than people who drink beer. However, all alcoholics have low folate levels, which could be the reason their homocysteine is high. If you drink regularly, keep your vegetable intake high and supplement your diet with a multivitamin.

Vitamin B_6 also helps lower homocysteine, according to the Framingham Heart Study, the lengthiest evaluation of heart problems and nutrients ever conducted. In this study, low folic acid and vitamin B_6 correlated with high homocysteine in people who had heart attacks. Vitamin B_6 is found in meats and whole grains, but the amount in food may not be enough to lower your homocysteine. Consider taking a multivitamin with 25-50 mg of B_6.

Vitamin B_{12} is also needed to keep homocysteine low, and this vitamin is lacking in a vegetarian diet. However, many vegetarians have sufficient B_{12} due to a healthy digestive system. The amount of B_{12} found in most multivitamins is sufficient to meet your daily needs of 5-8 mcg a day. In fact, one cup of black tea contains 9 mcg.

The primary problem with vitamin B_{12} is that it is absorbed in the large intestines. If you have digestive problems, including a lot of gas, you may not be absorbing this important nutrient, since a chemical called "intrinsic factor," manufactured in the large intestines, is needed for vitamin B_{12} absorption. This means you need to pay attention to your digestion as part of a homocysteine-lowering program. To correct digestive problems, begin by chewing your food well. Next, consider taking enzymes and/or hydrochloric acid. Check with your health-care practitioner about these supplements before taking them.

Check It Out!

You can have your homocysteine levels tested through a simple laboratory blood test. Talk to your doctor about this, and take the necessary dietary precautions for reducing homocysteine if yours is

---

Triglycerides and Heart Disease

Because heart disease is the number one killer for postmenopausal women, I think you'll be interested in knowing that two recent studies showed that women whose triglyceride levels were over 100 mg/deciliter had twice as many heart attacks as women whose levels were under 100. The higher the triglycerides, the greater the risk for heart attacks. Why? Because when levels exceed 190, the blood gets thicker, and less oxygen and other nutrients get into the heart muscle.

Fish, which contain a helpful fat called omega-3 fatty acids, may help reduce your triglycerides. But limiting alcohol and foods high in sugar is probably going to get you the fastest results. When we eat too much sugar, some of the excess is stored as triglycerides. Lower your sugar intake and triglycerides usually go down pretty quickly. If this approach doesn't work well enough for you, see your doctor for additional information.

"Studies lower ideal triglyceride levels," *New York Times,* November 12, 1996.

high. These dietary changes will contribute more to your health than simply lowering homocysteine. Bottom line: If your homocysteine level is high, you're not eating properly, or your lifestyle needs to be adjusted a bit.

What About Hypertension?

I'm constantly surprised to find that most of my female patients are more concerned about osteoporosis than high blood pressure and heart disease. They simply don't realize that heart disease is the leading cause of death for postmenopausal women in this country. Since 1984, deaths among women from heart disease have exceeded those in men. Sixty percent of Caucasian women, and 79 percent of African-American women over the age of 45, have high blood pressure.

Some women believe that hormone replacement therapy reduces the risk for heart disease. They are hoping a quick fix will work equally as well as changing lifelong habits. This is wishful thinking. Now we're finding out that hormone therapy may not be preventing heart disease. We just don't know for certain yet. What we do know is that if you're going to have to make changes either to prevent hypertension or to control it, you might as well prevent it. And as you'd suspect, it's much easier to prevent one of its risk factors —hypertension — than to control it. Although you just can't escape the fact that you're going to have to make some important lifestyle changes in any case. So the question is, what do you have to do and where should you start?

Understanding Blood Pressure

Let's begin by understanding just what high blood pressure, or hypertension, means. As you know, your heart pumps blood through your blood vessels and into your tissues. The force of this blood pressing against the walls of your arteries is known as blood pressure. The two numbers used to analyze your blood pressure are called "systolic" (the first number) and "diastolic" (the second number). Systolic blood pressure measures the force used by your heart to circulate through your blood vessels. Diastolic blood pressure measures the resistance to that force. The combination indicates how hard your heart has to work to circulate your blood.

If you have high blood pressure, it means that your heart is working harder than it should and your blood vessels may eventually become weaker. Then you're at an increased risk for cardiovascular disease, stroke, an aneurysm, congestive heart failure, kidney failure, and peripheral vascular diseases including phlebitis.

Your Weight Matters

Obesity is a risk factor for hypertension, as well as one of a number of conditions that it may lead to heart disease, congestive heart failure, and stroke. I've counseled many obese women during the 22 years I've been in practice as a nutritionist, and I know how difficult it is to lose weight. But even a 5 to 10 percent weight loss can reduce blood pressure if it's high. It can also reduce hypertension by 20%-50% if your blood pressure isn't very high.

Here's what I've found works best:

Surprise! Nuts Are Good for You

A 14-year study of over 84,000 women aged 34-59 explored the relationship between eating nuts and getting heart disease. Those women who ate nuts five times or more every week had a significantly lowered amount of coronary heart disease (CHD) as well as fatal and non-fatal heart attacks.

Nuts contain essential fatty acids (EFAs), the beneficial fats that support your immune system and help you burn fat faster. That's right, eating nuts in moderation won't cause you to gain weight. It could even help you lose it!

All nuts should be bought fresh. This means, buy them from a store that sells a lot of them. Store them in your freezer or refrigerator, and don't eat them if they're more than three months old. Their oils could be rancid.

Chew nuts very well. This fatty food needs all the help it can get from your digestive system. Keep the amount low, like adding four to five walnuts or almonds to your breakfast cereal, salads, or smoothies.

Hu, F.B., et al. "Frequent nut consumption and risk of coronary heart disease in women," *American Journal of Epidemiology* (SER Abstracts), vol 147, no 11, 1998.

A positive, determined attitude (not so easy, but it really does help). You need to decide you will find a way to lose weight and keep it off, and you won't stop until you do, no matter how discouraged you may become at any moment.

Address your emotional and physiological cravings. Find other ways to reward yourself, such as putting off unpleasant tasks or feeding an emotional void. Use emotional answers to emotional problems. Food is only a temporary fix.

Control your portions. Learn the difference between feeling stuffed and eating until you are no longer hungry. Reduce your portions and wait 15 minutes before taking seconds. If you're not hungry after eating less, stop.

Change your diet. Eat more dense foods that turn to sugar slowly, like beans. For a few months, concentrate on eating some protein (including beans and tofu) with each meal and lots of vegetables. Drink water throughout the day.

Exercise more. Even if you don't lose any weight, half an hour of mild to moderate aerobic exercise done for three to six days a week can lower your blood pressure. A brisk walk is enough. When the weather is bad, try walking through a local shopping mall. Do your half-hour walk first, and then take time for any shopping or window-shopping.

Watch your alcohol intake. Limit your alcohol consumption to 5 oz of wine, 12 oz of beer, or 1 oz of hard liquor a day. If you're overweight, consider drinking even less. These are empty calories. Instead, if you must drink, have a smaller drink or limit yourself to one drink a day on weekends only. Of all alcohol, red wine still comes up as being most beneficial in protecting against heart disease because of the antioxidants it contains. But if you don't drink, don't start.

Watch Your Minerals

Sodium: Some studies have shown that a low sodium diet can actually prevent hypertension. When you reduce your sodium intake to 2.5 grams/day (2,500 mg) or less, you are reducing your risk for hypertension — especially if you're over 60. Even a small reduction in salt can decrease blood pressure in people whose blood pressure is normal. Remember that canned vegetables, soy sauce, and MSG are all sources of high sodium. Some foods with a lot of sodium include most cheeses (Think about it. Cheese is made from milk, and milk isn't at all salty!), chips, and canned soups.

Potassium: Supplemental potassium may be helpful in preventing and reducing high blood pressure, but only take them if your health practitioner advises it. You want a diet higher in potassium than sodium, and many people eat the reverse. Potatoes, sweet potatoes, beet greens, and avocados are all high in potassium. Most fruits and vegetables contain potassium. Eat fresh vegetables twice a day and fruit at least once a day, to give you enough potassium with very little sodium.

Calcium: Calcium's role in preventing hypertension is uncertain. Some people with hypertension improve with calcium, but not all. Observational studies on calcium and hypertension that claim calcium supports lower blood pressure didn't measure sodium levels. The better-designed studies don't suggest that it is particularly beneficial. So don't increase calcium to help your blood pressure. One serving of dairy a day is the most you want. Calcium is also found in many dark green leafy vegetables and tofu.

Magnesium: In their book, *Encyclopedia of Natural Medicine,* naturopaths Murray and Pizzorno cite numerous studies that indicate a high magnesium intake is associated with lower blood pressure. This may be because magnesium activates a cellular membrane pump that pumps out sodium from the cells as it pumps potassium into them. Your diet, and supplements, should be high in magnesium. Take magnesium to bowel tolerance (too much causes loose stools), and eat high-magnesium foods like nuts, seeds, legumes, and whole grains.

Vitamin C: In the July 2000 issue of *Hypertension: Journal of the American Heart Association* (vol 36), a study was published indicating that vitamins C and E were able to reduce high blood pressure in rats. The theory was that these antioxidants might protect nitric oxide in the body. Nitric oxide is a molecule that relaxes blood vessels, making them more pliable. The scientists who conducted this study caused oxidative stress in the rats and their nitric oxide levels decreased as their blood pressure rose. When vitamins C and E were added to their diets, their blood pressure dropped to normal.

A diet high in whole foods with plenty of fresh fruits and vegetables, along with a good multivitamin/mineral, will give you enough vitamins C and E. But don't depend only on supplements. Since vitamin C is found in fruits and vegetables that also contain plenty of potassium, begin by eating more of them.

Won't Hormone Replacement Help?

Don't count on hormones to reduce your risk for heart disease. The Postmenopausal Estrogen/Progestin Intervention Trial took a close look at how hormones affect the risk for cardiac diseases. There was *no significant improvement* in women on hormones over those on placebos. Other trials are incomplete, and we'll have to wait and see, but so far it looks like hormones are not the "silver bullet" many people had hoped they'd be.

Pregnancy-Induced Hypertension

Some women become hypertensive after their fifth month of pregnancy. When this hypertension is accompanied by edema and protein in the urine (proteinuria) it can cause pre-eclampsia, a condition that can lead to convulsions (eclampsia). While magnesium has not been found to reduce high blood pressure alone, studies have found it reduces both pre-eclampsia and eclampsia and is not at all harmful to the fetus. It stands to reason, that if magnesium can help lower pregnancy-induced high blood pressure, it should be featured in your preventive diet and supplement program. A higher ratio of potassium to sodium is also helpful in controlling pregnancy-related high blood pressure.

Stress

What about stress as a contributing factor to high blood pressure? As anyone with normal blood pressure knows, your blood pressure can climb in stressful situations. If you are at the doctor's office waiting for a report on an exam, your blood pressure could be abnormally high, even when it is usually normal or low. Chronic stress is, of course, the most harmful, because it's not a temporary condition. To prevent stress-related high blood pressure, you need to set time aside to use some form of daily stress reduction like breathing from the diaphragm (See Murray & Pizzorno's book), meditation, or prayer. I'm not talking about dashing off a quick note to God to ask for calmness as you rush out the door. I'm talking about taking from 10-30 minutes a day to do some form of active stress reduction.

The Bottom Line

Hypertension can often be prevented, and when your blood pressure is normal your risk for serious health problems drops significantly. I know it's not easy. We live in a stressful world where fast foods are low in fruits and vegetables and high in fats, sodium, and sugar. We're in a hurry to do everything we need to in a day packed with too many tasks.

Eating fast foods, junk foods, and some of the less healthful

---

Lowering Cholesterol Easily

You can lower your cholesterol along with your LDL (the undesirable cholesterol) with a product found in most natural food stores: oat milk. Oat bran has been found to lower cholesterol, but now oat milk is showing promise. Oats contain three to five percent beta-glucans, soluble dietary fibers that appear to reduce cholesterol. In a small study, subjects were divided into two groups. One group had oat milk for a month, then soy milk for a month. The other group had oat milk for a month, then cow's milk for a month. Oat milk reduced cholesterol by four percent and the harmful LDL cholesterol by nine percent in this short period of time.

Of all "milk-like" products including soy, rice, grain, almond, and oat, I find oat milk tastes the most like cow's milk. You can use it in your cereal, to make soups creamier, and as a beverage. Oat milk comes in boxes that don't have to be refrigerated until after they're opened, making it easy to have on hand.

Onning, G., et al. "Effects of consumption of oat milk, soya milk, or cow's milk on plasma lipids and antioxidative capacity in healthy subjects," *Ann Nutr Metab*, 42, 211-220, 1998.

foods we grew up with and love to taste are fine every once in a while. But if you want to keep your blood pressure low and reduce your risk for heart disease and other problems, concentrate on a healthy diet along with stress reduction and regular exercise.

Chapter 9

Osteoporosis, Part 1: The Great Calcium Hoax*

Some 25 million Americans, 80 percent of them older women, suffer from osteoporosis, or "brittle bone" disease. Unfortunately, most women find out they have osteoporosis when it's too late — usually after a fracture of the wrist, hip or spine, loss of height, or curvature of the spine has occurred.

Like high blood pressure, osteoporosis is a silent, underlying condition, usually symptomless, with potentially devastating consequences. All of us lose some bone as we age, but people with osteoporosis lose an excessive amount. Their bones become fragile, and their skeleton is weakened to the point where even a minor fall can result in a fracture.

Osteoporosis leads to some 1.5 million spine, hip, and wrist fractures in the U.S. each year, of which about 40 percent are spinal, 25 percent are hip, and 15 percent are wrist. Spinal fractures will affect one out of every three women in their lifetime, while wrist and hip fractures will happen to one out of six.

Osteoporosis is like high blood pressure in another way, too. In many cases, it can be prevented and treated with a combination of lifestyle, diet, and therapeutic approaches.

Osteoporosis-related fractures can affect any bone in the body. But it is particularly critical to do everything possible to prevent hip fractures, because they can lead to loss of function and independence. A woman's frequency of hip fracture — three times that of a man's — is more serious than most of us realize. One hip fracture alone can total more than $30,000 in direct medical costs. Half of those affect-

*Reprinted from *The Giant Book of Women's Health Secrets*.

ed lose the ability to walk independently, and up to a third become totally dependent. Studies have shown that within one year, up to 20 percent of hip-fracture patients die from conditions related to the fracture or to fracture-related surgery.

Do We Have Enough Information?

Your risk of developing osteoporosis-related hip fracture is equal to your combined risk of developing breast, uterine, and ovarian cancer. Nevertheless, a survey of women between 45 and 75 showed that most are not aware of the widespread nature of the disease. Nearly three-fourths of the women thought they were knowledgeable about osteoporosis, but eight out of 10 didn't connect the disease with hip fracture. Yet, ask an older woman what she most fears, and chances are fracture will be high on the list.

Doctors themselves are often not knowledgeable about the disease. One study, for example, found that only four percent of a group of people entering long-term care were diagnosed with osteoporosis, although nearly all of them had it.

Steroids and Osteoporosis

The American College of Rheumatology admits that one out of every four patients who uses steroids to counteract the inflammation of arthritis and rheumatism eventually gets a fracture from thinning bones. In fact, bone wasting is most rapid during the first six months of steroid therapy. How much steroid contributes to osteoporosis? Just 7.5 mg of prednisone a day is enough to cause thinning, brittle bones, and eventual fractures.

Doctors are being told to use topical or inhaled steroids, rather than those that are ingested, whenever these forms are appropriate. We'd like to add that there are anti-inflammatory agents that do not have side effects of bone loss, like vitamin C and glucosamine sulfate. Explore with your alternative health-care practitioner other, safer, anti-inflammatory medications.

Some topical creams containing capsaicin, a chemical found in cayenne pepper, reduce the pain and inflammation from arthritis and rheumatism. They're either going to work for you — or not. But they won't cause bone loss.

McCarthy, Michael. "Guidelines issued for steroid-induced osteoporosis," *The Lancet*, vol. 348, November 2, 1996.

In addition, most doctors insist that high doses of calcium, hormone therapy, and the newer bisphosphonate drugs are the only effective ways to prevent osteoporosis. They are ignoring many of the more current studies, which indicate there are much more effective (and safer) options.

Bone: It's Not What You Think

Most people think of bone as a hard, permanent substance — the skeletal "infrastructure" of our bodies. But bone is living tissue that constantly undergoes remodeling — an alternating process of the removal, or resorption of old bone, and formation, the laying down of new bone. In healthy tissue, bone-removing cells carve out cavities in the bone's surface, while cells that form bone fill in these cavities. Thanks to this remodeling process, about a fifth of your skeleton is replaced each year.

During your first 30 years, more bone is formed than is lost. Sometime in your early 30s, peak bone density is reached, and the balance begins to shift to the loss column.

Bone loss is a natural part of the aging process. By age 70 or 80, women will have lost about a third to a half of their bone mass. (In men, bone mass also declines as a natural part of aging — about 20 to 30 percent by comparison — but the decline is slower and begins from a point of higher density.)

In osteoporosis, however, the loss is much greater. Too little bone is formed or too much is removed — or both. As a result, bones become fragile and break easily, leaving people vulnerable to pain and injury.

Osteoporosis and the Calcium Controversy

Since the 1950s, American women have been told by the medical profession that increasing the amount of calcium in our diets can greatly reduce the risk of developing osteoporosis. Advertisers and the media have emphasized the importance of this one mineral over all others — suggesting that calcium is enough to prevent bone loss. And as a result, sales of calcium supplements have skyrocketed and the consumption of dairy products has soared as well.

Still, a number of health problems that are the result of calcium-related imbalances, including premenstrual syndrome, arthritis, heart disease, and osteoporosis, continue to escalate.

Why?

We all need calcium for a variety of bodily functions including good colon health and building strong bones. But all recent studies do not agree that a high calcium intake has a positive effect on bone health. And it's no wonder. The more calcium one ingests at any given time, the smaller the percentage of calcium that is actually absorbed. And there is research that has shown that when we adapt to a low calcium diet, we actually excrete less of it in our urine and increase our absorption.

What's more, in 1988 the National Women's Health Network announced that women who lived in countries where calcium intake was low had less osteoporosis than women in this country who are on a high-calcium diet.

And indeed, a great number of studies support the idea that lowered calcium intake may benefit American women as well. A Dutch study published in 1960 was one of the first to caution that excessive calcium could result in soft tissue calcification, or arthritis, and one possible beneficial nutrient to help counteract this effect would be magnesium. Recently, a study published in the *Journal of Applied Nutrition* showed an increase in bone density in post-menopausal women who took more magnesium and less calcium than has been generally recommended.

Magnesium's Role in Preventing PMS, Arthritis, Osteoporosis, and Even Heart Disease

One greatly overlooked factor in calcium absorption is the importance of having enough magnesium.

When women take large amounts of calcium, either in supplements or by eating diets high in dairy products and low in whole grains and beans, calcium is elevated in the blood and stimulates the secretion of a hormone called calcitonin. At the same time, it suppresses the secretion of the parathyroid hormone (PTH). These hormones regulate the levels of calcium in the bones and soft tissues and are related directly to osteoporosis and osteoarthritis. PTH draws calcium out of the bones and deposits it in the soft tissues, while calcitonin increases calcium in the bones.

But the optimum execution of these two delicate functions is dependent upon having sufficient magnesium. Because magnesium suppresses PTH and stimulates calcitonin, it helps move calcium into our bones. This chemical action helps prevent osteoarthritis and osteoporosis.

A magnesium deficiency, however, will prevent this chemical action. And more calcium is not the solution, because while magnesium helps the body absorb and utilize calcium, excessive calcium prevents the absorption of magnesium. Taking more calcium without adequate magnesium — and what is adequate for one woman may be insufficient for another — may either create calcium malabsorption or a magnesium deficiency.

Only additional magnesium can break this cycle, as was demonstrated by a study reported in *International Clinical Nutrition Review*. Volunteers on a low magnesium diet were given both calcium and vitamin D supplements. All subjects were magnesium-deficient, and all but one became deficient in calcium, as well, in spite of the fact that calcium had also been added to their diet. When

---

HRT and Osteoporosis

While hormone replacement therapy (HRT) claims to improve bone density, there has been a dramatic increase in broken bones in women between the ages of 35 and 65 in those countries where HRT is routinely prescribed. This may be due to the nutrient-depletion side effects of hormone therapy. One measure of bone formation is serum bone alkaline phosphatase (ALP) activity. ALP needs particular nutrients: zinc, magnesium, and manganese, but its production is diminished with too much copper. Women who take synthetic hormones tend to have lower serum ALP along with abnormally high copper. At the same time, magnesium and other minerals associated with bone formation are lower. If you feel you need to be taking hormones, you may want to take extra minerals and have a blood test to check your copper levels. And be sure to take natural hormones.

McLaren-Howard, J., et al. "Hormone replacement therapy and osteoporosis: bone enzymes and nutrient imbalances," *J Nutr Envir Med* 8, 129-138, 1998. *Int'l Clin Nutr Rev*, January 99.

they were given intravenous calcium infusions, the level of calcium in their blood rose for the duration of the intravenous feedings. When intravenous calcium was stopped, blood levels of calcium dropped again. However, when they were given magnesium, their magnesium levels rose rapidly and stabilized, and their calcium levels also rose within a few days even though they had not been given any additional calcium.

In addition to helping move calcium into the bones to reduce the risk for osteoporosis, magnesium is helpful in battling premenstrual syndrome. That's because magnesium helps the body utilize

Don't Let New Fosamax Study Fool You

Drug-maker Merck is pleased with the results of the latest study on its non-hormonal osteoporosis prevention drug Fosamax. This popular drug, which 2.2 million women in this country currently take, produced an average bone density increase of 3.5 percent at the spine and 1.9 percent at the hip, in a study reported in the *New England Journal of Medicine* in February 1998.

That sounds great. Unless, of course, you know about the magnesium studies: In one study, which reduced calcium intake and increased magnesium intake, participants had an average increase in bone of 11 percent. In another study, in which only magnesium intake was increased, participant bone density was increased by an average of eight percent. I won't be fooled by the new Fosamax study and hope you won't be either. Before considering Fosamax or another bisphosphonate drug, try magnesium — up to 1,000 mg/day and enough to keep you regular. Get a moderate amount of weight-bearing exercise as well, and let me know in six months if your doctor isn't impressed with the results.

You will have saved yourself a lot of suffering and needless health risks, too. Fosamax is so disruptive to the gastrointestinal system that it must be taken at least 30 minutes before the first food, beverage, or medication of the day with a full glass of plain water. Then, you aren't supposed to lie down for at least 30 minutes and until after you've eaten. Fosamax actually works by interfering with the body's natural bone resorption process, and by doing so can lead to other serious health risks.

Rosen, Clifford J. "A tale of two worlds in prescribing etidronate for osteoporosis," *The Lancet*, November 8, 1997.

Gennari, L, et al. "Vitamin D and estrogen receptor allelic variants in Italian postmenopausal women: Evidence of multiple contribution to bone mineral density," *J Clin Endocrinol Metab*, 83(3) 939-943, 1998; *Intl' Clin Nutr Rev*, January 1999.

B vitamins, as well as inactivate excessive estrogens. And it is these conditions, low quantities of B vitamins and high estrogen to progesterone ratios, which have been found to contribute to premenstrual moodiness and irritability.

In most studies of women and heart disease, the magnesium factor is also being overlooked. In fact, magnesium may even be more important than calcium in reducing our incidence of heart disease. Consider this: Calcium causes muscles to contract. Magnesium, on the other hand, causes muscles to relax — and your heart is a muscle.

A recent randomized, controlled trial using magnesium in about 4,000 patients with acute myocardial infarction (heart attacks) showed that there were fewer deaths in people who were given magnesium than in those who did not take this mineral. The study recommends giving magnesium to all patients during acute heart attacks, and suggests this long-overlooked mineral may be beneficial when it is added to traditional medical treatments.

Postmenopausal women, those at highest risk of heart disease, would be wise to consider a diet higher in magnesium (whole grains and beans) and lower in calcium (dairy products). Nutritional supplements can be found that contain equal amounts of calcium and magnesium. Some, formulated specifically for postmenopausal women, already contain more magnesium than calcium.

Finally, high-calcium diets may actually increase the risk of stroke, another leading cause of death in women as well as men. A UCLA study recently reported in the *Journal of Clinical Investigation* suggests that artery wall cells are able to form bone tissue and high-calcium diets may contribute to such growth. In turn, this bone growth may contribute to the development of hardening of the arteries and blockages, which can cause strokes.

How Did This Trend in Magnesium Deficiency Begin?

Women's obsession with weight control may be at least partially responsible for much of our current magnesium deficiency. We have been assured that high quantities of non-fat dairy products, like milk and yogurt, were both safe and beneficial. But when you increase dairy products, even those without fat, you are upsetting your body's balance of calcium and magnesium.

The high protein content of dairy, especially when combined with other animal products, can pull calcium from the bones where it's needed. One study, reported in the *American Journal of Clinical Nutrition* of 1,600 women found that those who followed a vegetarian diet for at least 20 years had only an 18 percent loss of bone mineral by age 80, while meat eaters had a 35 percent bone mineral loss!

Also, dairy products contain nine times as much calcium as magnesium. If you have been eating a lot of dairy products, along with few or no grains and beans (which are rich in magnesium), you have probably upset your calcium/magnesium ratio even further.

In addition, most nutritional supplements contain twice as much calcium as magnesium. But again, because we've eaten so much dairy and so few grains and beans, our bodies have come to need as much magnesium as calcium, or even more. To bring yourself back into a chemical balance you would have to eat three cups of brown rice every day to compensate for one small serving of dairy. Because white rice has most of its magnesium removed, along with fiber and many other nutrients, you would need 10 cups to balance one portion of calcium-rich foods.

Restoring Your Calcium and Magnesium Balance

What can you do to help eliminate PMS symptoms, protect yourself against osteoporosis, heart disease, stroke, and reduce your risk of arthritis?

Begin with a magnesium-rich diet. Many of the foods we eat have been refined, and magnesium is one nutrient removed in the refining process and not added in "enriched" products. Increase your consumption of whole grains like brown rice, millet, buckwheat (kasha), whole wheat, triticale, quinoa, and rye, as well as legumes, including lentils, split peas, and all varieties of beans. A whole grain cereal or bread in the morning, a cup of bean soup at lunch, a snack of whole grain crackers, and a serving of brown rice, millet, or other grain with dinner should go a long way to help increase your magnesium intake.

Eat plenty of fresh vegetables, too. Fresh produce and whole grains will, in addition to calcium and magnesium, provide your body with many other essential minerals. And it's especially important for you to not overlook one vitamin or mineral for another, since all work together to supply you with the nutrients you need.

Reduce your consumption of refined sugar and alcohol as well, to prevent excessive magnesium from being excreted in the urine. You may think your chocolate cravings are due to a sweet tooth, but they may be an indication that you have a calcium/magnesium imbalance. Cocoa powder contains more magnesium than any other food, so you may be a chocoholic if your body needs more magnesium, less calcium, or both.

But don't rush out and stock up on candy bars and other chocolate-rich foods. If you do, you're creating even more of an imbalance. You already know that chocolate contains an excessive amount of sugar. Not only does sugar cause magnesium excretion, but it also causes calcium to be leached out of your bones. In this way, diets that are excessive in sugar contribute to premenstrual bloating and weight gain. When you increase your magnesium and decrease calcium, eventually the chocolate cravings will leave and chocolate will be more a flavor you enjoy than a craving that drives you.

Another extremely important step is to evaluate the amount of dairy in your diet. If it has been high — more than a serving or so a day at most — reduce it at the same time as you increase magnesium-rich foods. Oriental and Indian diets contain little or no dairy, and arthritis and osteoporosis are not major health problems in these cultures. By featuring greater amounts of green vegetables, grains, tofu (soy bean curd), and seafood, these diets contain twice as much magnesium as the average American diet.

In addition, keep your animal protein (chicken and meats) low, since a diet high in phosphorous, a mineral found in animal protein, can cause lowered calcium levels. Vegetable protein (grains with any beans) in any amount is safer, since a diet high in soy protein maintains calcium levels.

And if you've been taking vitamin/mineral supplements that

are higher in calcium than magnesium, you may want to reverse the proportions to take more magnesium than calcium.

Can Soft Drinks Promote Osteoporosis?

Yes — this is one of the unhealthful effects of soft drinks. Some of them, mostly colas, contain phosphorus (in the form of phosphoric acid) that is added to keep the bubbles from going flat. But unfortunately, too much phosphorus in the diet can cause calcium to be leached from bones — hastening the development of osteoporosis.

In one survey, soft drinks containing the highest amounts of phosphorus included Tab, Coke, Diet Coke, and caffeine-free Coke.

Asthma Inhalers May Cause Osteoporosis

Is there a connection between osteoporosis and asthma? There may be if you use inhalers with steroids, says a study published in *The Lancet.* Investigators studied 200 women who used steroid-based inhalers for an average of six years to treat mild asthma. Researchers estimated that the most rapid bone loss occurred in the first one to two years of using steroid inhalers. In fact, bone loss was five times greater than someone smoking a pack of cigarettes daily for 10 years!

While the amount of bone loss was small, this preliminary study is saying that someone using 200 mcg of steroids in their inhaler for one year will have minimal bone loss. Someone using 2,000 mcg of steroids a day for seven years would have measurable bone loss (one ST, or standard deviation). Over a period of decades, the use of high doses of steroids could impact on bone density. If you're using inhalers, you may want to check with your doctor to see how much you're taking and how much you really need.

Be aware that asthma may originate from emotional disturbances or from food sensitivities. Foods containing histamines (wine, beer, cheeses, fish, and pickled cabbage) can cause asthmatic incidents. Try locating the food or foods that trigger your symptoms. One study, reported by Melvyn R. Werbach, MD, in his database, *Nutritional Influences on Illness,* found that nearly 60 percent of the patients with food intolerances and asthma had considerable improvement after just one month of eliminating these foods. Explore every possible cause of your asthma that you can. Finding the cause could help you get away from steroids all together. Don't, however, stop using any medication without consulting your physician.

Werbach, Melvyn R., MD. *Nutritional Influences on Illness,* Third Line Press, Tarzana, CA, 1998.

Phosphorus-free soft drinks included Pepsi Free, Diet Pepsi Free, 7-Up, and Mountain Dew. Others are low in phosphorus.

It's a good idea to limit any soft drinks that contain phosphorus to one a day. An excellent alternative is carbonated mineral water. The only phosphorus it contains is found naturally in water — and therefore, an amount more appropriate for human consumption.

How Much Magnesium?

How much magnesium does your body need? According to Dr. Mildred Seelig, executive president of the American College of Nutrition, we need about 200 milligrams more than we get in an average diet. She suggests that geriatric patients on a good diet take between 700 and 800 milligrams of magnesium supplements each day. This is considerably more than the Recommended Daily Allowances (RDA) of 350 milligrams per day for women of all ages.

Can you take too much magnesium? It's unlikely, according to Melvyn R. Werbach, MD, author of *Healing Through Nutrition* (Harper Collins, May 1993) and *Nutritional Influences on Illness,* a health practitioner's reference book. His research into medical studies has not found any cases of magnesium toxicity from taking it in the form of oral supplementation.

Guy E. Abraham, MD, a research gynecologist and endocrinologist in Torrance, California, has given postmenopausal women from 200 to 1,000 mg of magnesium a day to strengthen their bones. He based the amount he gave each woman on bowel tolerance — enough magnesium to cause soft stools, but not diarrhea. These women showed an average bone density increase of 11 percent in one year, by adjusting their diets to increase magnesium (600-1,000 mg/day) and lower calcium (500 mg/day).

Another study touting the benefits of magnesium for postmenopausal women, this one from Israel, also suggests that it is magnesium, not calcium, that protects our bones from the thinning characteristic of osteoporosis as we age.

In the Israeli study, 31 postmenopausal women were given from 250 to 750 mg of magnesium each day for two years. In almost 75 percent of the women, their bone density actually increased — in some, as much as eight percent. Women who refused additional magnesium had a loss of bone density from one to three percent — an expected decrease according to most medical doctors.

Most studies on the effect of increasing the amount of calcium in the diet show that calcium merely slows the rate of bone loss by an average of around 50 percent, but does not prevent or reverse osteoporosis.

For many women, getting sufficient magnesium is the missing link to reducing the risks of osteoporosis, heart disease, and arthritis, as well as eliminating PMS symptoms.

Calcium, Aluminum, and Kidney Failure

While calcium citrate is an easy-to-absorb form of calcium, we have said many times before that increasing your calcium without sufficient magnesium could lead to problems like PMS, muscle spasms, and even bone loss.

Now a South African study brings up another concern. As little as four grams of calcium citrate increases the absorption of alu-

---

Calcium and Kidney Stones

Small amounts of calcium are normally stored in the kidneys, but large amounts, in the form of calcium oxalate crystals, can result in problematic kidney stones. Now a 12-year study of over 90,000 women shows that dietary calcium decreased the risk of stones, while calcium supplementation may have increased them.

The theory for this phenomenon is that dietary calcium reduces the absorption of calcium oxalate in the intestines, so it can't get trapped in the kidneys.

Once again, Mother Nature triumphs. By getting your nutrients from foods you get balanced nutrients. Harmful substances may be contained in a food, but blocked from being absorbed. Can you get enough calcium from food alone? Yes, if you count broccoli (1 cup = 178 mg), tofu (1/2 cup = 258 mg), and white beans (1 cup = 121 mg). Even a cup of butternut squash has 84 mg of calcium. Whole grains and beans also contain both calcium and magnesium, the mineral that helps get calcium into your bones, where you want them.

"News in brief," *The Lancet,* April 5, 1977, p. 1002.

minum, a mineral that has lead to kidney failure and is suspected to be linked to Alzheimer's disease. Calcium citrate can be found in some antacids, effervescent calcium, and buffered vitamin C supplements.

Are you safe if you take calcium citrate and are not taking any of these products that may contain aluminum? Yes. It's an excellent form of an essential mineral. Just be sure you're not cooking in aluminum pots and pans or using a deodorant with aluminum.

The Estrogen Puzzle

The rapid bone loss many women experience as they go through menopause is due to the drop in estrogen, a hormone that regulates menstrual periods and plays a role in our bones' ability to absorb calcium from the bloodstream. Women who choose estrogen replacement therapy often do so for symptomatic relief of such menopause-related symptoms as hot flashes, vaginal dryness, and depression.

Studies have shown that estrogen intervention, particularly in the years immediately following menopause when the rate of bone loss can be as high as five percent a year, can decrease the risk of hip fracture by 25 to 50 percent and vertebral (spinal) crush fractures by perhaps as much as 50 to 75 percent. Estrogen, which blocks the process of bone resorption, has been shown to increase bone density three to five percent in the first year. In the long run, however, studies show that estrogen merely slows the rate of bone loss by an average of around 50 percent.

Although some studies strongly suggest that estrogen also provides protection from cardiovascular disease, there are as yet no definitive answers. Heart disease in postmenopausal women may come, in part, from increased calcium intake. Preliminary results from a study currently in progress show blood clots and heart disease actually developed in women taking estrogen, but not their placebo counterparts. It's very possible that doctors and drug companies jumped too early, concluding that since estrogen tends to lower cholesterol, it also lowers heart-disease risk. Not necessarily!

There is also evidence that synthetic estrogen replacement therapy increases the risk of breast and endometrial cancer as well as stroke and gall bladder disease. Many women, such as those who have had breast cancer, or whose mothers had breast cancer, should not take synthetic estrogen. Others choose not to for a variety of reasons.

Side effects, which may be difficult to tolerate, can include migraine headaches, breast soreness and swelling, bloating, mood changes, and cramping. Women on estrogen therapy report that ERT increases weight and contributes to the body's thickening, but medical doctors tend to deny this phenomenon.

In women who do take estrogen and have not undergone a hysterectomy, taking progesterone may offset the increased risk of endometrial cancer. The estrogen-progesterone combination, referred to as hormone replacement therapy (HRT), usually results in menstrual bleeding, which some women regard as a disadvantage.

Many women are reluctant to undertake hormone therapy, including progesterone, because the research on long-term effects is so limited. Their health-care providers cannot give them clear and definitive answers, positive or negative.

We do know long-term synthetic estrogen use significantly increases breast-cancer risk. A Harvard study reported in the *Journal of the American Medical Association* found a 71 percent increase in breast-cancer risk among women aged 60-65 who had taken estrogen for five years or more! (There is also a disturbing lack of long-term safety studies for natural estrogens and progesterone.) Many physi-

---

Q: Ever since menopause I've had migraines every 35 to 40 days. I'm now currently taking 800 mg of magnesium and 500 mg of calcium and the headaches are improved. Do the high amounts of magnesium collect in the body the way calcium does? — *R.M.H., Englewood, NJ*

A: No. Magnesium actually helps calcium get into your bones. It also relaxes all muscles (including your heart). Tense muscles can contribute to headaches. Several studies have shown magnesium to be helpful for migraines. Because it's such a safe supplement, and so inexpensive, it's worth trying if you suffer from any headaches. Magnesium may be taken to bowel tolerance. This means as much as you need to have comfortably loose stools without diarrhea.

cians advise that women limit therapy to seven to 10 years. Others recommend it for longer, depending on a woman's individual situation. It is important for women to understand that once therapy stops, the increased rate of bone loss that marks the early postmenopausal years resumes. There is no carry-over in protective effect.

Although studies show that women who take estrogen for at least seven years between menopause and age 75 reduce their risk of fracture by half during that time, recent studies show little difference after age 75, the period when women are most at risk. When women over the age of 75 who had taken estrogen for 10 years following menopause were compared with women who had not taken estrogen, there was only a two-percent difference in bone density. This suggests two types of bone loss — estrogen-dependent in earlier years and age-dependent later on.

Better Than Estrogen

A new type of plant estrogen, called isoflavonoids, has been so successful in trial studies in Europe that a drug containing this substance, Ipriflavone, is now an accepted treatment for osteoporosis in Italy, Hungary, and Japan. Since the drug is a derivative of a naturally occurring substance, women in this country should know that natural isoflavonoids can be found at their local markets. Soy products are high in this natural estrogen, making soybeans, tofu, and miso soup (the soup found in Japanese restaurants) desirable foods for women concerned about bone loss.

It's interesting to note that the lower incidence of osteoporosis in Japanese women has been attributed in part to their high consumption of soy products. If you aren't familiar with soy foods, we recommend Earl Mindell's *Soy Miracle* ($12, Fireside Books) for ideas on easy ways to incorporate them into your daily eating and a wide variety of recipes.

Estrogen Alternatives for Osteoporosis Prevention

Begin at the beginning: Have good digestion. You need acid to help break down and absorb calcium. Your stomach, when digestion is normal, produces enough hydrochloric acid (HCl) to help utilize calcium. With poor digestion, or if you're taking acid-neutralizing antacids, you may have low production of HCl, or the HCl may be neutralized, and the result is poor calcium absorption. Signs of poor digestion include anemia, lack of appetite for protein, feelings of constant hunger, tiredness, and gas or bloating after eating. To improve digestion, eat slowly while sitting down, chew foods well, and drink fewer liquids with meals. Then, if you still think your digestion may need improvement, try taking the digestive enzyme Beano (sold in most food stores) before meals — or talk to your health practitioner about taking HCl supplements.

Increase your magnesium: Several studies, including one from Israel, show that higher magnesium levels increase bone density. Magnesium is high in whole grains and legumes (all beans). Increase your dietary sources of magnesium and consider taking 250 to 1,000 mg of magnesium a day. The side effect from taking too much magnesium is loose stools. Postmenopausal women who are constipated may find they are improving their health in more ways than bone density by increasing their magnesium intake. Dr. Guy E. Abraham, who has published numerous articles on PMS and osteoporosis, believes postmenopausal women should take magnesium to bowel tolerance. That is, however much you need to not be constipated and without creating stools that are uncomfortably loose.

Specific fats protect your bones: Essential fatty acids, like

Be Wary of Tums!

An article in the *American Journal of Epidemiology* (vol 145, 1997) published the results of a two-year study of over 9,000 women aged 65 or older. They found "no important associations between dietary calcium intake and the risk of any of the fractures studied." In fact, taking calcium supplements proved to increase the risk of hip fracture. What about Tums? Again, an increase in bone breakage. The authors conclude that they can find no benefit of calcium on the risk of fractures. If your doctor insists you take calcium, or Tums, refer him or her to this study. And make your own decision.

Cummings, R.G., et al. "Calcium intake and fracture risk: results from the study of osteoporotic fractures," *Am J Epidemiol* 1997;145:926-934.

omega-3 fats found in fish oils, protect against osteoporosis. You can take fish oil capsules (one or two, twice daily) or add fatty fish like salmon to your weekly diet. If you are a vegetarian or not a fish lover, essential fatty acids are also found in high amounts in flax seeds (grind one to three tablespoons in a coffee grinder and add to your cereal or breakfast drink) and walnuts.

It's soy good for you! The plant estrogen called isoflavonoid found naturally in soybeans is very similar to synthetic phytoestrogens and tamoxifen, chemicals that have been shown to reduce bone loss. Lowered osteoporosis in Japanese women has been attributed to their high consumption of soy products like green soybeans, dried soybeans, miso soup, and tofu. In Europe, a drug containing isoflavonoids is accepted treatment for osteoporosis. In this country, many natural progesterone creams contain progesterone extracted from soybeans.

Increase your consumption of soy products. Try a soy-based protein powder if you make a breakfast drink. Or you can take low-fat tofu (Mori-Nu brand comes in little waxed paper boxes that don't have to be refrigerated until after you open them. And they have some that are one percent lite rather than 50 percent fat, like most tofu). Blend it in your blender and add it to your soups, stews, sauces, and salad dressings. Soy has very little taste. It takes on the flavors that surround it.

Hot Flashes and Your Hypothalamus

If you have uncomfortable periods of menopausal hot flashes, chances are it's because your hypothalamus is having a difficult time adjusting to your new levels of hormones. The hypothalamus is part of your brain and sits above the pituitary gland. It regulates body temperature, sleep patterns, your stress reactions, metabolism, moods, and libido — and it releases pituitary hormones, as well. To work properly, your hypothalamus needs substances called endorphins.

Athletes think of endorphins as "feel good" chemicals, because when you exercise your body produces more of these chemicals that bring a feeling of well-being. They act as natural antidepressants (when you're feeling low, get out and exercise!) and relieve pain. They also allow the hypothalamus to work properly.

Exercise, diet, and certain supplements can help balance the hypothalamus. Or you can use ERT. What if you do nothing? Will Mother Nature balance your hypothalamus? Of course it will. But why be hot and sweaty longer than necessary? Here are some safe and effective ways to speed regulation of your hypothalamus.

Natural Solutions for Hot Flashes

Fats and sugars increase body heat. So keep your dietary fats low and reduce your sugar intake. Decrease heat-provoking spices like cayenne and other hot peppers. At least temporarily lower the spiciness of the foods you eat one or two notches.

Eat foods high in phytoestrogens (plant estrogens). They help balance your hormones. Fennel root and fennel seed are high in phytoestrogens. So are celery and parsley. Try adding these to a vegetable juice or just increase their use in salads and soups. Soy products eaten on a daily basis have been shown to lower hot flashes in Japanese women. (In fact, menopause is such a non-event in the lives of Japanese women that the word "menopause" doesn't exist in the Japanese language.) Tofu wieners (Smart Dogs are one tasty variety) and soy-based veggie burgers (I love fat-free Boca Burgers — juicy and flavorful and in most frozen food sections of supermarkets) may decrease your hot flashes while their animal-based varieties increase the heat.

Vitamin E and evening primrose oil have both been used to reduce hot flashes. Eight capsules daily of evening primrose oil (take four in the morning, four at night) or 800 IU of a dry or water-soluble vitamin E for best absorption. Reduce your vitamin E to 400 IU after your hot flashes have subsided.

One of my favorite solutions to hot flashes is a flavonoid found in citrus fruits called hesperidin. Hesperidin appears to act directly on the hypothalamus, turning off the "hot" switch in your brain. I have seen a great deal of success with women taking 500 mg of HMC hesperidin (hesperidin methyl chalcone — another flavonoid from citrus) twice a day. Michael T. Murray, ND suggests hesperidin be added to 1,200 mg of vitamin C a day. While vitamin C with bioflavonoids does usually contain hesperidin, the amounts are too small to be effective in this form. Check your health food stores for this safe answer to hot flashes.

Herbs have also been used to reduce menopausal symptoms including hot flashes: Dong quai (Angelica sinensis), licorice root (Glycyrrhiza glabra), chaste berry (vitex agnus-castus), and black cohosh (Cimicifuga racemosa). In the Orient, where herbs have been used extensively, herbal combinations have been found to be more effective than taking any one of them individually. These four herbs appear to have mild estrogenic effects on the hormone system. Remifemin, an herbal remedy for hot flashes and other menopausal symptoms, contains a standardized amount of black cohosh and has scientific studies to back up its effectiveness. All of these can be found in health food stores.

Vaginal Dryness

As we age, our tissues begin to thin. This includes the vaginal lining, which is called atrophic vaginitis, and is another reason many women take estrogen replacement. However, soybeans will give you the same results. Michael T. Murray, ND, says that one cup of soybeans contains about 300 mg of isoflavone. This is equal to about 0.45 mg of conjugated estrogens or one tablet of Premarin. The difference is that soybeans will not increase your risk for cancer like Premarin. If you're troubled by vaginal dryness during intercourse, a personal lubricant will usually help.

The New Osteoporosis Drugs: Bisphosphonates

This new family of drugs acts to decrease bone loss by preventing bone resorption. These drugs, called bisphosphonates, are mineral compounds whose structures have been altered to act selectively on bone. Two popular bisphosphonate drugs go by the trade names Etidronate and Fosamax.

In a double blind placebo controlled study of Etidronate therapy in 135 postmenopausal women without osteoporosis, at the end of seven to 10 years, women taking the drug showed a 3.42 percent increase in lumbar spine bone mineral density, compared to a .38 percent decrease among the placebo group.

What about Fosamax? Five controlled clinical studies, involving more than 1,600 postmenopausal women with osteoporosis, showed that patients treated with Fosamax experienced 29 percent fewer fractures of the hip and other bones (excluding the spine), compared to patients who took a placebo. Fosamax was also shown to reduce the incidence of new vertebral fractures by 48 percent.

In two, three-year trials with 994 postmenopausal women with osteoporosis Fosamax built bone. Women taking Fosamax had an increase in bone mineral density of 8.2 percent at the spine and 7.2 percent at the hip, compared with patients treated with a placebo, in whom bone mineral density decreased by between .065 and

---

Q: You suggest that women should take twice as much magnesium as calcium. If I take 1,000 mg of calcium, I need to take 2,000 mg of magnesium. Won't that cause diarrhea? — *A.B., New Orleans, LA*

A: That much magnesium could certainly cause loose stools or diarrhea. We suggest women take magnesium to bowel tolerance —whatever amount you need to have comfortably loose, but not runny, stools. (This makes magnesium supplements a healthy remedy for constipation, too.) Some women may need twice as much magnesium as calcium, others do well with just a little more magnesium.

Dr. Guy E. Abraham, a research gynecologist, in a small controlled study, found that women who took 500 mg of calcium and between 600-1,000 mg of magnesium had an average 11-percent increase in bone density after one year. His study suggests we don't need to take as much calcium as most doctors say.

Remember, you need magnesium to get calcium into your bones. Dairy products contain very little magnesium. Beans, nuts, and seeds, tofu, and whole grains generally have a better balance of both minerals. The amount of calcium, magnesium, and other nutrients you take includes those nutrients in the foods you eat. A healthy balanced diet with no more than one serving of dairy a day should provide you with sufficient nutrients, along with a balanced vitamin/mineral supplement (we like those that contain 500 mg calcium and 500-600 mg magnesium).

1.16 percent.

Like many popular prescription drugs, the long-term safety of bisphosphonates has yet to be established.

Current advice from the manufacturer, Merck, is that patients with low levels of calcium in their blood, severe kidney disease, or who are pregnant or nursing should not take Fosamax. The manufacturer also urges that caution be used when Fosamax is given to patients with active upper gastrointestinal problems. Apparently Fosamax can irritate such problems. The most commonly reported drug-related side effects in patients taking this drug are musculoskeletal and abdominal pain, and other digestive disturbances such as nausea, heartburn, and irritation or pain of the esophagus.

The severity of the digestive disturbances should not be underestimated. Fosamax users frequently complain of horrible burning that wasn't helped by either Tums or Maalox. The manufacturer is very aware of this and has made the unprecedented move of distributing special drug warning stickers for pharmacists to adhere to prescription bottles. The stickers warn patients to take Fosamax 30 minutes before breakfast with water (coffee, orange juice, and other acidic beverages will contribute to digestive problems) and not to lie down for at least 30 minutes after taking the drug (this also can aggravate digestive problems).

In the absence of long-term safety testing, these dramatic digestive problems may very well be the body rebelling against even greater unknown threats. Nausea, for example, can be a warning sign for potential liver damage. Beware!

Users should also be aware of how these drugs work — by inhibiting bone resorption. This process, in which calcium moves into and out of the bones to other parts of the body, helps maintain healthy levels of calcium elsewhere throughout the body for important functions, including nerve cell communication, contraction of muscle cells, blood-clotting efficiency, enzyme function, and production of certain proteins. If calcium is not allowed to move around freely in its normal manner, will any of these functions be adversely affected? Currently lacking long-term studies may provide an answer. The fact that patients with low levels of calcium in their blood are presently advised not to take Fosamax might be an early clue to a yes answer.

In view of these concerns, taking bisphosphonates to prevent osteoporosis may be a much riskier proposition than doctors and drug companies are letting on. It might be wisest to reserve use of these drugs for cases of advanced osteoporosis, when other safer therapies aren't enough, or in temporary conjunction with other therapies when circumstances require fastest results.

Etidronate and Osteoporosis

Today, many doctors are prescribing the drug etidronate to prevent osteoporosis, and for good reason — at least at first glance. Two studies published in 1990 showed that etidronate increased bone density and decreased new fractures in the spine after being used for just two years. But, unfortunately, a three-year follow-up study finds no difference in spinal fractures in women who did or did not take the drug.

And that's not all. Etidronate use has been associated with osteomalacia. This means that your bones get softer. More dense, maybe, but we want strong, not soft bones. After this follow-up study, the FDA gave approval to another drug, alendronate, that didn't cause soft bones. It produces even greater bone density than etidronate. But now the most recent studies are indicating that fracture prevention is not necessarily associated with the increase in

---

Q: How does magnesium make bones more flexible? — *M.W., Hobbs, New Mexico*

A: Bone contains both calcium and magnesium, which are necessary components in the formation of the mineral crystals that make up its structure. When magnesium is lower, these mineral crystals are larger and more perfect in shape. However, smaller crystals with irregular shapes join together to form stronger, more flexible bones. Magnesium helps make bones strong and flexible by creating the smaller structures.

Nutrition Reviews, vol 53, no. 3, March 1995.

bone density. A research gynecologist, Dr. Guy Abraham, says that bone fractures are controlled in part by bone flexibility. Magnesium, not calcium, helps bones stay more supple.

Researchers at the Maine Center for Osteoporosis Research and Education are now asking for a large, randomized, placebo-controlled study of postmenopausal ·women with osteoporosis to find out just what's really going on. But they know this is unlikely to happen because the FDA is getting ready to approve still more drugs.

Do Statins Increase Bone Density?

Scientists in England may have stumbled upon an answer to osteoporosis — at least for some people. They noticed in a 12-year trial of more than 1,000 women that the women who were taking statins (cholesterol-lowering drugs such as lovastatin and simvastatin) had significantly higher bone density in their spine and hips than women who didn't take them. Statins inhibit the production of an enzyme that is needed by the body to make cholesterol. The researchers say this same pathway is involved in the production of bone.

It's too early to suggest that people use statins to reduce osteoporosis, especially since there appear to be other methods with no side effects — such as 10-minutes daily of specific isometric exercises with the OsteoBall, and taking an equal amount of magnesium with calcium. And there are side effects and interactions that come with taking medications. Grapefruit and grapefruit juice, for example, should not be ingested by anyone taking statins. They greatly increase the absorption of these drugs, and you could be taking much more than is safe or needed.

Steroids and Osteoporosis

The American College of Rheumatology admits that one out of every four patients who uses steroids to counteract the inflammation of arthritis and rheumatism eventually gets a fracture from thinning bones. In fact, bone wasting is most rapid during the first six months of steroid therapy. How much steroid contributes to osteoporosis? Just 7.5 mg of prednisone a day is enough to cause thinning, brittle bones, and eventual fractures.

Doctors are being told to use topical or inhaled steroids, rather than those that are ingested, whenever these forms are appropriate. We'd like to add that there are anti-inflammatory agents that do not have side effects of bone loss, like vitamin C and glucosamine sulfate. Explore with your alternative health-care practitioner other, safer, anti-inflammatory medications.

Some topical creams containing capsaicin, a chemical found in cayenne pepper, reduce the pain and inflammation from arthritis and rheumatism. They're either going to work for you — or not. But they won't cause bone loss.

Steroids and Hip Fractures

Corticosteroids, like cortisone and prednisone, alter the way your bone repairs itself and contribute to bone loss. In fact, bone density declined two or three times faster in people on steroids than

---

Q: For more than 12 years my blood test showed elevated calcium levels. My doctors didn't think this was unusual. In 1972, I had radioactive iodine treatment for a goiter problem. Apparently, this lead to a parathyroid problem, which resulted in osteoporosis. I had parathyroid surgery and my calcium count became normal. Now what can I do about my osteoporosis? The endocrinologist at the Mayo Clinic told me to take Tums and Premarin and I'd be fine. — *C.M., Tucson, AZ*

A: According to our sources, high levels of serum (blood level) calcium can be caused by a number of factors: an underactive thyroid, overactive parathyroid, heavy metal toxicity, and too much vitamin D, just to name a few. Any consistent high levels of calcium found in blood tests should be investigated. It can be an indication of a problem.

Just because the calcium level in your blood is high doesn't mean bone calcium is high as well, as you found out. Concerning your osteoporosis, I've mentioned before that for calcium and magnesium (needed to get calcium into the bones) to be absorbed, you need acid in your stomach — like the hydrochloric acid your body makes naturally when you eat. Tums neutralizes stomach acid, making the calcium in Tums unabsorbable. Unabsorbed calcium can get into joints and become arthritis, or in arteries and cause atherosclerosis. I'm disturbed that a doctor at the Mayo Clinic would suggest Tums, but I'm not surprised either.

those who didn't take this form of anti-inflammatory drug. But until recently, it was not known if this decline in density resulted in more hip fractures, or merely weakened arms, legs, and the spine. Researchers from the Study of Osteoporotic Fractures Group looked at more than 8,000 women over the age of 65. Those who used steroid inhalers for asthma also took steroids orally. The average amount of steroids used was five milligrams of prednisone daily.

Among the women who didn't use steroids, there was a 2.8 percent incidence of hip fracture. In the group that used oral steroids, this figure nearly doubled. Women on oral steroids also had more rheumatoid arthritis, exercised less, and were less active in general. This rather large study confirms previous ones that have shown more broken bones in women taking steroids. But the authors are still not certain whether or not this data applies to people using nasal inhalers for asthma. Probably because so many of them also use the oral form.

Attention to Prevention

More and more of us are finding out how much we benefit from exercise. Young women reap the greatest benefit, since they can build bone mass up until their 30s. After that, exercise is critical to maintaining bone mass or slowing the rate of loss.

Exercise that forces the body to work against gravity (weight-bearing exercise) like jogging, walking, aerobics, dancing, and team sports, strengthens the skeletal system. Non-weight-bearing activities like cycling and swimming do not strengthen bone, but are important for cardiovascular health.

You don't have to train like an athlete — in fact, it's better if you don't. A good guideline is 30 to 60 minutes of exercise three or four times a week. Impossible? Even three 10-minute walks over the course of a day help.

As we age, we lose muscle mass as well as bone. Weight training can improve muscle strength and tone, which contributes to bone health, as well. There have been studies in the past that suggested heavier women have greater bone density than thinner women. A more recent study, however, now suggests it's not a person's weight, but the amount of muscle, that is the determining factor.

A group of nearly 250 healthy premenopausal women had their bone density examined. Those who had the highest amount of both fat and muscle had the densest bones. Those with flabby muscles had low bone density — whether they were heavy or thin.

While it's possible to say that bones that are dense before menopause will continue to remain strong and healthy after menopause, this study strongly suggests that weight alone will not protect you against osteoporosis. All women, whether heavy or light, should increase their muscle mass through regular weight resistance exercise.

You're never too old to benefit from exercise, either. One study that appeared in the *New England Journal of Medicine* compared mobility and strength of 100 nursing home residents between the ages of 72 and 98. Half the seniors participated in a 10-week weight resistance training program. At the end of this short time, their muscle strength had increased by an average of 113 percent, compared to the non-exercisers. Significant improvement in mobility was also seen, which made these seniors less prone to bone-breaking falls — a very significant achievement in view of the fact that 80 is the average age of persons suffering hip fractures.

Exercise is essential to good bone health, but it is far more effective when coupled with absorbed calcium. For women entering menopause, however, it is important to note that reduced estrogen, not calcium, is the primary cause of bone loss in the first five years beyond menopause. Women who do not get enough calcium (less than 400 mg/day), however, may lose even more bone mass.

When coupled with vitamin D and magnesium, calcium has shown tangible benefits. One study showed a reduction in hip fractures in a nursing home population whose average age was 85.

Another study published in the *Journal of Applied Nutrition* showed a reversal of osteoporosis in postmenopausal women who adjusted their diets to increase magnesium (600-1000 mg/day) and lower calcium (500 mg/day). These women showed an average bone density increase of 11 percent in one year.

Although this and other similar information has appeared in medical publications, most doctors still ignore it and attempt to frighten their patients into taking 1,500 milligrams of calcium a day. The majority of nutritional supplements contain twice as much calcium as magnesium, perpetuating the myth that calcium prevents osteoporosis. Numerous studies, however, show that most of this calcium does not get into the bones.

Boron and vitamin D are also necessary for calcium absorption. Many older people need vitamin D since it is harder for them to absorb calcium. Many housebound older adults get less sunlight — the major source of this essential vitamin — and consume fewer vitamin D-rich foods, such as fatty fish, liver, and egg yolk.

Recommended daily amounts of vitamin D are 200 to 400 IUs (international units) but no more than 800. A good quality multivitamin/mineral may have both, and offers good insurance toward having adequate quantities of many other important nutrients your body needs to maintain optimal bone health.

In the future, health-care providers may have a test to determine who is genetically at risk for developing osteoporosis. Recently, Australian researchers discovered that women with two copies of the variant of the gene for the body's vitamin D receptors reached a "fracture threshold" eight years earlier than women with two copies of the normal gene.

Are You at Risk?

Why do some of us develop osteoporosis? We need much more research to understand the causes, but some factors have been identified.

• **Loss of estrogen**. Women are most vulnerable to osteoporosis when they go through menopause, whether it occurs naturally or is surgically induced. During these years, the body is changing the way it makes estrogens and as the amount of estrogen produced declines, bone loss increases significantly. This is particularly true in the first five to seven years after menopause when we can lose from two to five percent of bone mass each year. After that the annual rate of loss slows to about one percent.

• **Cessation of menstrual periods.** Hormone imbalance, often characterized by lack of menstrual periods, may also contribute to bone loss. High-performance athletes are at risk. One study found that 40 percent of competitive women skaters do not have a menstrual period. Many young women who diet excessively or suffer from eating disorders like anorexia are at similar risk.

• **Smoking and alcohol.** Researchers have found strong links between smoking and reductions in bone mass, resulting in a deficit of five to 10 percent in some cases. Because it decreases levels of calcium and vitamin D in the body, moderate to heavy alcohol use can also reduce bone mass.

• **Diet.** Women may also be more vulnerable to osteoporosis in midlife if their calcium absorption has been low since childhood. The recommended amounts for children and young adults range from 800 to 1,500 mg/day. Vulnerability increases even more in later years as our bodies become less able to absorb this essential mineral.

Although as we age we have more difficulty absorbing calcium, doctors and the media still insist we increase our intake, both in our diet and supplements. This increase in unabsorbed calcium often leads to heart disease (the biggest killer of women past menopause) and arthritis.

Calcium, Bone Loss, and Caffeine

It takes more than calcium and other minerals to prevent or reduce osteoporosis (bone loss) in women who are past menopause. You need to also take a look at how much caffeine you're drinking. A study in the *American Journal of Clinical Nutrition* showed that women who drank two to three cups of brewed coffee or more (450 mg of caffeine) could have increased bone loss from their spines, especially if their calcium intake was less than 800 mg a day.

It would be interesting to determine in a medical study whether or not women who take additional calcium are absorbing it, since calcium absorption is inhibited as we age and our stomachs produce less acid. Antacids contribute to calcium malabsorption. Perhaps it is not the amount of calcium but our body's ability to absorb it that is the major factor. Still, it is important that women understand that more than one cup of brewed coffee may contribute to bone loss. Instant coffee and tea (especially green tea) have less caffeine per cup.

Diets high in sugar, protein, phosphorous (found in colas), and caffeine cause calcium to be excreted from the bones, contributing to osteoporosis. Some nutrients help the body absorb calcium into the bones, helping to prevent osteoporosis.

Magnesium contributes to calcium absorption. It is found in abundance in whole grain foods such as brown rice, oatmeal, corn tortillas, and whole grain breads, as well as legumes such as split peas, lentils, soy products, and beans.

Lack of vitamin D, which also helps the body absorb calcium, is a critical factor, particularly for older people who may not get enough sunlight, a primary source of the vitamin, and do not take vitamin supplements which include this vitamin.

In general, the better *all* nutrients in your diet are balanced, the more your bones will benefit.

• **Immobility**. Use it or lose it. People who are bedridden or in a cast for any length of time show evidence of bone loss from lack of use. An example of this is the astronauts who spend time in a weightless environment and get osteoporosis from their time in space. Women who exercise too little lose bone strength as well, placing them at greater risk for osteoporosis-related fractures.

• **Ethnicity and body type**. Caucasian and Asian women are more likely to develop osteoporosis than members of other ethnic groups. Although studies show that fewer African-American and Hispanic women experience the disease, they are still at risk and should take the same preventive measures. Thin, petite women are also more vulnerable. Although heavier women produce more estrogen and are thus better protected against osteoporosis than thin women, they also need to take their risk for the disorder seriously.

• **Medications**. Some medications given for other disorders may cause osteoporosis. The most common are glucocorticoids (steroid medicines), generally prescribed for diseases such as arthritis, asthma, and ulcerative colitis. As research progresses, we are learning that other medications, such as high doses of thyroid hormone, may also increase bone loss. Ask your health-care provider if any of your medications fall in this category and what, if anything, can be done about it.

Bone Density and Heredity

One important, and often overlooked, risk factor for osteoporosis is genetics. If you listened to the general media talk around the subject, you'd believe that just taking more calcium and walking daily will prevent this condition. Not so. While calcium metabolism and exercise are important, the major risk for osteoporosis appears to be genetic. Different genes are necessary for bone mineral density, including some that regulate the activity of bone cells, and others that regulate your body's balance of calcium, vitamin D, and other minerals.

If you have a family history of osteoporosis, you may have to work harder to prevent or slow down your own loss of bone minerals. In this case, having a health professional evaluate you for good digestion (you need enough hydrochloric acid in your stomach to break down and use calcium), dietary mineral balance, stress reduction, and exercise. If your family has a low incidence of osteoporosis, this doesn't give you license to eat poorly, ignore your mineral balance, and not exercise. Certain people may have a greater or lesser tendency for osteoporosis than others, but this is only a tendency.

Why Calcium Makes Bones More Brittle

Would you like your bones to be as brittle as chalk or as strong as ivory? You may have a choice in this. In fact, without realizing it, you may be opting for exactly what you don't want — brittle bones. This section addresses bone flexibility versus brittle bones, and answers a number of other questions relating to osteoporosis prevention and reversal.

The husband of one of our readers used to drink two gallons of milk every week, thinking that it would keep his bones strong. Then he developed definite signs of osteoporosis. He stopped drinking milk and is now taking magnesium to help the calcium in his diet get into his bones better.

She wanted to know why magnesium sometimes causes loose stools. Which is the best form of magnesium to take? And whether or not it should be taken with calcium or alone? She also asked what causes magnesium to make bones more flexible and less prone to fracture.

An Expert Says...

The media is bombarding you with appeals to consume massive quantities of calcium. I say ignore this hype and concentrate on a high magnesium intake, and this will actually enable you to absorb more calcium into your bones. Who should you believe?

To help better convince you of our position, I called on one of the country's leading experts on the subject, Dr. Guy Abraham. Dr. Abraham is a research gynecologist and endocrinologist in Southern California where he heads Optimox, Inc., a small supplement company that designs some of the most often copied nutrients on the market: Optivite PMT, a formula that has been shown to eliminate PMS; and Gynovite, a multivitamin/mineral that has been shown to reverse osteoporosis in a small but significant study.

Yes, he does have a vested interest in selling his products, but not in whether or not women (or men) use more magnesium and less calcium in general. He just advocates magnesium over calcium because he and others have found through scientific studies that it makes the most sense. He's an expert in the field who is always happy to give me general information I can pass on that's based on sound scientific studies.

First, why might magnesium cause loose stools? Because it's not well absorbed. Unabsorbed magnesium that enters your large intestine causes diarrhea. So you want to be able to utilize this mineral before it gets to your gut. This means you need enough hydrochloric acid (HCl) in your stomach to begin breaking it down. Antacids neutralize stomach acids. Taking antacids along with magnesium is counterproductive and can contribute to loose stools. Just as taking an antacid prevents calcium (which is in some antacid tablets) from being absorbed, it prevents magnesium absorption as well. Chew your food well to stimulate your body's natural production of HCl, and remember that as you age, your body produces less of this digestive juice, so don't overeat.

Next, find a well-absorbed form of magnesium such as magnesium citrate, aspartate, or chelate. If you get loose stools from taking even 100-200 mg of magnesium, try switching to another form of magnesium oxide. If another form causes loose stools you might want to try Dr. Abraham's. (Optimox, Inc., 800-223-1601). According to Dr. Abraham, a well-absorbed form of magnesium should be tolerated at levels of around 600 to 800 mg/day.

When you want to increase the bone-strengthening effect of magnesium, take it alone, not with calcium. You may have a supplement that contains both minerals, but which has insufficient magnesium to meet your requirements (several studies have shown that 500 mg of calcium and 600-1,000 mg of magnesium can reverse osteoporosis). In this case, take additional magnesium alone.

Chapter 10

Osteoporosis, Part 2: Kiss Frailty Goodbye!*

The closer Clara Hough got to the century mark, the harder it became for her to do the normal, everyday tasks she had done all her life.

Her legs weren't able to hold her steady any longer and the steps outside her mobile home seemed to get tougher to transverse every day.

She had given up the one thing she loved to do the most, gardening, several years earlier and she could tell her days of walking about without a cane or walker were quickly coming to an end. Her daughters were having to do more and more for her, including meal preparation, which was especially troublesome — she had always prided herself in her cooking.

Sadly, Clara's situation is not uncommon for women (and men) who are in the latter part of their golden years. Even women in their 70s find they can't do as much as they could just 10 or 15 years earlier. And if you have arthritis, rheumatism, back injuries, sore knees, a frozen shoulder, or have had a heart attack, you may feel frail at 50!

Frailty is a huge factor of aging. By age 70, most people have at least 20 percent less muscle than they did at age 30. *About 70 percent of elderly women are too frail to lift just 10 pounds, and 60 percent cannot perform such household work as vacuuming.* About 35 percent of men are equally frail.

The good news, though, is that you're not destined to become frail. And if you're already so frail you can't do the things you really enjoy, there's even more good news — frailty doesn't have to be part

*Portions reprinted from *The Giant Book of Women's Health Secrets*

of your life. In fact, studies have found that even 90-year-olds can rebuild lost muscle and bone structure with some careful exercise.

What Determines Frailty?

The three main factors related to frailty are muscle and bone deterioration and balance. (Other factors, such as ligament and cartilage damage, also contribute, but not to the same degree.) While most people are aware that muscles are strengthened by exercise, few people realize that bones are also strengthened by exercise.

Bones are tissues that can grow or shrink, depending on how well you take care of them. If you've ever broken a bone, you've seen firsthand how bone tissue grows to heal the fracture.

In order for your muscles to grow in strength and help you keep your balance, you have to subject them to a certain degree of stress. Your bones are no different. The difference comes in the type of stress each responds to. While your muscles respond to contractile stress, your bones must undergo bending, compression, and twisting to experience stress. As with muscles, you can overdo the stress on your bones, which is when you suffer breaks and stress fractures.

On the other extreme, if your bones and muscles don't undergo at least a minimal amount of stress on a regular basis, they begin to atrophy. The adage "use it or lose it" definitely applies here.

The degree of stress your bones and muscles must experience in order to grow is called the minimal essential strain. This is the point that if surpassed often enough will cause the bone or muscle to call in help to deal with the stress. This help comes in the form of osteoblasts, which migrate to the area being stressed and help build more muscle and bone tissue.

As we age, our muscles and joints tighten, arthritis often sets in, and years of neglecting our body begins to take its toll. The exercise we know we need gets harder and harder to do, so a sedentary lifestyle sets in (or continues). Let's face it, very few of us enjoy getting out of our comfort zones, especially when it hurts.

But that inactivity is a prime cause of frailty.

Setting Some Standards

I've discussed many times how necessary it is for women to have a regular exercise program, regardless of how old you are or how strenuous the exercise program. And I'm not the only one spreading the news. Hundreds of magazines and TV and radio programs have confirmed what I've been reporting for years. So by now, you're probably as convinced as I am of the necessity to exercise.

But before you begin an exercise routine, you need to find out what kind of condition you're in right now. This helps you determine what type of exercise you can begin with, and it sets a standard you can use to see how you're improving.

To help you in this process, researchers have come up with a way to check your "frailness factor."

Roberta Rikli, PhD, a professor at California State University, Fullerton, led a study of 7,000 Americans ages 60 to 94 that established a set of tests to help you determine your fitness standards. That's an impressive number of subjects and lends credence to the project.

If the tests signal you're at risk of becoming too frail, "we can do something to try to prevent that," Dr. Rikli said. The exercise tests are simple enough that many people could try them at home, but I think it's best to do the exercises with your doctor, so you won't be tempted to overdo it.

Rikli and her colleague Jessie Jones devised the following simple tests:

• How many times in 30 seconds can you rise from a straight-backed chair without using your arms to push yourself up? This measures lower body strength.

• How many times in 30 seconds can you lift a weight — five pounds for women, eight pounds for men — in a "biceps curl." This measures upper body strength.

• How many yards can you walk in six minutes, to measure aerobic fitness?

• How long does it take you to rise from a chair, walk eight feet, and return to a seated position, to measure mobility?

Rikli found that fitness declined with age, on average, one percent a year. Regardless of age, people who got moderate physical activity at least three times a week were the most fit. "Our main interest is in keeping people mobile and staying physically independent as long as possible," said Rikli.

Some doctors already use similar but experimental tests to assess elderly patients' limitations. "They're very powerful predictors" of who will wind up disabled, said Dr. Jack Guralnik of the National Institute on Aging.

Getting Started With Resistance Exercises

Once you've done the simple tests above, it's time to start "stressing" your muscles and bones. This will help strengthen your muscles, contribute to their ability to help keep your balance, and help build bone density. It's extremely important that you start out slowly and not hurt yourself while you're trying to improve your condition. Most exercise regimes I've seen are lengthy and difficult to do if you have any chronic pain — and most of us do, at least at times. We need an exercise program we can keep doing even when we have a sore shoulder, pains in our knees, and an achy back. That's why I personally like the idea of specific resistance training.

Some months ago, I talked with rheumatologist Robert Swezey, MD. Dr. Swezey had been looking for a way to increase range of motion as well as build bone density in his arthritis patients. What he discovered has great implications not only for people with arthritis, but folks who have had heart attacks or who have hypertension.

Dr. Swezey found that when you stress your muscles at the place where they attach to the bone, your body builds denser bones as well as strengthens your muscles. Let me give you an example. If you want to build strong biceps, you can do a "biceps curl" and strengthen your upper arm. What you're doing is stressing your biceps in the middle of your upper arm. But Dr. Swezey found that if you stress the biceps at its attachments — to your elbow and shoulder — then you encourage your bone to grow at those sites. So, which would you prefer? Do you want a big bulging muscle in the middle of your upper arm, or would you rather have nice muscle tone and stronger bones?

Dr. Swezey went through the body and came up with exercises that build bone not only in the legs and arms, but the hips and spine as well. He found that the easiest way to do these exercises was with a partially inflated ball. The ball could be used with very specific exercises to increase a person's range of motion as well as strengthen muscles. And the end result was denser bones.

So Dr. Swezey tested his theory and published his findings in the *Journal of Rheumatology 2000*. Then he wrote out the exercises he found worked and had a ball with handles manufactured that he called the OsteoBall. By the way, Dr. Swezey also found that resistance exercises may be even better than weight-bearing exercises such as walking to prevent osteoporosis.

But I think what I like most about the specific resistance exercises Dr. Swezey has come up with is that they can not only reverse osteoporosis, but reverse frailty. You see, you're not "stuck" with poor balance. You can improve your bone density. And you can strengthen your muscles throughout your body even if you have physical limitations that prevent you from walking, running, or using heavy exercise equipment.

Oh, yes, and the rest of the good news is that Dr. Swezey's program takes only 10 minutes a day (or 20 minutes every other day). For more information on how to purchase an OsteoBall, please call 800-728-2288.

Get Hip to Fracture Prevention*

Let's face it. Broken bones just aren't hip. In fact, hip fractures, which affect 17.5 percent of white North American women over 50, and six percent of similarly aged white North American men, are not only inconvenient; they also kill, disable, and substantially increase medical costs. Studies have found that up to 20 percent of those who suffer a hip fracture die, and at least half of those who survive are less able to perform activities of daily living for at least a year. In other words, these fractures — usually the result of osteoporosis — carry a high price. To avoid paying that price, consumers need to take action to prevent hip fractures. But how?

A study reported in the *New England Journal of Medicine*

---

* Parts excerpted from *People's Medical Society*

sheds some light on the subject. The study examined potential risk factors for hip fracture in 9,516 white women 65 or older, confirming previously discovered factors, identifying several new ones, and disproving others. This information can be used to identify people at risk for hip fracture, inform them of that risk and help them reduce it. It can also be used to help people in general reduce their risk of fracturing a hip.

According to the study, the risk factors for hip fracture include:

Maternal history: Women whose mothers had a hip fracture had twice the risk of having a hip fracture than women whose mothers did not. The risk increased to 2.7 percent if the mother fractured her hip before age 80.

Lack of weight-bearing exercise: Women who spent four hours per day or less on their feet had twice the risk of women who spent more than four hours per day on their feet. And women who walked regularly for exercise had a 30 percent lower risk of hip fracture than those who did not walk regularly. And their risk decreased as the distance they walked increased.

Caffeine intake: As caffeine intake increased, so did the risk of hip fracture.

Other factors found to increase risk are:
- A history of hyperthyroidism.
- Use of long-acting benzo-diazepines (tranquilizers) or anticonvulsant drugs.
- Poor depth perception.
- Poor contrast sensitivity (ability to distinguish visual contrast).
- A fast resting pulse.
- The inability to rise from a chair without using one's arms.
- A history of fractures after age 50.

On the positive side, several factors previously suspected of increasing the risk were found not to increase risk. They include: hair color, ethnic ancestry, a maternal history of fractures other than hip fractures, the timing of menopause, past smoking status, cataracts, the use of short-acting benzodiazepines, and a low dietary intake of calcium.

The study found that women with multiple risk factors, which may reduce bone density or increase the risk of falls and those with low bone density itself, are at high risk of fracturing a hip and should focus on preventive efforts. An accompanying editorial said these findings may also be helpful in designing strategies to prevent hip fractures in general.

For example, the study adds to the evidence that customary physical inactivity among elderly women increases the risk for hip fractures. The editorial said, "Women who are able should be advised to walk for exercise or spend four hours a day on their feet, and that if this practice is followed, the incidence of hip fracture in the general population should be reduced. In addition, there will be additional cardiovascular and psychological benefits, and the intervention is culturally acceptable as well as relatively inexpensive and safe."

The study also supports the finding that modifying the risk factors for falls may reduce the risk of hip fracture. Medications that increase the risk of falling should be curtailed; exercise programs, which may improve neuromuscular coordination, should be undertaken; and improvements to the home should be made, including the elimination of hazards such as loose rugs and the installation of structures such as grab bars and stair rails, which help prevent falls.

Other methods for reducing hip fractures include: Increasing physical activity in general; avoiding long-acting sedative-hypnotic drugs; reducing caffeine intake; quitting smoking; treating and preventing impaired vision, particularly conditions like cataracts, diabetic retinopathy, and glaucoma, which impair depth perception and contrast sensitivity; and maintaining bone density.

Hip Fracture Risk-Reduction Checklist

- Increase your level of physical activity.
- Walk for exercise.
- Spend at least four hours a day on your feet.
- Engage in exercise that may improve your coordination.
- Decrease your caffeine intake.

- Avoid long-acting sedative or hypnotic drugs.
- Quit smoking.
- Get regular eye exams and treat visual problems.
- Secure loose rugs, electrical wires and other falling hazards.
- Use light-colored carpet, paint, or other finish on stairs to increase depth perception visibility.
- At night, use a small, plug-in night-light to light up path from bed to bathroom.
- Install grab bars, stair rails, and other structures that can help prevent falls.

Making Bones Strong: Chalk vs. Ivory

Let's address the subject of bone flexibility, since this may be the determining factor in whether or not your bones break when you fall as you get older. The more flexible your bones, the less likely you are to break them. Bone density is only one part of osteoporosis — the part we can now easily measure. Bone flexibility may be even more important, though. And we have no sophisticated tests to let us know whether or not our bones are brittle. This is why doctors only talk about how dense your bones are.

As I discussed in the previous chapter, calcium contains properties that makes bones brittle, while magnesium binds to protein in your bones and keeps them supple. Take a look at two substances in nature with relationship to these properties of suppleness and brittleness: chalk and ivory. Chalk is pure calcium carbonate, the stuff they put in mineral supplements to help you meet your daily requirements. Take a new piece of chalk and drop it. Watch it break. Then compare it with a piece of ivory the same size taken from an elephant's tusk. The ivory is a combination of calcium and magnesium. Now, which do you need, more calcium or more magnesium?

Dr. Abraham believes we can get sufficient calcium from our foods without taking additional amounts in supplement form. His supplements, which have been shown to improve bones, are lower than most in calcium. I suggest you may need more magnesium to make your bones more like ivory and less like chalk. And that you find a product that will allow you to increase your magnesium to

600-800 mg/day while limiting calcium supplements to around 500 mg. You'll get even more calcium as well as magnesium in whole foods like whole grains (millet is especially high), beans, nuts and seeds, dark green leafy vegetables, as well as tofu and soy products. The minerals you take are not just in pills. They're in your food, as well.

So when your doctor suggests you take more calcium or consider taking hormones or other prescription drugs to increase your bone density, ask him or her what they suggest to make your bones more flexible. If they don't have an answer, tell them about magnesium.

Beware of Bone-Density Testing!

Doctors' offices across the country are being filled by a new breed of diagnostic machines. These new machines measure your bone density and they sound like a good idea — especially if you're interested in preventing osteoporosis.

But watch out! If you're old enough, you're virtually guaranteed that one of these machines will convince your doctor that you have, or are at dangerous risk of developing osteoporosis. Then, before a meaningful discussion can take place, your doctor will likely write you a prescription for one or more osteoporosis drugs — such as Fosamax or Premarin. But is this the best course of action?

It used to be that osteoporosis was diagnosed when an older person with brittle bones actually suffered a fracture.

In recent years, however, the definition of osteoporosis has changed. In 1991, a panel of medical experts, in a report that appeared in the *American Journal of Medicine*, redefined osteoporosis as: "A disease characterized by low bone mass and microarchitectural deterioration of bone tissue, which lead to increased bone fragility and a consequent increase in fracture risk." In plain English, this new definition of osteoporosis simply means you have an increased risk of fracture, not that you had a fracture or will definitely get a fracture.

But doctors are now diagnosing osteoporosis by completely disregarding your bone's flexibility, fragility, and micro-architec-

ture (in the aforementioned definition), and instead are heavily relying on bone density, which can be easily measured using various
machines. Some of these machines are more accurate than others,
though there are accuracy problems with all of them.

In addition, many are inadequate for precisely monitoring
your progress, including the results of any therapy you are using to
prevent osteoporosis. Yet doctors persist in using these machines for
this purpose as well. Urine tests, which measure the rate of bone
breakdown as reflected in various markers, are also problematic.
They can produce day-to-day variations of up to 40 and even 50
percent. Unfortunately, there are no tests to measure bone flexibility vs. fragility.

In addition, bone density is not always the same throughout
your body. A high or low density reading in one area, say the heel
or lower spine, doesn't necessarily mean you have similar density
elsewhere in more critical locations such as your wrist, hip, or upper
spine, where fractures are most likely to occur.

Finally, to complicate matters even more, deposits of unab-

Irritable Bowel and Strong Bones

Can you have strong, healthy bones if you have Crohn's disease or
Irritable Bowel Syndrome (IBS)? The authors of a recent study published in
the *Journal of Pediatric Gastroenterology Nutrition* say, probably not.
Using blood samples from children ages seven to 16 years of age who had
either Crohn's disease or ulcerative colitis, there was poorer bone formation
and more bone loss in all of them than in the controls who had normal bowel
function.

It appears that inflammation in the bowel produces substances,
pro-inflammatory cytokines, which prevent bones from absorbing nutrients.
Ultimately, the authors say, this leads to bone loss. Further studies will need
to be performed to give additional information. For now, just realize that
bowel problems should, if at all possible, be treated. Often, an elimination
diet, beginning with avoiding sugar, dairy, wheat, and other grains, is sufficient. Speak with your medical or alternative doctor for additional suggestions for your particular case.

Hyams, J.S., et al. "Alterations in bone metabolism in children with inflammatory bowel disease: an in vitro study," *J Pediatr Gastroenterol Nutr* 24(3), 289-95,1997.

sorbed calcium — perhaps from arthritis — can result in overreads, in which machines report higher density than actually exists.

The bottom line on test results is this: Don't make assumptions. Instead, get straightforward answers from your doctor about the accuracy and real meaning of any bone-density and bone-loss testing.

Impossible Standards Are Also Deceptive

One reader recently wrote, "I am trying to decide which estrogen to take. My bone density is at 85 percent, and I'm 55 years old."

It's easy to understand how, upon first hearing that your bone density is 85 percent or even 60 percent or another percent less than 100, you might be concerned. But when we take a closer look at exactly what these numbers mean, it's easy to see that (even if test results were completely accurate) their value and importance is still limited.

That's because all test results are compared to the peak bone density of a typical premenopausal female, not other women in your own age group, including the ones who are actually getting fractures. This is akin to telling postmenopausal women they are estrogen-deficient and, therefore, diseased simply because their estrogen levels are not comparable to those of premenopausal women. This is ridiculous. Estrogen levels do decrease after menopause. Bones do lose some of their density. But this doesn't mean they are going to break.

Rather than taking age-related differences into account, however, doctors compare your bone density to premenopausal peak levels to determine your T score, in which the T stands for fracture threshold. Now here's the catch. According to the bone-mass chart, which the National Osteoporosis Foundation was kind enough to send me, by age 80 nearly every woman will have bone density below the fracture threshold. Once your bone density falls below this fateful line, you are deemed to be at increased risk of fracture, and therefore are diagnosed as having osteoporosis.

Dr. Susan Love, a leading authority on female health care, summarizes the predicament this way: "The level of bone density that [now] defines osteoporosis has been set rather high, with the result that most older women will fall into the 'disease' category — which is very nice for the people in the business of treating disease."

Osteoporosis Is Now Big Business!

In spite of the fact that only 39 percent of older women will ever suffer a fracture....

Or the fact that the large majority of these fractures will be minor and have no permanent long-term consequences (most people who suffer osteoporosis-related fractures recover and return to their normal lives)....

Or the fact that a combination of frailty, weakness, and other considerations such as slippery or poorly lit walking surfaces, poor balance, and a lack of mental alertness (often a side effect of prescription drugs), also frequently contribute to the occurrence of disabling or life-threatening fractures....

Most researchers now advocate that women whose bone density is nearing or already below the fracture threshold need treatment — which usually includes prescription drugs.

Is it possible that health-conscious women are being marketed a disease that requires them to load up on lots of expensive doctor's appointments, diagnostic testing, and prescription drug treatments?

Merck, the maker of the popular osteoporosis treatment drug Fosamax, wrote in its 1995 Annual Report that, "We have been aggressively working to educate consumers about the disease and the importance of early diagnosis and appropriate treatment with organizations such as the National Osteoporosis Foundation, the Older Women's League, and members of the European parliament. We have established the Bone Measurement Institute, a non-profit organization, to increase the accessibility and affordability of bone measurement technologies. Merck has also provided funding for the first world summit of osteoporosis societies."

This excerpt basically says that Merck is helping to fund the distribution of bone-density testing machines around the country. So wherever you are, it will be easier for you to get to one of these machines, get diagnosed with osteoporosis, and maybe even start taking Merck's drug Fosamax. (Remember that annual reports are about profits, not public service.)

What's more, during the next two years, you might not have to go out of your way at all to get your bone density measured. As I was writing the above paragraph, I received a phone call and long fax from a public relations firm being paid to tell me about a newly formed group called The Osteoporosis Business Coalition, and the new osteoporosis public awareness campaign this coalition is launching. The campaign will offer free bone-density testing at work sites, as well as other locations including the National Association of Realtors State Conventions and Dress Barn clothing outlets.

More prominent members of this coalition include Wyeth-Ayerst Laboratories, the maker of today's best-selling estrogen supplement (Premarin), which happens to slow bone loss and Proctor & Gamble Pharmaceuticals that is getting ready to launch a new osteoporosis treatment drug called Actonel. (I'll report the scoop on Actonel after it gets final FDA approval.) In other words, here are more businesses promoting bone-density testing that stand to profit when women are found to have low bone density. And the National Osteoporosis Foundation is in cahoots with this coalition, as well.

In the midst of current and coming propaganda that plays on our fears of becoming disfigured and disabled with osteoporosis, it will become increasingly easy to get the idea that if your bone density is low, you're destined to become a hunched-over little old lady who eventually falls, breaks a hip, and spends the remainder of her days in a convalescent home. Although this serious and life-threatening, worst-case scenario does indeed happen, it's not as likely to happen to you as vested interests would like you to believe.

For a more realistic perspective, take a closer look at the older women around you in your community and your family. What do you see? Few, if any, women stooped over with dowager's humps, and probably a good number of healthy, active older women. What's more, there's a lot more you can do — besides taking potentially harmful drugs — to help ensure you have healthy bones in your senior years, even if you're already in them.

Here's a parting thought on the importance of bone density that you might share with your doctor: Asian women are living proof that bone density is of highly limited value in determining fracture risk. Their bone density averages are so low that simply being Asian is frequently listed as a risk factor for osteoporosis. Yet Asian women have far fewer hip fractures than Caucasian women. Asian women also consume little, if any, dairy foods.

To Prevent Fractures, Prevent Falls

For persons with reasonably good health, a good diet (emphasizing magnesium instead of calcium), a moderate amount of exercise, and a healthy lifestyle are the best ways to keep bones healthy.

But what if your general and/or bone health is declining, putting you at a greater risk of bone fracture?

Fortunately, there are additional steps you can take to help prevent fractures. Even those of us with excellent bone health can benefit from reading this — because most women eventually become caretakers of someone who is at increased risk of fracture.

Make Balance a Top Priority

One of the most critical considerations for such persons is balance. After all, the better your balance, the less likely you are to fall and, in turn, suffer a fracture. Other key factors that affect balance and the risk of falling are strength, mental alertness, and vision.

So the first line of defense for protecting bones in persons at increased risk of fracture is to protect and, if possible, improve balance, strength, mental alertness, and vision.

A general fitness and exercise program can work wonders for balance and strength, which are closely related. Increased strength can improve balance. And practically everyone can increase his or her strength and overall fitness. Even assisted-care settings often offer physical fitness programs. Limited-ability fitness classes and video exercise tapes can also be helpful. The bottom line here is that fitness improvements can help a person avoid a fall, and even speed recovery if a fracture does occur (the better your health, the better you heal).

An exercise program can also improve mental alertness, by improving circulation, metabolism, oxygen to the brain, etc. Many medications, on the other hand, have side effects that dull alertness. Work with your doctor to possibly eliminate, or reduce dosages of any medication that is having this effect. Also look into doing the same with other medications that might make you feel dizzy, weak, cause blurred vision, or any other side effects that might impair your ability to walk.

To maximize vision, get your eyes checked regularly and update glasses prescriptions as needed. When you get a new pair of glasses, take it extra easy until you get used to the new lenses. If glasses are interfering with your depth perception as you walk, work with your ophthalmologist or optician to get the problem resolved. And if your depth perception is better without your glasses, remember to remove them when walking on uneven surfaces or going up or down steps.

Fall-Proof Yourself and Your Home

There are also a number of ways, beyond fitness improvements, to fall-proof yourself. For starters, wear shoes with soles that have a good, gripping tread.

Also use a cane or walker at all times, if doing so improves your stability. A surprising number of seniors are reluctant to do so. Yes, walking aids can be bothersome, but a severe hip fracture can be life threatening, and the worse your health, the more so.

Dr. Susan Love suggests frail seniors wear protective padding. And if doing so prevents a fracture, you'll have the last laugh! You may be able to rig up your own system, using a regular girdle as the foundation. A wide range of ready-made protective clothing is also available at your local sporting goods store. Ask about football girdles, which pad the hips and tailbone (which can also be vulnerable to fracture), and work so well even NFL pros wear them. Make the extra effort to find padding that's comfortable, so you'll wear it on a regular basis.

Last, don't leave home without reminding yourself to be extra careful every step of the way in unfamiliar places — especially on steps and stairs, and when getting into and out of cars, busses, trains, and planes. If you're on a long trip, take periodic brief walks if possible or do some in-seat exercises to make sure your legs are warmed up and ready to walk when it's time. Then proceed slowly with extra care and caution. Finally, don't hesitate to ask for a wheelchair or other assistance. After all, everyone wants you to have a safe trip.

Just as important as fall-proofing yourself is fall-proofing your home by making changes that would decrease your risk of falling. Make sure walking surfaces (inside and out) are level, and carpets and rugs are secured in their places. All steps and stairwells should be well lit, plus have side rails to hold onto when ascending and descending. Outside steps and smooth walkways that get wet may need abrasive strips to provide more secure footing. The path from your bed to the bathroom should be well lit and free of clutter and other objects on which you might trip.

In addition, consider using handicap aids in your bathroom. These can include raised toilet seats, sturdy grab-bars beside the toilet, and in all bath and shower stalls. Stall and bathtub bottoms should also have adhesive stripping or a large, top quality bath mat. Also consider using a chair or stool in the bath and shower and at the sink.

Drugs: A Last Line of Defense

If you know your bone density is extra low, well below the fracture threshold, or you've already suffered a fracture, or have another reason to believe that you're at exceptional risk of incurring a fracture, taking a bone-building prescription drug may be a good idea. Proceed with caution in your decision-making, however, because they all have adverse side affects. Ask your doctor to review them all with you. Plus, discuss with your doctor the actual short- and long-term results you can expect from any osteoporosis drug.

Thoroughly reviewing with your doctor what you stand to gain vs. the side effects you risk with currently available osteoporosis drugs, may make other fracture-prevention measures — such as increasing magnesium (and lowering calcium) intake, get-

ting more exercise, and fall-proofing yourself and your home —
suddenly seem much more attractive. In addition, by covering these
bases first, you might be so impressed with the results; you decide
you don't need to risk taking drugs to prevent a fracture.

It's Never Too Late!

A six-month study of two dozen women over the age of 75
(the average age was 79), reports that exercising an hour a day twice
a week can improve balance, other muscle coordination, and muscle strength. The exercise included warm-up, light aerobics, and
calisthenics.

Loss of balance as we age is one of the most predictive risks
for falls and broken bones. While more frequent exercise could
improve your heart, preventing falls and broken hips ranks high on
our "to do" list. Consider starting before you're 75! Join a gym if
you're not disciplined, or buy a videotape or two for bi-weekly
workouts.

Chapter 11

Why Women Get Breast Cancer*

W e're losing the war on breast cancer and it looks like it's getting worse. So is environmental pollution and the cumulative
effect of pesticide residues in our food.

Is there a connection? I think so, and so do many others.

Doctors at the Universite Laval in Quebec, Canada have said
"The upward trend in breast-cancer risk parallels that of the historical pattern of organochlorine accumulation in the environment."
Organ ochlorines, found in many pesticides, act like estrogen in our
bodies and promote the common estrogen-receptor positive form of
breast cancer and contribute to testicular cancer. They're affecting
our hormone balance.

Fifty years ago, one in 20 women got breast cancer. Thirty-five
years ago the risk increased to one in 15. Today, the figure
has jumped to one in eight. Look around you at a school meeting for
parents, in church, or at a play or concert. Look around you at the
supermarket. One out of eight women in the room with you is likely
to get breast cancer. That's frightening. When you include yourself in
this equation, it's terrifying. And when you realize that you may be
passing along this risk to your unborn children, it becomes unthinkable. But unless we think about a problem and face it, we can't
change it. Fortunately, even with incidents of breast cancer increasing, there is something you can do about lowering your risk.

According to Liane Clorfene-Casten in her book, *Breast
Cancer: Poisons, Profits and Prevention* (Common Courage Press,
1996, $18.95), 30 percent of women who contract breast cancer are

*Portions reprinted from *The Giant Book of Women's Health Secrets*

affected by the amount of estrogen they produce in their bodies, along with the length of time they produce it. The longer a woman's body is exposed to estrogen; the more she is at risk. Beginning menstruation early with a late onset of menopause and having no children (to interrupt your estrogen producing years) increases the risk for breast-cancer. That's the genetic component to breast-cancer risk, but it's the smaller percentage of women who contract the disease.

It is now more widely believed that 70 percent of women who get breast cancer are very likely getting it from increased exposure to chemicals in the air and water, and foods contaminated with pesticides that act like estrogen in their bodies. These chemicals, called organochlorines, can cause cells to grow abnormally and often lead to cancer.

Organochlorines are found most commonly in many pesticides and insecticides. They get into the foods we eat, the air we breathe, and the water we drink. They are present in particularly high quantities in breast milk, where they accumulate in fat cells, so

Women Ignore Tamoxifen Results

A chilling letter written by a number of English doctors, was recently published in *The Lancet* (October 10, 1998). It points out that every one of the 4,500 women enrolled in a study using tamoxifen to prevent breast cancer are remaining in the study, even after American researchers conducting a similar study showed that tamoxifen resulted in higher incidents of endometrial cancer and embolisms.

The American trial was stopped, but in an English trial, comprised of women in the UK, Europe, and Australia, all have opted to continue. Almost one-third of these women were concerned about the toxicity of tamoxifen, but all wanted to continue as participants. Scientific studies often turn out to give false results, but we believe we should all err on the side of caution.

While tamoxifen, as a preventive agent, may decrease a woman's risk of breast cancer by a whopping 45 percent, the risk of other life-threatening illnesses should be taken into account. I am astonished that not one woman has dropped out of this study.

Hutchings, Owen, et al. "Effect of early American results on patients in a tamoxifen prevention trial (IBIS)," *The Lancet,* vol 352, October 10, 1998.

if your exposure to these chemicals is high — such as eating non-organic foods high in pesticides (grapes, strawberries, lettuce, and artichokes are among the most heavily sprayed) — you may be unknowingly storing up and passing along potent carcinogens to any infant you are breast-feeding. Still, I don't advocate you stop breast-feeding. The benefits of giving your baby a stronger immune system through breast milk outweigh the dangers. What you can do is to become more aware of your exposure to these chemicals and reduce it by eating more organic or unsprayed foods.

Liane Clorfene-Casten talks about the role of these environmental carcinogens in great detail in her book. I can only touch on them here. What she proclaims is that the operative word when it comes to an increased risk for breast cancer appears to be "estrogen." Not just the stuff found in hormone replacement therapy (HRT), although this needs to be assessed along with your total lifetime exposure. But the estrogen that comes from chemicals that mimic this hormone in your body — the organochlorines found in pesticides.

When the Diagnosis Is Cancer

There's a lot of money to be made in cancer therapies. Some have good track records — excellent doctors with real data of remissions, or beating the odds in length of survival and quality of life. Some, on the other hand, are just ways to get you to trade your money for hope.

To complicate matters, cancer therapy is a highly individual issue. Not all cancers are alike. And people differ tremendously in their biochemical makeup. This makes it easy to get confused when you hear about the results others have gotten with various treatments. Just because something worked for someone else doesn't mean it will work for you.

Fortunately, there are people who do nothing but research different types of cancers, talk with scientists and doctors around the world, and prepare reports on your specific kind of cancer. These reports range from 20 to 40 pages, are packed with information and suggestions, and can help take a lot of the guesswork out of selecting a course of treatment.

Types of Breast Lumps

Pseudolump: Breast tissue approaching one inch in diameter that has formed into a lump, such as a pocket of dead fat or scar tissue that resulted from trauma caused by surgery or injury. Can also include pieces of silicone.

Lumpiness: Consists of little lumps that are approximately an eighth of an inch in diameter. Some doctors still needlessly alarm patients by diagnosing this condition of general lumpiness as fibrocystic breast disease. In reality it is harmless, perfectly natural, and has not been linked to later development of breast cancer.

Cyst: Most common in women between ages 30 and 55, these lumps are fluid-filled sacks. Near the surface, cysts feel squishy. Those that are more deeply embedded in breast tissue feel harder because overlying tissue obscures the squishiness.

Fibroadenoma or fibroid: A lump ranging from approximately half an inch to two-and-a-half inches or larger in diameter. A rare cancer, called cystosarcoma phylloides, occurs in about one

---

Colon-Cancer Marker

I've talked about a high-fiber diet and magnesium as solutions to constipation. Now we find that frequent constipation can be a marker for colon cancer. In a study of over 800 people, half of whom had colon cancer, it was found that those who were chronically constipated had a higher risk for getting colon cancer. For people who were constipated more than 52 times in a year, the risk quadrupled. Using laxatives did not contribute to colon cancer, say the researchers. It's the production of cancer-causing chemicals, released during fermentation in the intestines that sit around too long when a person is constipated.

Still, if you've been constipated over a period of time, you do want to check with your doctor to rule out any problem. In the people participating in this study, colon cancer followed after two years of constipation. Many people are constipated much longer than this.

A high-fiber diet and taking extra magnesium is a good way of moving food through the intestines. So is regular exercise and drinking water throughout the day.

Jacobs, E.J. and E. White. "Constipation, laxative use, and colon cancer among middle-aged adults," Epidemiology 9 (4), 1998. *Int'l J Clin Nutr,* April 99, 111.

percent of all fibroadenoma lumps (usually the larger ones). This type of cancer is relatively harmless because it doesn't spread.

Cancer lump: By the time a cancerous lump is large enough for you to feel, it has usually grown to about half an inch in diameter. If a cancerous lump is much smaller, you won't feel it. This is because in the early stages, a lump of cancerous cells feels like normal tissue. Once this lump of cells has grown big enough for the body to react to it, scar tissue will form around it that makes it detectable by touch. In this way, a cancer lump can appear suddenly. It will not change with menstrual cycles and is rarely painful.

Prevention Is Often Possible

New findings on the preventive value of exercise alone, reconfirm that breast cancer can indeed often be avoided. A while back, a detailed study of more than 1,000 women by Dr. Leslie Bernstein of the University of Southern California School of Medicine in Los Angeles, found that women who exercised 3.8 or more hours a week were less than half as likely to develop breast cancer as inactive women. Among the most active women who had experienced at least one full-term pregnancy, the risk was reduced by an impressive 72 percent.

Additionally, researchers from the University of Tromso and the Cancer Registry of Norway in Oslo found that women who exercised at least four hours a week were 37 percent less likely to get breast cancer than the least active women. Even greater reductions were seen in lean women under 45 who had been exercising regularly for three to five years. This study was based on 25,000 women who were followed an average of 14 years. Why such a dramatic difference between exercisers and couch potatoes? Exercise decreases estrogen production, enough so that, over a lifetime, it can significantly decrease breast-cancer risk. What's more, there are many excellent ways to boost your chances of not getting breast cancer (or having a recurrence) — and these simple strategies will be well worth a little extra effort since they will also lower a multitude of other serious health risks.

Good Food Is Good Medicine, Too

An article in the *Journal of the National Cancer Institute* also recently reported that breast-cancer risk was cut in half for pre-menopausal women who ate the highest amounts of vegetables. Fruits did not reduce their risk. The article goes on to say that no single dietary factor explained why breast-cancer risks decreased so much when women ate more veggies. It may be years before science understands the protective effects of nutrients other than major vitamins and minerals, and the interactions between nutrients that boost our health.

Essential Fats

The threat of breast cancer sits quietly in the recesses of our minds, jumping out to alarm us when we hear about a friend or family member who has just been diagnosed.

High-Dose Chemotherapy

Original studies on high-dose chemotherapy for breast cancer patients indicated that it might be an effective form of treatment. But that was what non-randomized studies showed, and it was only part of the picture.

Unfortunately, before any large, randomized studies were completed, results of the first studies leaked out. We're desperate for a solution to breast cancer, and it's only natural that we look for answers promised in the media. But sometimes these results are premature and can cause more harm than good. This is one example.

While consumer groups argue that women should be able to use whatever resources are out there, including high-dose chemotherapy, the National Breast Cancer Coalition disagrees. It is convinced after looking at all the data that high-dose chemotherapy often destroys bone marrow, resulting in a need for a bone-marrow transplant. It also points to a 7.4 percent treatment-based mortality cited in one study.

In Europe, cancer specialists are reluctant to routinely use high-dose chemotherapy for breast cancer. We need to consider not only patient's rights, but the effectiveness of any treatment and its risks over a period of time. To make decisions based on preliminary studies can be counterproductive and may even be dangerous.

Editorial, "Chaos surrounds high-dose chemotherapy for breast cancer," *The Lancet,* Vol 353, May 15, 1999.

We feel frightened and powerless. And yet, we have more power than we exert. Fear can be paralyzing and cause us to retreat into denial. "This won't happen to me. It can't." Unfortunately, it can. Let's look at some of what you can do to promote healthy breasts and reduce your risk for breast cancer. Previously I discussed the importance of substituting foods exposed to organochlorines for organic foods. Now I'd like to expand on other avenues you can explore to support your total health and reduce your risk for breast cancer.

Consume More EFAs

The type and quality of the fats and oils in your diet may be either increasing or decreasing your risk for breast cancer. Perhaps the most widely respected authority on this subject is Udo Erasmus, PhD, who wrote the book *Fats That Heal, Fats That Kill* (Alive Publishers, Vancouver, 1993).

After being poisoned by pesticides, Erasmus researched the subject of dietary fats and health. He found that omega-3 fatty acids, one type of essential fatty acids (EFAs), inhibit tumor growth. The other type of EFA, omega-6 fatty acids, has other health benefits. When they're combined, they help the body make hormone-like substances called prostaglandins that help nourish the heart, digestive system, kidneys, and hormone production and metabolism.

Now here's the problem with many oils. EFAs are destroyed by heat. Most oils you buy in supermarkets have been extracted by harsh acids, like Drano, along with bleaches, and are then heated to high temperatures to remove any odors. This changes them from being a healthy, protective source of good fats to interfering with the beneficial functions of EFAs. The oils you buy should always be cold-pressed.

Which Oils to Use

For cooking, use extra virgin olive oil. Erasmus advises against sautéing with any oil, especially if you have had breast cancer, since frying damages all oil. If you do want to use an oil, use a small amount of olive oil, or a little butter. Butter fries at a lower temperature than vegetable oils. Most importantly, don't eat foods that have been commercially deep-fried. The oils have become rancid and carcinogenic. This occurs whenever an oil is reheated or reaches a high temperature.

Finding EFAs in Food

Cold-water fish, like salmon and tuna, and flax seed oil, are among the healthiest forms of beneficial fats. Flax contains lignans, a chemical that is antifungal, antibacterial, antiviral, and anticancer. You can use a good quality flax oil (I suggest either Barleans or Spectrum) on salads or added to a meal of cooked vegetables with rice or pasta. You can also grind flax seeds (found in health food stores) in a small seed or coffee grinder, and add it to your breakfast shake or sprinkle it over cereal. One tablespoon of flax seed equals

Eat the Right Stuff

In my opinion, the most alarming news about our breast-cancer risk is this: Women who consume Western diets, such as a typical American diet, have the highest rates of breast cancer worldwide. Women who consume traditional Mediterranean diets have an intermediate risk, relative to the rest of the world. And women who consume traditional Asian and Hispanic diets have some of the lowest rates of breast cancer in the world. In fact, the breast-cancer rate of American women is eight times higher than that of Korean women and 22 times higher than that of Thai women.

This is no genetic coincidence. Asian and Hispanic women who move to the U.S. and other Western nations, and abandon their traditional diets in favor of a Westernized diet, soon catch up with Western women in terms of breast-cancer risk.

Since diet has been strongly linked to breast cancer incidence, your first line of defense against breast cancer should be dietary — adjusting your diet to more closely resemble the breast-cancer fighting characteristics of Asian and Hispanic diets. And at the same time, avoid the breast-cancer promoting foods (such as animal fat and high-sugar foods) found in Western diets.

This translates into an anti-breast cancer diet that consists mostly of whole grain foods, legumes (or beans), vegetables, fresh fruits, and little, if any, meat, poultry, and dairy foods.

one teaspoon of the oil. The amount of flax oil to take each day varies with individuals and their health conditions. A minimum of one teaspoon a day would be a good beginning. If you'd like a book of delicious recipes using flax oil, pick up *Flax for Life* by Jade Beutler (Progressive Health Publishing, Encinitas, CA, 1996).

Other foods high in EFAs include pumpkin seeds, walnuts, and soy products. Because soy is high in these good fats, it's not necessary to eat low-fat soy products.

Eat More Soy

A study conducted on 600 women found that soy products protect against breast cancer. This is how: Soy contains plant-based estrogens called phytoestrogens. Unlike synthetic hormone replacement therapy and organochlorines, this type of estrogen doesn't promote tumor growth. It does the opposite. Friendly bacteria in your intestines work on these plant hormones and change their activity so that they actually inhibit hormone-dependent cancers. To make this happen, you need two things: soy in your diet, and friendly bacteria like acidophilus and bifidus (from yogurt and other fermented foods) in your intestines.

In addition, the phytoestrogens block harmful estrogens from getting into breast tissue. Eating a diet high in soy can actually help

---

The Irony of Progress

Everything appears to be carcinogenic, even anti-cancer drugs, it seems. We're constantly learning new things about old substances. The U.S. National Toxicology Program's current publication, *Eighth Report on Carcinogens,* has just added 14 chemicals to its list of known or suspected carcinogens. Included in this list are Cyclosporin, used to boost the immune system, and Thiotepa. Never heard of Thiotepa? Well, it's used to treat breast and ovary cancers as well as lymphomas. Why a drug that promotes cancer is being used to fight the disease is totally confusing to me. We know all drugs have side effects, but this doesn't make sense, unless these two drugs are taken off the market. It could happen, but don't hold your breath.

"New human carcinogens named," *The Lancet,* Vol 351, May 23, 1998. From http:// eis.niehs.nih.gov.

prevent breast cancer! Soy also inhibits the growth of cancer cells and changes them back into normal cells.

How much soy is enough? Many people believe that half a cup a day will give you the beneficial nutrients. You can add tofu to salad dressings, tomato sauce, and soups (blend all of them for creamy results), or just add chunks of tofu to stir-fried or steamed vegetables. Other forms of soy that have more flavor include tempeh (found in health food stores) and green soybeans (edamame). Edamame can be found in the frozen sections of Asian markets and look like small lima beans. They have been boiled and just need to be thawed or lightly cooked (three to five minutes). They make a delicious, nutty snack or addition to meals. Some edamame are sold in their pods (not edible), some out of the pods. They are worth looking for!

Estrogen Mimickers

I'm concerned here with your exposure to the total amount of estrogen and estrogen-like chemicals, since they have a cumulative effect in your body. And exposure to small doses of synthetic estrogen over a long period of time can make your tissues more sensitive to them. So let's take a look at some environmental estrogen-mimickers and see how you can lower your exposure.

One of the most potent chemicals that acts like estrogen in your body is DDT. As it breaks down, it forms another carcinogen: DDE. But DDT is outlawed in this country, and has been since 1972. It's still a problem, says Liane Clorfene-Casten, who points out that the half-life of DDT is seven years. That means that it lasts, at half its original potency, for seven years. Then it breaks down into another estrogen-mimicking chemical: DDE. It takes up to 30 years to get DDE out of our air, water, and soil. So by the year 2012, we would theoretically be free from these chemicals — except that they're still manufactured in various parts of the world and make their way back into our country in the form of imported foods.

Testicular cancer is also increasing greatly. Some researchers believe it is because DDE causes abnormalities in the sexual development of males. Studies in Scandinavian countries are finding a link between high concentrations of DDE in breast milk and these abnormalities. They believe this is one reason why we're seeing more testicular cancer. Men, as well as women, are getting hormone-related cancers from environmental toxins.

In Israel, a strong association was found between pesticides and breast cancer. Three chemicals linked to breast cancer — DDT, BHC, and lindane — were finally banned in the late 1980s after a great deal of public pressure. High concentrations of these pesticides had been found in cow's milk, which then contaminated human breast milk, as women continued to eat a diet high in dairy products.

Immediately after the ban, breast-cancer rates dropped. But Israel was the only country out of 28 that had a significant drop in breast cancer 10 years after the ban went into effect. What does this mean to future generations? Probably a lot, since infants and children are particularly sensitive to toxic chemicals. Their young bodies are constantly growing, using nutrients (and storing poisons) that they ingest from food and the environment. If a substance is

Breast Cancer in Young Women

Breast cancer is a difficult illness for any woman to face, but for young women, it can be especially difficult to overcome. Now we may know why. It appears that when young women have estrogen-receptor positive breast cancer, the type of treatment they get can often predict their outcome. A study published in *The Lancet* (May 27, 2000) indicates that chemotherapy alone is not as effective as chemotherapy with tamoxifen or surgical removal of the ovaries. Apparently, young women with estrogen-receptor positive breast cancer are more sensitive to the presence of estrogen than those with estrogen-receptor negative breast cancer or postmenopausal women with either type.

Relapse occurred more frequently, and earlier, in women under the age of 35 than those who were older. Whether you choose allopathic medicine, complementary medicine, or a combination, I strongly advise any young woman with estrogen-receptor positive breast cancer to consider an aggressive treatment plan that goes beyond chemotherapy.

Aebi, et al. "Is chemotherapy alone adequate for young women with oestrogen-receptor-positive breast cancer?" *The Lancet,* May 27, 2000.

harmful to an adult, the same exposure is obviously much more harmful to a child.

Exposure to estrogen-mimicking chemicals will most likely impact most on an increased incidence of breast cancer in young women who were exposed as babies to contaminated breast milk and foods containing high amounts of pesticides. Unfortunately, young women with breast cancer have the worst prognosis for survival.

If you are concerned about your exposure to these chemicals, don't rush to detoxify yourself from some of them. Dr. Joseph Pizzorno, a naturopathic doctor, cautions against this in his book *Total Wellness* (Prima Publishing, 1996): "When patients suffering from significant contamination with fat-soluble toxins, such as DDT, fast, so much DDT is released into circulation that it can reach blood levels toxic to the nervous system." If you decide to detoxify, work with someone — a nutritionist, naturopath, and acupuncturist — who knows how to help you do this slowly and safely.

Dioxins

Tiny quantities of dioxin are also toxic and can damage cells. In fact, dioxin is one of the most toxic man-made chemicals ever

---

Q. In one of your articles on green tea you say that drinking it reduces breast tumors. Just what do you mean by this? Do existing tumors shrink or is the incidence reduced? — *S.L.C., New York, NY*

A. I apologize for not being more specific. Studies at Case Western Reserve University, under the direction of Professor Hasan Mukhtar, have shown that green tea contains five major polyphenols that inhibit one or more steps in the development of cancer cells. One of Dr. Mukhtar's studies on mice showed a reduction of lung and stomach cancers that ranged up to 90 percent when the mice consumed the equivalent of four cups of green tea a day.

Studies conducted on laboratory animals do not always translate into human results. But these studies are promising and indicate that in some cases, green tea polyphenols have been shown to inhibit the growth of tumors, while in other cases they have reduced the size of tumors.

CWRG: *The Magazine of Case Western Reserve,* May 1993.

made. It attacks the immune system and acts like an environmental hormone.

Most dioxins are a by-product of burning chlorinated wastes and are found in medical and city waste disposal incinerators. These dioxins are then carried in the air and water and find their way into our soil and plants. The plants are then eaten by animals, which store them in their fat cells, which we then eat and absorb. Due to this pathway, there is more dioxin stored in the fat cells of the animals we eat than in the plants we eat. Why? Because dioxin can be washed off plants. In all food preparation, produce is washed. However, the grasses on which dairy cattle graze are not.

Fish retain 159,000 times as much dioxin as the water they swim in. The higher up the food chain, the more dioxins that are likely to accumulate. This is one reason why it may be helpful for you to move closer toward a vegetable-based diet. Or at least to reduce the amount of animal products you eat, and make sure that whatever can be organic — like dairy products — is.

Some pesticides, banned in this country because they are known to be so toxic and contain organochlorines, are aggressively marketed to other developing countries, where they are used to raise crops that are imported back into the United States for sale and consumption here. This is referred to by some as the Circle of Poison. It means you need to be watchful of the quality of imported produce you eat and eat more locally produced, organic foods.

There was an accident that occurred in Italy in 1976 that brought the effects of dioxin to the public's attention. Several kilograms of dioxin spilled in a little village. Nine months after the accident, twice as many girls were born than boys. Studies then showed that when both parents were exposed to dioxin, more girls than boys were born. But I'm not concerned that there will be too many girls to go around. The implications are far greater. This incident suggests that dioxin changes hormonal balance in fetuses. It is possible that the reason twice as many girls as boys were born is that some male fetuses were miscarried due to this hormonal imbalance. Scientists are following the children born after this dioxin spill to maturity. In time, we'll learn more about the long-term effects of dioxin. The question is, how much time do you have to wait?

Begin Anywhere! Begin Today!

We have so much exposure to estrogens and chemicals that act like estrogen in our bodies that anything you do will help reduce this total amount. The first step is to become more aware of the situation. We all need to pay closer attention to the quality of the foods we buy for ourselves and our family. Organic foods may be the best, least expensive investment you can make in your future health.

The second step is to take some kind of broader action. This means everything from making these suggested dietary changes to writing letters or making phone calls when bills are being considered to allow unsafe waste disposal, or when contaminants are spilling into our waterways. It means standing up for more stringent

---

So Can Tamoxifen Even Prevent Breast Cancer?

Apparently not, according to preliminary results of the Breast Cancer Prevention Trial reported in the *The Lancet* (July 11, 1998) and a randomized five-year trial conducted in Italy. Tamoxifen blocks estrogen, and it's of interest to note that the Italian study found that while women on tamoxifen or a placebo had no difference in the frequency of breast cancer incidents, women who took tamoxifen along with hormone-replacement therapy had less breast cancer. Go figure.

Due to these results, however, the FDA decided not to allow the pharmaceutical company that manufactures tamoxifen to market it for breast cancer prevention. Since the Italian study showed a "significantly increased" risk of vascular disease and high triglycerides with women who took tamoxifen, I support their decision. I have just one question: If tamoxifen does not prevent breast cancer, why is it used to prevent a recurrence of breast cancer in women who have had the disease? More studies may reveal a stronger connection between breast cancer and tamoxifen. For now, I suggest that eating a diet high in plant-based estrogen, like soy, will block the uptake of harmful estrogens in a safer way than tamoxifen. It's something to consider, and to talk over with your physician.

Veronesi, U., et al. "Prevention of breast cancer with tamoxifen: preliminary findings from the Italian randomised trial among hysterectomised women," *The Lancet*, vol 352, July 11, 1998.

laws to keep pesticides out of our food and to stop manufacturing these chemicals for export — when we will be the ultimate recipients of them in the future. And it means buying safer, cleaner goods in all areas, from durable goods, such as carpeting (which outgases toxic chemicals) to cleaning supplies to personal care products and even paper products (such as unbleached toilet tissue, paper towels, tampons, sanitary pads, diapers, etc.).

In addition, eating a lot of meat — a high-fat, iron-rich diet — enables your body to store estrogen in your fat cells and can promote tumor growth. You may not be able to do much about the amount of hormones your body produces, but you can do something about the hormones you take in through contraceptives, synthetic hormone-replacement therapy, your diet, and more.

The Value of Organics

Since many pesticides act like estrogen in our bodies, the only way we can prevent our increased exposure to environmental estrogens is to buy the most natural, organic products we can find. There is no price you can put on the lives and health of your family and yourself. I believe it is more important than ever before to buy the most natural products you can find (including organic pesticides and fertilizers for your own lawn and garden).

One book you may want to get is called *Safe Food: Eating Wisely in a Risky World,* by Michael F. Jacobson, PhD and staff, published by the Center for Science in the Public Interest (Living Planet Press, 1991, $9.95). It will help you choose the foods you buy more wisely, and is written in an easy to understand language.

Another extremely helpful book is *Home Safe Home,* by Debra Lynn Dadd (Tarcher/Putman books, $18.95). Our environment and our food may be more polluted than ever, but we can do a lot more than sit and wait in fear or pretend we're not going to be affected. Big changes are necessary, and possible, when you get headed in the right direction. Begin taking a small step today, by buying organic foods whenever available.

Breast Cancer Clusters

If you live in Hawaii, you have a 32 percent lower risk of dying of breast cancer than the national average of women. If you live in Washington, D.C., your risk is 28 percent higher than the national average. In fact, a report from the National Cancer Institute has found that women who live on the east coast from New York City to Philadelphia are living in an area where breast cancer incidents are higher than in the rest of the country. It's called a cancer cluster. Smaller clusters on the east coast include northeast New Jersey, central New Jersey, Philadelphia, and Long Island, N.Y. On the west coast, the San Francisco area has a very high incidence of breast cancer.

What does this mean to you if you live in any of these areas? I think it means you may want to take extra steps to reduce your risk for breast cancer. Here are a few suggestions. Put a chlo-

---

More on Mammograms

There is still a controversy over mammograms. Who needs them, how often, and are they as beneficial as mainstream groups suggest? This is a decision each woman must make for herself, and one which is highly influenced by family history, and length of estrogen production (the longer you menstruate — years, not days per month — the higher your risk, it is suspected, for breast cancer). The National Women's Health Network has a few additional comments on mammograms.

First, remember that a clear mammogram does not mean you have no tumors. Although the American Cancer Society says that mammograms won't miss finding tumors, this is not true, especially in women with dense breast tissues. In fact, mammograms miss 10 percent of the tumors in women over 50, and nearly 25 percent in women in their 40s. At best, mammograms are only part of a breast cancer prevention program.

Do regular breast self-exams. The breast exams, along with mammograms if you choose, offer a much better screening than mammograms alone. Get to know your breasts and how they feel. Touching your breasts regularly is not taboo. It is smart preventive medicine.

Whenever possible, have any previous mammogram films sent to the radiologist(s) for comparison.

Pearson, Cynthia. "Mammography controversy," *The Network News,* March/April 1997.

rine-removing filter on your shower to reduce your exposure to this carcinogenic material that is absorbed through the skin (call 800-728-2288 for more information). Eat more organic produce to reduce your exposure to organochlorines, chemicals that act like estrogen in your body. Eat more soy products to increase the beneficial plant estrogens (phytoestrogens). Do regular breast self-exams and check in with your doctor regularly for any follow-up exams.

Evaluate Your Need for ERT

Women who take synthetic hormones after menopause are frequently taking estrogen as part of their program. Estrogen replacement therapy (ERT) is often suggested for postmenopausal women by gynecologists and other physicians. But menopause is not an estrogen-deficiency disease. Some women may need ERT, especially those who have had an early, natural, or surgical menopause. If you do, make sure the hormones you take are identical to those your body produces. These are the safest. For many-women, there are other safer solutions to menopausal symptoms, including reducing your risk for osteoporosis — if you're willing exercise regularly and eat a protective diet.

Before deciding to take ERT, take a look at your options. Some herbs, like black cohosh, reduce menopausal symptoms. HMC hesperidin, a bioflavonoid (part of the vitamin C complex), can eliminate hot flashes in doses of 500 mg twice a day. And soy products can give you a safe source of estrogen.

When to Call Your
Doctor About Self-Exam Findings

If you haven't been doing regular self-exams, getting started might produce more questions than answers. Don't be embarrassed to have your doctor double-check anything unusual or suspicious. With time, your self-exam expertise will grow and you will become increasingly adept at spotting any potentially adverse changes — which you'll definitely want to report to your doctor as well.

Update on Estrogen and Breast Cancer

For years, I've been harping on the fact that higher estrogen levels are one of the only known risk factors for breast cancer. I've also offered just about every last suggestion under the sun for keeping your estrogen levels healthfully low. This may turn out to be especially important for the 40 percent of women who researchers now estimate carry a gene called CYP17. It controls estrogen production and may double the risk of breast cancer, causing 30 percent of all cases.

Lung Cancer, a Bigger Threat for Women

Although women fear breast cancer most, the incidence of lung cancer among women has been increasing for decades, and in the '80s it became the leading cause of cancer death among females. Since then, more research has been completed on women and lung cancer.

One study recently reported that the risk of lung cancer is higher for women than men, even when differences in age when started smoking, number of cigarettes per day smoked, and body size were considered. Women were 20 percent to 70 percent more likely than men to develop lung cancer. It is estimated that approximately 80 percent of all lung cancers are due to smoking, so the best way to avoid lung cancer is not to smoke. Women who haven't managed to do so might be prudent to avoid other risk factors associated with lung cancer, including breathing (especially their own) second-hand smoke by smoking only outside or in well-ventilated areas, poor dietary and other lifestyle habits, and inhaling chemical fumes.

Japanese men are notorious for being heavy smokers. Yet they have the lowest heart-disease rate in the world, and a lower-than-average rate of lung cancer. Most experts contribute this to their extra-healthy diet — lots of green tea, soy foods, fish, and vegetables.

One study also found that non-smoking housewives had higher rates of lung cancer, and the researchers suspected breathing the fumes of toxic household cleaning products may have increased their risk.

Another survival tip for female smokers is to consider regular chest X-rays. Lung cancer survival rates are very poor, in part, because relatively few cases are diagnosed in the earlier, more treatable, stages. Regular chest X-rays offer the advantage of early diagnosis, and in this case, the benefit might outweigh the risks of radiation.

Zang, E.A. and E.L. Wynder. "Differences in lung cancer risk between men and women: Examination of the Evidence." *J Natl Can Inst* 1996;88:183-91.

The research on which this estimate is based was conducted by Dr. Brian E. Henderson and his colleagues from the University of Southern California, and presented in late March at a conference sponsored by the American Cancer Society. In contrast, the breast cancer genes BRCA1 and BRCA2, may raise the risk of breast cancer 20 times, especially in younger women, but account for only about four percent of all cases.

More research is needed on the CYP17 gene, however, to confirm Dr. Henderson's initial findings, which we will report as they become available.

In the meantime, please keep following the *Women's Health Letter* breast cancer prevention program. It includes:

• Exercise, preferably four or more hours per week.

• Avoid chemical-laden foods, personal care products, household products, and tap and shower water. Many of these contain environmental estrogens — chemicals like chlorine that increase our estrogen levels.

• Eat plenty of whole grains and beans, especially soy foods. These contain beneficial phytoestrogens that mimic our own estrogen and therefore reduce our own estrogen production. Keep dietary fat around 20 percent of total calories.

• Don't use birth control pills and standard synthetic estrogen supplements such as Premarin, unless absolutely medically necessary. Natural estrogens are safer.

Tamoxifen for Early Breast Cancer?

There have been over 50 trials using tamoxifen to reduce early breast cancers, but the drug appears to work only on specific kinds of tumors: those that are estrogen-receptor positive (ER-positive). This makes sense, since tamoxifen is an anti-estrogenic drug. It blocks estrogen and removes a source of nourishment from these tumors. In this way, tamoxifen has been shown to improve the 10-year survival of women with ER-positive tumors.

A study published in the *The Lancet,* (vol 351, May 16, 1998) gives an overview of these studies and breaks down the benefits, both long- and short-term, into categories (age, menopausal status, recurrence of cancer, length of use of tamoxifen). In our opinion, it is a valuable report for you and your doctor to read if you are on or considering using tamoxifen therapy for breast cancer.

Basically, the authors say that if your tumor has been shown through reliable tests to be completely ER-negative, tamoxifen may not be for you. If it has some detectable ER, then taking tamoxifen for five years could be beneficial. Longer than that may produce negative results. Women who plan to take tamoxifen for more than 10 years should read this overview study carefully to assess whether or not the drug is likely to produce more harm than good. Like all drugs, herbs, and modalities, tamoxifen has its place. Be sure it's your best choice.

What's a Good Test?

You don't have to look very hard to find scientific studies to back up any point of view. That's what makes it so difficult for all of us to know what to do. One day we hear about a study that tells us a substance is harmful, the next day another study says it's not. Wait long enough and you might even find one that touts its benefits. No wonder we're confused.

Last year, scientists on the United Kingdom's Coordinating Committee on Cancer Research, part of an annual seminar on National Breast Cancer Trials, met to discuss their work. They agreed that there have been too many small trials, and not enough large, simple, well-organized ones. With pressure to get information to the public quickly, small, quick studies may be giving us false information. Richard Gray, a researcher from Birmingham, UK, said that in order to either confirm or deny a small improvement in breast cancer survival, at least 3,200 women need to participate.

Until enough time has gone by for such studies to be run and published, we need to read between the lines and do the best we can with the information we have. We tend to forget, however, that there can be severe limitations in the data that comes out of small or poorly designed studies. This is why we're so confused. In an attempt to simplify the amount of conflicting information being given by the media, we look at the numbers of participants in the studies we report about, and examine them in light of the criteria mentioned at this conference.

Bradbury, Jane. "Simple cancer trials best, say UK experts," *The Lancet*, vol 352, December 5, 1998.

Tamoxifen Side Effects

Tamoxifen is being used as an estrogen-blocker for some women with breast cancer. Like all drugs, there can be side effects. A recent finding out of Japan indicates that 40 mg of tamoxifen, taken for three to five years, caused an increase in liver enzymes in half of the women studied. Most changes occurred within 18 months of taking the drug. Elevated liver enzymes is a sign of a fatty liver, which is related to cirrhosis of the liver.

The researchers of this study believe that tamoxifen may be causing a dysfunction of fat metabolism leading to a fatty liver. If you're on tamoxifen, ask your doctor to check your liver enzymes through a simple blood test (SGOT and SGPT) to make sure your liver is not being adversely affected.

The findings of a placebo-controlled follow-up study of healthy women raises additional concerns about tamoxifen, the controversial anti-estrogenic drug commonly prescribed to help prevent breast cancer recurrence. Now tamoxifen appears to induce significant loss of bone density in premenopausal women, according to Dr. Trevor Powles and a presentation given at the American Society of Clinical Oncology. Dr. Powles reported that premenopausal women experienced a two percent annual loss of bone density in the lumbar spine for the first two years of taking tamoxifen. The study

If Your Father Had Breast Cancer

While less common than in women, some men do get breast cancer. We suspect that daughters whose mothers had breast cancer may be at an increased risk for the disease. But what if your dad had breast cancer? One genetic link to breast cancer, the BRCA2 gene, has been found in daughters of men with breast cancer in both Danish and Icelandic studies. The incidents of cancer were more than twice those expected, and none of these daughters had mothers with breast cancer. The daughters who came down with breast cancer were all under the age of 40. Sons of these men were not at an increased risk. If your father had breast cancer, you may want to consider being tested for the BRCA2 gene.

Storm, Hans H. and Jorn Olsen. "Risk of breast cancer in offspring of male breast-cancer patients," Lancet, vol 353, January 16, 1999.

also confirmed previous findings that tamoxifen prevents bone loss in healthy postmenopausal women not taking hormone replacement therapy. It appears that the body recognizes tamoxifen as an antiestrogen in women with higher estrogen levels, and as an estrogen in women with lower estrogen levels.

Evista: The Good, the Bad, and the Ugly

If you've been reading my ongoing reports on tamoxifen, you know it is used primarily to prevent the recurrence of breast cancer. Still, a U.S. tamoxifen study to investigate tamoxifen's ability to prevent breast cancer was halted last year because it significantly increased the incidence of endometrial cancer and embolisms. Clearly, there are big problems with tamoxifen. In addition, after five years of use, the lower breast cancer recurrence risk with tamoxifen ceases; and continued use appears to increase risk, especially after 10 years of tamoxifen use.

Why is this relevant to a discussion of Evista (also known by its trade name Raloxifene). Because Evista and tamoxifen are close cousins. Both are SERMs (selective estrogen receptor modulators), a class of drugs with anti-estrogenic activity.

Evista, however, is being marketed to doctors and their patients as an ideal alternative to estrogen replacement therapy. Unlike estrogens such as Premarin, Evista doesn't cause breast tenderness or bleeding. It also hasn't been shown to increase the risk of breast cancer, more about that later. What Evista does do is help fight osteoporosis, and this in fact is the use for which the FDA approved it and the key reason doctors are recommending it. That's the good news.

Here's the bad news. Evista does nothing to relieve menopause symptoms. Neither has it been proven to reduce the risk for heart attack, stroke, and other cardiovascular events (remember here that heart disease is the leading cause of female death).

And now for the ugly news. Recently reported results of an ongoing trial (the Multiple Outcomes of Raloxifene (MORE) Trial), reveal that a 3.5-fold greater relative risk of deep vein thrombosis and pulmonary embolus has been found with Evista. That's a statistically significant increase in life-threatening outcomes, but not surprising since Evista's cousin tamoxifen also causes embolisms. What's more, there's an excellent chance that like tamoxifen, long-term use of Evista will eventually be found to increase breast-cancer (and recurrence) risk since the required long-term testing to settle this question has yet to be done. In addition, long-term testing could reveal other adverse effects.

For now, though, all we can say is that Evista is closely related to tamoxifen, and behaves very much like it in significant ways, and this in itself should be considered a big red flag against using this drug. But are there exceptions, such as women whose osteoporosis risk is especially high? Could using Evista for five years or less (giving consideration to tamoxifen's behavior with respect to breast-cancer risk) be beneficial for such women? Maybe. But be forewarned, you might not get as much bang for your buck, as you'd expect. Evista is only about half as good as Premarin at decreasing bone resorption and increasing bone density. That translates into a heck of a lot of risk for little in return.

Healing After Radiation Therapy

If you've had radiation treatments for breast, head, neck, or other cancers, you know that the exposed skin tissues that lie just beneath the skin become thicker and more fibrous. A study published in the *Journal of Clinical Oncology* showed that a combined treatment of 1,000 IU/daily of vitamin E, along with the drug pentoxifylline (Trental, 800 mg/daily), used for at least six months, significantly improved the affected tissues. Pentoxifylline thins the blood and increased blood flow, enhancing tissue oxygenation. Historically, it has been used for peripheral vascular disease. Vitamin E is also a blood thinner.

The study compared the combined therapy with both single therapies. The combination of Vitamin E with pentoxifylline was considerably more effective. If you have changes in your tissues due to radiation therapy, or if you're planning on having radiation, you may want to bring this study to the attention of your doctor to see if it's appropriate for you.

Delanian S; et al. "Striking regression of chronic radiotherapy damage in a clinical trial of combined pentoxifylline and tocopherol," *J Clin Oncol* 1999;17:3283-3290.

Townsend Letter, February/March 2000.

In wrapping up here, let me mention that a reader with whom I recently spoke inspired this article. She impressed me with her knowledge of health care issues and her dedication to making sound health care decisions for herself. We talked at length about her osteoporosis risk and her doctor's recommendation to take Evista. I asked about her diet and she described excellent eating habits, including consuming a fair amount of soy foods. Next we discussed taking magnesium supplements (to bowel tolerance). Doing so has been proven to outperform prescription drugs, both in terms of bone building ability and safety. One study found that simply increasing magnesium intake in this way resulted in an average eight percent increase in bone density within a year. Another study found that female participants, who, in addition to increasing magnesium

Radiation and Thyroid Cancer

If you're between the ages of 52 and 62, and drank a lot of milk when you were young, you're at a higher risk for thyroid cancer than other Americans. If you lived in Colorado, Montana, Utah, Idaho, or South Dakota during the 1950s and 1960s, when nuclear bomb testing was going on, your risk may be higher yet.

The National Cancer Institute (NCI) estimates that 70 percent of thyroid cancer cases from exposure to radioactive iodine from these tests have not been diagnosed.

During the time of nuclear testing, people across the country received about two rads of radiation. Naturally occurring radioactivity exposes us to annual doses of about 0.1 rad a year. But people living in the states where the most radioactivity exposure occurred, received from 9-16 rads, and much of that was from milk coming from cows and goats that ate contaminated grasses. The younger the person was during this exposed time, the smaller their thyroid glands. Children who drank a lot of milk may have received three to seven times as much radioactivity as people in the same area who drank little milk and ate little dairy.

If you believe you may have been exposed to higher levels of radioactivity, be sure to have your thyroid checked annually. It may be years before government agencies develop protocols for doctors along these lines. Take responsibility for your health and check this out with your doctor.

McCarthy, Michael. "Nuclear bomb test fallout may cause many U.S. cancers," *The Lancet*, August 9, 1997.

intake, also lowered calcium intake, experienced an average increase of 11 percent within a year.

But perhaps the most important question I asked was, "Do you walk?" Well, no, she didn't. So we talked more about walking for exercise, and about how, living in a high-tech information age might have the effect of over-focusing our attention on the newest, latest high-tech health care solutions, like Evista. Newer isn't necessarily better, though, especially when it comes to bone health. There's no substitute for exercise for maintaining it. And well-toned muscles are the best indicator of well-toned bones underneath. Oftentimes, backaches and back-muscle strains are indicators of poor muscle tone. In these cases, ask your doctor or other health care provider, perhaps a physical therapist, to teach you exercises to strengthen your back muscles. Doing so can help improve and even restore back health, plus keep vertebra strong, supple, and more resistant to osteoporosis-related fracture.

Not exercising and staying inactive, is in effect, inviting early deterioration of your entire body, including your bones. A study that appeared in the *Journal of the American Medical Association* (vol 279, No 6.) tracked 16,000 sets of healthy twins for an average of 19 years. It found that those who exercised regularly by taking at least two brisk 30-minute walks per week reduced their risk of dying by 44 percent. That's a lot of free prevention. And you can be sure that maintaining your ability to walk like this not only benefits overall muscle and bone tone, it also reduces your risk of falling (due to weakness or poor balance), and therefore reduces the risk of fracture even more. Some weight-bearing exercise will further strengthen muscles and bones, and improve overall agility. If these exercises aren't appropriate for you, do what you can.

Until then, if your doctor thinks taking Evista might be good for you, ask to discuss the bad and the ugly news on Evista as well.

New Soy-Based Breast Cancer Drug on the Way

If preliminary studies are an indication of the powerful way a drug can target and destroy breast cancer cells, we may be looking at an answer to this serious problem within a few years. An answer that begins with soy.

Recently, researchers out of Wayne Hughes Institute in St. Paul, Minn. formulated a drug comprised of a hormone, EGF (epidermal growth factor), and genistein (a plant chemical found in soy).

Here's how the drug EGF-Genistein works, according to the senior author of the study, Dr. Fatih Uckun. The hormone part of the drug, EGT, binds itself to a substance on the surface of breast cancer cells. Then the synthetic genistein enters the cell and shuts down its survival mechanism, and the breast cancer cell dies. In addition to being effective, EGF-Genistein has been found to have no known toxicity at this date, even using larger than necessary amounts. Sound promising? It is. And the possibilities are exciting.

But before you ask your doctor how to get this new drug, understand that so far the studies done with EGF-Genistein have been done only on mice. The authors are now applying for status to begin phase-1 and phase-2 clinical trials with people. At the end of the trials we'll know how well it works. For now, EGF-Genistein is not available to the public.

I am concerned that media hype will give you the impression

How Much Tamoxifen?

If you're taking tamoxifen as protection against breast cancer, you may be taking more than you need. Tamoxifen is a drug that binds to estrogen receptors. These estrogen receptors, in turn, regulate various biomarkers including how blood clots and triglyceride levels. Researchers from the European Institute of Oncology in Milan, Italy, found that the dose of tamoxifen greatly affects these biomarkers. The best results were obtained when women were given 10 mg of tamoxifen every other day, rather than 20 mg every day.

The daily dose of 20 mg, they say, comes from "clinical intuition" rather than evidence-based studies. Lowering tamoxifen may reduce a woman's risk for blood clots and high triglycerides, two negative effects of the drug. Andrea Decensi, who headed this Italian study, suggests that less tamoxifen can still protect against tumor activity and have less toxicity as well.

Bonn, Dorothy. "Doses of tamoxifen used to prevent breast cancer may be too high," Science and Medicine, *The Lancet,* vol 354, September 4, 1999.

that eating soy products will give some of the same results. They won't. Genistein is only one chemical component of soy, and while Dr. Uckun admits that Asian women who eat a high soy diet have a lower incidence of breast cancer, and have more genistein in their urine than American women, he stresses that this drug is not the same as the naturally occurring genistein in soy. It is a synthetic drug made in a pharmaceutical laboratory based on some, but not all, of the features of genistein.

EGF-Genistein contains only small amounts of synthetic genistein because that's all it takes for the drug to work. Using genistein alone was not effective. Dr. Uckun says that genistein can damage the DNA in genes. One study he participated in using this manufactured form of genistein without the EGF hormone gave poor results, while the combination drug was found to be more than 1,000 times more potent than plain genistein.

Soy products containing all the chemicals found in the plant, many of which have been shown to be protective against breast cancer, are still a good idea, suggests Dr. Uckun. He recommends a healthy diet containing soy products, regular physical exercise, and a healthy lifestyle in general as our most sensible approach to protect ourselves against breast cancer.

In the future, EGF-Genistein may be found to be protective as well. Mice that carried breast-cancer genes and given this experimental drug as "teens" did not go on to develop breast cancer. Maybe this will be an answer for the children of the future. It's too early to say. Mice inoculated with tumor cells and then given EGF-Genistein 24 hours later had their tumors decrease by 50 percent or disappear entirely. In a handful of years, we may find this drug to be the answer to some cases of breast cancer.

But for now, if you hear about companies selling pills or tablets of genistein claiming it has been shown to protect against breast cancer, be cautious. The information is premature and such a statement is inaccurate. The difference between such a product and EGF-Genistein is more than one being synthetic and one being "natural." Soy genistein does not attach itself to breast cancer cells without EGF. Like all nutrients, the best form of genistein for you and me is found in foods, where all chemicals are in balance with one another. Taking too much of one ingredient could adversely affect your nutrient balance, be ineffective, or even be harmful.

Mammogram Limitations

Everything has limitations, even mammograms. Maybe I should say, especially mammograms. Researchers at the Harvard Pilgrim Health Care, an HMO associated with Harvard Medical School, studied 2,400 women for 10 years. During this time they had regular mammograms and breast exams. Here come the statistics:

Almost one in two women who have mammograms for 10 years will have a false-positive result. This means you will be told you have breast cancer when you don't. After 10 years of mammograms, the figures get lower. At this point, only one in four women will get a false-positive result. But after a total of 10 mammograms the cumulative risk of being given a false-positive scare is nearly 50 percent!

Along with this, remember that women with large breasts often get a clean slate when, in fact, a mass can't be seen by mammography. We're not saying mammograms are worthless. We just think their risks and limitations should be common knowledge. Too many women are falsely alarmed or relieved by their results. Nothing takes the place of regular self-breast examination. Put mammograms in perspective. Don't rely on them exclusively.

When to Have a Mammogram

If you've decided to have a mammogram and are still menstruating, consider this: Your breasts tend to be less dense during the first two weeks of your cycle than right before your menses, which would make it easier for the mammogram to "read" your breasts. Many women have tender breasts before menstruating, but not all. Still, their breast density can change enough to affect the results of this test.

An article in the *Journal of National Cancer Institute* (vol 90, 1998) suggests that by having your mammogram when your breasts are less dense could improve the accuracy greatly. This may be one factor in some of the "false positive" test results that only lead to fear and confusion. Give yourself the best opportunity for an accurate mammogram by taking into account its timing with your menstrual cycle.

Unnecessary Mastectomies

National health statistics show that 71 percent of women with early-stage breast cancer undergo mastectomy — removal of an entire breast — while only 28 percent have a lumpectomy, a breast-conserving option that involves removal only of the cancerous lump, followed by radiation therapy. However, a recently released national survey reveals that women's preferences are almost exactly the reverse of those numbers. After receiving a full description of both treatments and their outcome rates, 63 percent would choose a lumpectomy with radiation therapy and only 20 percent would select mastectomy.

Update on Ovarian Cancer Risks

Too much sun significantly increases the risk of skin cancer. Yet too little sun can increase other health risks, including breast and intestinal cancer risks. Now a new study has linked a lack of sun to increased risk of ovarian cancer. Apparently, women between the ages of 45 and 54 who live in the northern U.S. were five times more likely to die from ovarian cancer than women in sunnier, southern states, according to findings by researchers at the University of California at San Diego. They believe these increased risks are due to lower vitamin D intake, resulting from less sun exposure. Vitamin D has also been linked to lower rates of osteoporosis since it helps the body absorb calcium into the bones. If you live in an area that doesn't get much sun, you might consider vitamin D supplements, especially during the winter.

In another study, this one by researchers at Boston's Brigham and Women's Hospital, tricyclic depressants such as Elavil, and benzodiazepine tranquilizers such as Valium and Halcion were found to increase the risk of ovarian cancer twofold. Women who used these drugs before age 50 had an increased risk of up to 3.5 times higher. This was a preliminary study, so more research on this will likely be underway soon.

The survey of 800 women, aged 35 and older, strongly suggests that women need more information from physicians (or other sources) in order to choose the most appropriate and less radical form of treatment for early-stage breast cancer. The survey also found that women age 65 years and older were even less informed of treatment options than women in younger age groups. Daniel Perry of the Alliance for Aging Research noted: This survey confirms that older women also need to know their options because they too would choose lumpectomy with radiation therapy over mastectomy when both treatment options are fully described. The importance of doctors communicating clearly with their patients about their treatment options cannot be overemphasized.

An increasing number of women are also skipping radiation treatment, and sometimes even surgery, in order to pursue alternative treatments. For a well-documented and comprehensive review

Sunscreen and Melanoma

Don't rely on sunscreen to prevent skin cancer, say dermatologists. Mark Naylor, MD, at the University of Oklahoma, reports that there are current theories that sunscreen may actually be a cause of melanoma by making individuals feel so complacent they don't practice good skin hygiene.

Ultraviolet (UV) light exposure is a known risk factor for melanoma and other skin cancers, and this light is present year-round not just in hot summer months. If you've been exposed to intense sunlight in the past, you want to protect yourself now. And if there's a history of skin cancer, or your skin is particularly light in color, you can't ignore UV light.

Practices that can save your skin include wearing a hat, wearing a shirt with long sleeves whenever possible when you're outdoors, and putting on a shirt and hat after swimming. Also, simply staying out of the sun or enjoying warmer weather outdoors but in the shade, especially between the peak burn hours which are from 10 a.m. to 2 p.m. Some doctors advise wearing a tee shirt while you're swimming. Tightly woven natural fiber clothing filters out the sun's harmful rays, reflects heat, and keeps you cool. Finally, examine your body for any changes in moles or any suspicious lesions, and get to your doctor quickly if you find anything. Good protection can protect your skin and save your life.

Naylor, M.F., MD, K.C. Farmer, PhD, "The case for sunscreens," *Archives of Dermatology,* September 1997.

of breast cancer treatment options, see *Breast Cancer: What You Should Know (But May Not Be Told) About Prevention, Diagnosis, and Treatment,* by Steve Austin, ND and Cathy Hitchcock, MSW (Prima Publishing).

Sometimes, women discover they have breast cancers that are too large to be removed by lumpectomy. Then their doctors usually suggest mastectomies. A study of over 1,500 women with primary breast cancer given one of two chemotherapy agents: doxorubicin and cyclophophamide. Some received the drugs before surgery, some afterward. Eighty percent of the women who were given these drugs before surgery had their tumors shrink at least in half — sometimes more. Many were able to have lumpectomies, rather than mastectomies.

In addition to shrinking tumors, pre-operative chemotherapy reduced the positive nodes by 59 percent; post-operative chemo reduced them by 43 percent. If your breast tumor is small, lumpectomy may be sufficient. If it's large, you may want to consider chemo first, then see if it has shrunk to a small enough size for a lumpectomy.

If not, you might still be a good candidate for a kinder, gentler mastectomy called "skin-sparing mastectomy." Cancer surgeons and plastic surgeons at the University of Pennsylvania Medical Center are using this new breast-conservation technique. It removes breast tissue through an opening made by removing only the nipple and surrounding areola, leaving an envelope, which is

---

Please Pass on the Sugar

Several studies have linked high sugar consumption to increased breast-cancer risk. This is not surprising when you consider the massive amounts of glucose cancer cells need to thrive — 10 times more than normal cells.

An epidemiologic survey reported in the *Journal of Medical Hypothesis* reviewed breast-cancer rates for 21 countries. Based on their findings, the researchers concluded that high sucrose (sugar) intake is a major risk factor for the development of breast cancer in women over 45.

then filled with the patient's abdomen and/or back tissue and mus-cle. This eliminates the need to heal before beginning reconstruc-tive surgery. Also, by keeping the original breast skin, shape is bet-ter maintained, and the patient's ability for sensation is improved. Women who don't opt for reconstruction will still have a more nat-ural-looking breast.

"Recurrence with this type of surgery is extremely low because all the breast tissue has been removed. Also, the ability to leave the hospital after surgery with a totally reconstructed breast provides many psychological benefits for the patient. This is the direction in which medicine is headed," says Louis P. Buckey, MD, and assistant professor of surgery at Penn's Center for Human Appearance. Not all patients with breast cancer are candidates for skin-sparing mastecto-

---

Don't Forget the Phytoestrogens

Another important dietary prevention step is to include plenty of phy-toestrogens (plant estrogens) in your diet. These are estrogens that nature intended us to have — consumed as part of our daily diet. They are natural hormones with just the right strength. Too weak to cause, yet strong enough to protect against, health problems such as breast cancer.

Phytoestrogens are found in whole grains and legumes. The lower breast-cancer rates among Asian women may be explained, in part, by the fact that soy foods (such as soy milk, tofu, and miso, which are made from soybeans, a legume) and rice are staples of most Asian diets. Hispanic women consume lots of rice, beans, and tortillas, which are made from corn or wheat. All of these foods are rich in phytoestrogens.

These hormone-like substances may help prevent the growth of hor-mone-dependent cancers such as breast cancer by behaving like the drug tamoxifen in the body — but with no side effects.

Soy is also the only known source of genistein, a phyto-estrogen that has been shown in test tube and animal experiments to block the growth of breast-cancer cells, so eating soy foods regularly may protect you against breast cancer.

Soy products may contain as much as 50 percent fat, however, so choose tofu, soy milk, soy cheese, soy mayonnaise (called nayonnaise) and other soy products that are no-fat or low in fat. You can find them in many health food stores. If you buy canned refried beans, choose fat-free. And for tortillas, choose corn or whole wheat.

my, however. To find out more about the procedure, you or your doctor can call Dr. Buckey's office at 215-662-4286.

Research: A Good Starting Point, a Good Investment

Just as no responsible firm commits to a major new project without preliminary research to justify the course, cancer treatment should be guided by research. Here are some ideas that will help get you started:

Author Ralph Moss, PhD, one of the most highly regarded cancer treatment researchers, writes the *Moss Reports* and numerous books on alternative cancer therapies. He is the first American to become an honorary member of Germany's Society of Oncology and is on the National Institutes of Health Cancer Advisory Panel. Moss worked in the public affairs department of Memorial Sloan-Kettering's cancer hospital, and was fired after he refused to cover up research data on the benefits of laetrile.

For $275, Ralph Moss sends you a lengthy report on treatments for your type of cancer. Reports are updated whenever new information is available, and scientific studies are given that back them up. The fee includes follow-up sessions with Dr. Moss' assistant, Anne Beattie, who speaks daily with Moss and gives out his replies to your questions or concerns. How long can you use this service without paying anything more? Indefinitely, says Beattie, who encourages people to ask questions and understand their condition and options. To contact Moss' office you can call 718-636-4433 or e-mail mail@ralphmoss.com.

Another highly respected cancer-treatment report comes from cancer researcher Patrick McGrady, Jr., who has a service called CAN-HELP out of Port Ludlow, Washington 360-437-2291. McGrady's report isn't cheap; it costs $425. But you get a lot of personal attention and information for your money. He looks at all your records, evaluates each practitioner he thinks could help you, and begins his report with the people he feels can, based on past results, help you the most. He explains each treatment, its cost, and even talks with some of the doctors on your behalf. In one case, he spoke with a doctor in Germany, explaining the client's condition in detail, and got information on just what direction this German doctor would take. With a CAN-HELP report, you're paying for McGrady's recommendations and evaluation, not just a listing of people throughout the world who deal with your kind of cancer. You can also speak with McGrady personally if you have any questions about his recommendations.

I looked at reports from each source on the subject of ovarian cancer, and each report had different information that was valuable, making both of them good investments for anyone who's been diagnosed with cancer. Both reports are skewed toward alternative therapies that are frequently not covered by health insurance policies. But then, many effective treatments aren't covered by insurance.

Q. I would like to know about taking proper nutrients after breast cancer. I am now taking Vitality and notice a difference in my energy level. I would like to know what to take with it. — *B.J., Internet Correspondent*

A. Glad to hear Vitality has perked you up. In addition to a top quality daily multiple, an excellent nutritional supplement for breast-cancer prevention and healing is calcium d-glucarate. It is a natural substance found in many foods, that binds itself to harmful toxic materials that get inside our bodies, along with excess steroid hormones (like estrogen), then carries them out of the body. Recent studies show that glucarate appears to protect against breast cancer.

Remember also that nutritional supplements are not intended to take the place of a good diet. In her book *Total Breast Health: The Power Food Solution for Protection and Wellness,* Robin Keuneke outlines a very thorough breast cancer prevention and healing diet. It includes 125 recipes and discussions on essential fatty acids and soy foods. Although it was written with breast health in mind, it's also an excellent general diet.

More specific supplement information for you is difficult to offer, since all cases are unique. But please don't try to treat yourself. Work with a knowledgeable doctor or nutritionist to help develop an individual supplement regimen for you. If you have difficulty finding one in your area, I consult with clients nationwide by phone. My office number is 707-824-1123.

Still, it's often preferable to pay out-of-pocket for the therapy of your choice. Insurance coverage can still be extremely valuable for what it does cover, especially expensive diagnostic tests. Many individuals choose complimentary courses of treatment — those that combine alternative and traditional therapies — in which case traditional therapies are covered by insurance and alternative therapies usually aren't.

Nothing beats personal attention in the area of alternative cancer therapies. Still, numerous books on the subject also have a lot to offer.

Perhaps the most important book for every cancer patient to read is *Questioning Chemotherapy* by Ralph Moss (Equinox Press, 1995). This book gives a lot of information on specific chemotherapy agents and which ones might be appropriate for you to consider. It also serves as an excellent companion to your doctor's suggestions and brings you face to face with the hard reality that in many (but not all) cases chemotherapy simply doesn't work. Dr. John Cairns of the Harvard University School of Public Health has said that about five percent of cancer patients are helped by chemotherapy. Perhaps this is because the toxic substances used to

Best Tests After Breast Cancer

The last thing a woman who has had breast cancer wants is to have the cancer recur. In an attempt to catch tumors early, many doctors suggest bone scans and chest X-rays. Now new guidelines from the American Society of Clinical Oncology (*J Clin Oncol,* 1997;15:49-56) say that these costly tests are unnecessary. Only one out of nine women who have abnormal bone scans actually have bone metastases. And X-rays for women who are symptom-free have not proven to show early tumors. In fact, the detection rate has been zero to five percent.

The doctors suggested that monthly self-examinations would be smart, along with a doctor's exam every 3-6 months for three years, every 6-12 months for two years, and then once a year. They also advocate annual mammograms. I suggest you look at the pros and cons of mammograms and make that decision for yourself.

McCarthy, Michael. "Costly tests are not the best after breast cancer," *The Lancet,* vol. 349, May 10, 1997.

destroy cancer also destroy the immune system.

Herbs, however, can both destroy cancer cells and support the immune system and Moss has a second book on this topic. *Herbs Against Cancer* (Equinox Press, Inc., Brooklyn, NY, 1998) gives you an easily understood overview of numerous herbs from around the world used in cancer treatment, including Essiac tea, the Hoxey formula, cat's claw, and Hulda Clark's protocol. Instead of running off and trying every herbal therapy you hear about, you may want to take a look at this book first for guidance.

A final cancer therapy essential is good nutrition. If you need help in putting together tasty, nutritious meals, you may want the *Cancer Survivor's Nutrition & Health Guide* by Gene Spiller, PhD and Bonnie Bruce, RD (Prima Publishing, 1997). In addition to giving plenty of easy to prepare recipes, this book contains valuable information on what to do if you have difficulty swallowing or chewing, if you lose weight, or if foods don't have much taste.

Q. I heard about a study done in 1998 in Uruguay that found essential fatty acids were not protective against breast cancer and, in fact, exacerbated tumor or cancer growth in the breast. Do you have any information regarding this subject? — *M.L., Pueblo, CO*

A. I called Jade Beutler, co-author with Dr. Michael T. Murray, ND of *Understanding Fats & Oils* (Progressive Health, 1996) and author of numerous articles on unrefined flaxseed oil. He was familiar with the study you cited. The Uruguay study appears to be inconclusive and most likely flawed. Women with breast cancer in Uruguay have a very high intake of saturated (animal) fats, and a low intake of the fatty acids found in flaxseed. Jade supplied me with information on numerous well-designed studies that indicate it is most likely no one fatty acid that either prevents or promotes cancer, but the proportion of all fats. Omega-3 fatty acids, found in freshly-ground flaxseed and in flaxseed oil, are very low in Americans. If you are using flax products, the evidence I've examined indicates you're helping your health, not hurting it. The company I found that has some of the best unrefined organic flax products is Barlean, found in the refrigerated section of your natural food store.

Popular Alternative Therapies That Lack Research

Both Moss and McGrady debunk therapies with claims that can't be substantiated.

For example, naturopathic doctor, Hulda Clark who wrote *The Cure for All Cancers,* speaks with authority about how all people with cancer have a liver fluke parasite called *Fasciolopsis buskii.* She claims that proplyl-alcohol, which is in cosmetics, hair sprays, rubbing alcohol, decaffeinated coffee, white sugar, and other products, render the body's immune system helpless against destroying these flukes. This has caused thousands of people to avoid contact with propyl alcohol, and to buy Clark's Zapper, a machine that allegedly destroys these parasites.

When the Centers for Disease Control (CDC) looked for parasites in stool samples of more than 200,000 people, only one had F. buskii. Clark claims than everyone who has cancer, is about to get cancer, and most that have had it in the past, has this parasite.

Statistics don't prove her right. Neither do the statistics showing that people in Mexico (where she practices) have less cancer and more parasites than people in the United States. Perhaps Clark is using different methods to find and test the cancer therapy she uses — the Zapper and an herbal formula. If this is so, other practitioners who use her methods should be able to scientifically document their success in the near future.

Another product that both Moss and McGrady would pass on is shark cartilage, sold in huge quantities after a book, *Sharks Don't Get Cancer,* appeared in bookstores. A 1997 study sponsored by the company that manufactures shark cartilage and published by the American Society of Clinical Oncology, showed there was no anti-cancer activity in the product. Dr. Judah Folkman, MD, of Harvard, experimented with shark cartilage. He used more than one ton of shark cartilage to get a few millionths of a gram of the protein that supposedly has anti-cancer properties. He found the protein was too large to get into the bloodstream. There are no good clinical trials with shark cartilage, according to McGrady, and no reason, other than hearsay, to spend money on it.

Therapy That's Right for You

Following the diagnosis of cancer, rather than taking someone else's path, takes the time to find your own way. With the help of Ralph Moss and Patrick McGrady, an individualized program is possible. With the help of a computer, you can also search the Internet for additional information. The American Cancer Society even has a Web site now with a section on alternative and complementary therapies (www.cancer.org/alt_therapies/) with information about diet, herbs, Chinese medicine, homeopathy, and naturopathic medicine.

Most important, find a health practitioner who's experienced in working with cancer patients, will assist you in decision-making (including making time to discuss issues of concern to you), then monitor your program and your progress. Don't skip around and try everything you hear about. You won't always know what's working. Instead, it's often necessary to stick with one or two treatments over a longer period of time to get results. And in the meantime, remember to pay attention to the rest of your life. Living life fully can help your body function at a higher level, opening the door to additional healing opportunities.

When Timing Makes a Big Difference

A study recently reported in *The Lancet* investigated the suggestion that breast cancer survival rates among premenopausal women are higher if surgery is performed during the last half of the menstrual cycle. The researchers discovered that women who had surgery during the luteal phase of their cycles, or days 15 to 36, had over 19 percent fewer recurrences than women whose surgeries took place during the first half of their cycles. The benefits of luteal phase surgery were even more significant for women whose cancer had spread to the underarm lymph nodes. The rate of recurrence for these women was lowered by over 33 percent. With findings like this, it's hard to believe many doctors continue to disregard menstrual cycle timing when scheduling breast-cancer surgery.

Press release, Alliance for Aging Research

Cancer Salves Work!

Last year, a friend who is well acquainted with herbs, told me of using a salve to treat a malignant tumor on a dog's lip. The owner used a topical salve of bloodroot, chaparral, and zinc chloride. Over a period of a month, the tumor slowly detached from the dog's lip, leaving a crater where blood vessels could be seen. Eventually, this crater healed. The tumor was gone.

This story impressed me, so we called around looking for a source of salves.

An oncologist friend, retired from private practice, had the information I was seeking. He used to prescribe herbs and nutritional supplements for his patients with a very high rate of success and knew about yellow and black salves for drawing out malignant tumors. He had found them to be extremely effective. After reading his detailed instructions on their use, along with their warnings, we decided these salves were nothing to play around with. If a tumor was being drawn out of the body, you wanted someone with a lot of knowledge to be able to tell you what's happening and to intervene if necessary. A doctor, nurse practitioner, or other health care specialists skilled in the use of cancer salves should administer them.

Ingrid Naiman, author of *Cancer Salves: A Botanical Approach to Treatment* (Seventh Ray Press, Santa Fe, NM, 1999) agrees. But instead of providing one or two sheets of information on how to use cancer salves, she has written a well-researched, complete guide to their history, formulations, and use. It is an excellent treatment guide for practitioners and offers explanations of various options open to cancer patients. In this book, Naiman has a quote from an unnamed doctor who has treated 10,000 patients with yellow and black salves successfully. It turns out, he is my retired oncologist friend.

Cancer Salves Are Potent

Most people are unaware that there are salves that can actually draw malignant tumors out of the body, providing them with alternatives to surgery, radiation, and chemotherapy. Surgery is not the only method for excising tumors.

However, this information is not new. Cancer is known to exist for thousands of years. Before surgery, caustic salves were used to remove tumors. Cancer salves have been used for 2,500 years. In the 12th century, Hildegard of Bingen, a German mystic, used a combination of violets, olive oil, and billy goat tallow successfully on cancerous tumors, bringing salves into early medicine. Since then, numerous doctors have worked with various formulas, many of which originated with Native American tribes. Many of these salves contain zinc chloride and bloodroot (Sanguinaria). But more complicated formulas have been found useful, as well.

Naiman's book is divided into three sections: a historical overview of cancer salves; use of cancer salves (when they're appropriate and what to expect from using them); and various methods of treating cancer with salves, diet, and ingesting herbs. This fascinating book provides little-known information in an easy-to-read format. It does not suggest using any of these salves on your own, but instead to find a practitioner skilled in using them. Barring this feat — and Naiman admits that not many practitioners exist who do know a lot about them — the book can serve as a guide to

It's Soy Good for Every Body!

Soy foods contain phytoestrogens. These are hormone-like substances that may help prevent the growth of hormone-dependent cancers, such as breast cancer, by behaving like the drug tamoxifen — but with no side effects.

In one study, premenopausal women in their 20s were given 60 grams of soy protein a day. The effect on their hormones was similar to that found in women on tamoxifen, a controversial anti-estrogenic drug, which is used to prevent development, as well as recurrence, of breast cancer.

Soy is also the only known source of genistein, a phytoestrogen that has been shown in test tube and animal experiments to block the growth of prostate and breast-cancer cells.

The lower breast-cancer rates among Asian women may be explained, in part, by the fact that soy foods (such as soy milk, tofu, and miso) are staples of most Asians diets.

any responsible medical practitioner who is willing to work with salves and monitor their patients closely.

Don't Self-Medicate With Salves

Some cancer salves fall into a category called escharotic salves, which means they have caustic substances that cause itching and burning on tissues. They work by increasing circulation around the site of the tumor, creating heat and blistering. This can be painful. Some people won't have any major reaction, while others will find the skin around the tumor gets red, blisters, and then changes color numerous times. Eventually, a crust develops and the tumor, which hangs on by a thread, drops off leaving a crater that eventually repairs itself. There may be a discharge of a clear fluid or pus. Cancer salves can remove all traces of malignancy or just some of a tumor. This is another reason why you want a highly skilled health practitioner working with you. An untrained eye cannot tell whether or not any malignancy remains, and the choice of salve along with length of treatment is highly individualized. Don't attempt to use cancer salves on your own.

While some cancer salves work by burning and irritating, some work by destroying tumors or separating them from healthy skin. Still others draw tumors up and out of the skin. Then there are salves used to help heal the craters that have been left when tumors are excised. By reading Naiman's book, you and your doctor can choose an appropriate treatment plan.

Various Methods Have Been Successful

Dr. Frederic Mohs, MD, at the University of Wisconsin, developed a system for treating skin cancer with a paste of bloodroot, zinc chloride, and stibnite (made from ore of antimony). Both he, and Ralph Moss, PhD, a cancer researcher I talked about in the March 1999 issue of *WHL*, claims a 99 percent success rate with all primary basal cell carcinomas. The technique used by Dr. Mohs is called chemosurgery, a combination of salves and surgery. He has used this technique on various types of cancer, and his method has been studied on tens of thousands of patients.

Drs. John Pattison, Eli Jones, and the more popular John Christopher all have different methods of removing cancers using salves, diet, homeopathics, and herbs. There are detailed explanations of each of their methods, along with the formulas they used, allowing anyone to make salves similar to the ones they used. But it should be remembered that these doctors had years of experience treating patients and observing the changes that came from their treatment plans. While it may seem simple to think of putting a salve over a spot on your body and getting rid of the cancer beneath, a great deal of knowledge is needed to know what treatment to use and when to change it.

In this age of over-information, we're looking for "magic bullets" — quick fixes to our problems. By using a salve, an herb, a nutritional supplement that eliminates our symptoms, we're ignoring the underlying problem that caused the symptoms. Ingrid Naiman knows this. She understands that we need to explore our emotional past and present, look at the way we view ourselves and the world, and change our lives to improve our health. Cancer salves are not "magic bullets." They may, however, be part of a treatment plan that not only eliminates tumors, but their cause(s).

Still, if you're going to use salves, they must be used respon-

---

Q. My husband and I both developed flat, soft lumps. The doctor said they were "fatty tissues." A specialist agreed and said not to worry about it, so I didn't. My husband's has disappeared with no treatment, but mine is still there. It isn't bothering me at all, but I'd like it gone in a natural way ... no surgery. What can I do? — *E.A., Blackwood, NJ*

A. It sounds like you have a lipoma, a cluster of fat cells that forms a blob of fatty tissue. Lipomas are benign fatty tumors, are very common, and usually cause no problems. They are occasionally absorbed back into the body, as with your husband. Most often, though, they just sit where they are. Lipomas can easily be removed surgically, and as long as the entire encapsulated mass of fat tissues is removed, it may not grow back. Sometimes, however, it does. The doctors we spoke to say the reason lipomas grow is unknown. But they do not seem to be a sign of illness.

Ref: C. Evans, MD.

sibly. Ingrid Naiman's book provides cancer patients and their health providers with the information they need to use them. It gives people an option that goes beyond surgery, radiation, and chemotherapy. This book should be in the library of every health care practitioner and physician interested in cancer therapies, whether or not they use them.

Start Making Changes Now!

After reading this chapter on breast-cancer causes and preventives, you may feel a bit overwhelmed by the dozens of prevention strategies. And it can be overwhelming if you envision implementing everything at once. Instead, remember that prevention is a long-term proposition. More important than doing everything at once is to try taking one step at a time.

The opportunities to do so will often present themselves in the course of your normal activities. For example, the next time you go grocery shopping, put salmon instead of beef steaks in your shopping cart. Or the next time you're buying personal care items, choose chemical-free, environmentally friendly formulas. The more prevention strategies you manage to implement, the lower your breast-cancer risk will drop.

If you are persistent, after a while many prevention strategies will be at work for you — with little or no extra effort or sacrifice.

Chapter 12

Down With Diabetes

Diabetes is not only on the rise, it's exploding! (*The Lancet,* end of year review, vol 352, 1998).

I'm not talking about type I diabetes, an autoimmune disease that often begins in childhood, but type II diabetes, an often-preventable disease that affects adults. According to Dr. Kathi Head, ND, naturopath and author of *Your Natural Guide to Diabetes* (Prima Communications, Inc., 1999), 90-95 percent of diabetics have type II.

Worldwide, type II diabetes is expected to double in the next 10 years from over 100 million people to 221 million. Some people have a genetic predisposition for this form of diabetes, but genetics is not why diabetes is doubling. We're getting more type II diabetes because we've become obese and lazy.

That's right. Obesity and lack of physical activity are two major causes of diabetes in later years. In fact, an article in *Diabetes Care* published in 1985 concluded that type II diabetes could be reduced by as much as 50 percent by preventing obesity!

Still, other studies have shown that few overweight people actually lose weight. If you've had problems with weight loss, you may have some biochemical imbalances that stand in your way. One book that addresses both the physiological and emotional aspects of overeating is my book, *Overcoming the Legacy of Overeating* (Lowell House, 1996). When you look at both parts of the problem, weight loss is possible! As you change your diet to include more beans and vegetables, you'll lose weight without restricting food quantities or feeling deprived.

It's important to keep in mind that the more risk factors you have, the greater your risk for diabetes. If you're obese but exercise, your risk is lower than if you're an obese couch potato. And the more obese you are, the more likely you are to become diabetic. The Pima Indians, a population with the highest prevalence of both diabetes and obesity in the world, brought this connection to the attention of the medical community.

What Is Type II Diabetes?

Type II diabetes is often called non-insulin dependent diabetes mellitus (NIDDM), or adult-onset diabetes. A common dietary cause comes from the production of too much insulin due to a diet high in sugar or in carbohydrates that turn into sugar quickly. Typically, people who get type II diabetes are over the age of 40 and are overweight. While some diabetics can regulate their blood sugar through diet, exercise, and nutrient therapy, others require insulin in daily injections or oral medication.

Nutritionist and author Nancy Appleton, PhD, in her book *Lick the Sugar Habit* (Avery Publishing, 1997), talks about how the pancreas in people with diabetes becomes overworked, exhausted, and finally stops functioning properly. It either can't keep secreting insulin in sufficient quantities or the insulin is too weak to work well. The result is that instead of being able to use the glucose from your foods, sugar levels remain high in your bloodstream. High blood sugar that can't be regulated equals diabetes.

Understanding Insulin

Insulin is a hormone made in the pancreas that is secreted when you have too much sugar in your blood. It prevents sugar from flooding the bloodstream. Your body naturally secretes insulin after eating meals, especially when those meals are high in sugar and simple carbohydrates. Almost everything we eat eventually turns into sugar, so your pancreas has a lot of work to do constantly, but some foods trigger this insulin response more than others. Insulin drives nutrients from the blood into cells of the liver, muscle, and fat tissues. It also stops your liver from producing glucose, and this also helps keep your blood-sugar levels normal.

With type II diabetes, a person's body develops resistance to insulin. This means that even if your pancreas is producing sufficient quantities of insulin, it is not able to regulate your blood sugar. You see, insulin can't just fasten itself anywhere on your cells and do its job. It has to attach itself to specific areas on cells called receptor sites. These are places reserved for insulin. In effect, these receptor sites are like parking slots where only insulin can park. Once attached, insulin can then activate various processes inside the cell and regulate blood sugar. Dr. Head points out that as your weight increases, the number of receptor sites for insulin decreases. Fewer parking places means less insulin is available to your body for blood sugar regulation. Fortunately, when you lose weight, you regain some of these insulin receptor sites.

Diabetic Symptoms and Complications

Interestingly, some people with type II diabetes don't have any symptoms at all and can only be diagnosed through a fasting blood test. If glucose levels are higher than 126 mg/dl, you may have diabetes. An even more specific blood test, glycosylated

---

Hypoglycemia and Caffeine

Medical doctors don't agree about hypoglycemia (low blood sugar). Some maintain it doesn't exist, and the symptoms attributed to it — afternoon fatigue, dizziness, feeling spacey, having difficulty concentrating, waking up exhausted in the morning — are all in you mind. But thousands of people, mostly women, experience these symptoms regularly. They know something physiological is going on.

Hypoglycemia responds to a diet of frequent meals high in whole grains, beans, and vegetables. Symptoms are made worse by eating refined sugar and drinking alcohol. Now, a study published recently in the *Annals of Internal Medicine* indicate that caffeine contributes to hypoglycemic symptoms, even when the blood-sugar level is not low enough to be considered hypoglycemic by those doctors who recognize the disease.

The amount of caffeine that caused hypoglycemic symptoms was the equivalent of two cups of coffee. If you suffer from hypoglycemic symptoms you might want to reduce you caffeine to half a cup a day for a few weeks. And by drinking a small amount of caffeine you won't experience caffeine withdrawal headaches.

hemoglobin, or HbAIc, lets your doctor know how well your blood sugar has been regulated over a period of about three months. If you've been overweight for a number of years, it's a basic precautionary measure to have your doctor include this test in your yearly exam to rule out potential problems.

When symptoms of diabetes occur, they may include frequent urination, thirst, increased hunger, weight loss, and muscle wasting. Because some of these symptoms may indicate other health problems, it's important not to self-diagnose and medicate for diabetes, but to check it out with a physician. While the symptoms of type II diabetes are not life threatening, complications from diabetes are.

Diabetes frequently leads to other more serious health problems like heart disease, stroke, nerve damage (with resulting numbness or pain), kidney problems, and eye problems that can lead to blindness. When blood-sugar levels remain high, blood vessels can become damaged. The result may be hardening of the arteries and poor circulation in your legs. There are specific nutrients that can be used for complications of diabetes that I won't discuss here. I think with a little information and change in lifestyle, you may not need to address them. And each complication requires a different set of

---

Diabetes and Vitamin C

If you're diabetic, you need more vitamin C than other people, since insulin helps move vitamin C into the cells. Vitamin C deficiencies can lead to poor wound healing, bleeding coming from fragile capillaries, high cholesterol, and a low immune system.

A random double-blind study published last year on 56 diabetics over a nine-month period showed that when taking two grams of vitamin C a day (2,000 mg), the diabetics who did not need to be on insulin had improved fasting blood sugar, as well as lower cholesterol and triglycerides.

With so many women who are diabetic, it's important to realize the importance of taking enough vitamin C. If you have diabetes in your family, increase your vitamin C-rich foods like potatoes, bell peppers, and citrus fruits as insurance. Most fruits and vegetables contain vitamin C, and we should all be eating plenty of them daily.

Eriksson, J. and A. Kohvakka, "Magnesium and ascorbic acid supplementation in diabetes mellitus," *Ann Nutr Metab* 39:217-23. 1995.

controls. Fortunately, not all methods of controlling type II diabetes include taking insulin.

Not All Diabetics Need Insulin

The good news is that many people can control their blood sugar through weight loss, exercise, and a combination of diet and nutrient therapy. While this means making major changes in your lifestyle, remember that diabetes forces you to make major changes. They may as well be changes that allow you to live a healthy life, rather than adapt to limitations. The first step is to keep your blood sugar from getting too high and requiring your pancreas to secrete more insulin. Exercise can help, so begin by walking every day — even if it's for a few minutes. Then work up to half an hour or more daily. Next, take a look at your diet. You need to eat a good quantity of beans and soy products, because these foods are low on the glycemic index.

Changing Your Diet

What is the glycemic index? Simply put, it is a system that tells you how quickly various foods turn into sugar. The faster they become sugar, the higher they are on the glycemic index. Sugar is 100, fructose — fruit sugar — is 20. Beans are low on the glycemic index (from 15-30), while potatoes are 85 and both carrots and white bread are 71.

This doesn't mean you can't eat foods high on the glycemic index when they're "healthy" foods, like potatoes. It just means you should combine high glycemic foods with low glycemic foods. For instance, instead of eating a salad with fat-free dressing and a large baked potato, you could have a small baked potato filled with chili beans with your salad. The idea is to limit the amount of high-glycemic foods you eat at any one meal. See page 368 for a partial list of foods and where they are on the glycemic index. Use this as a guide for revising your eating plan.

The Zone diet: The Zone diet, devised by Barry Sears, PhD, who works in biotechnology, consists of eating 30 percent of calories from protein, 40 percent from carbohydrates, and 30 percent from fat. This diet will help control blood sugar, because when you combine a high-glycemic index food like a potato with fats or protein, the glycemic index of that meal is reduced. In other words, a 40-30-30 diet like the Zone makes it possible to eat foods that turn to sugar quickly. But it's not a safe diet. High fat diets often lead to digestive problems and both gall bladder and colon disease. While Sears suggests lower fat animal protein like turkey and chicken, the majority of people use the Zone diet as an excuse to eat more beef, dairy, and other foods high in saturated fats. The Zone is a quick, easy way to regulate your blood sugar. I think there are other ways that are healthier on a long-term basis that will give you the same

Sugar Alternatives

What's the best new sugar alternative on the market today, Sucanat or Florida Crystals? Neither, if your energy soars after eating refined sugar and then drops. Neither, if you have any yeast infection and don't want to feed the bad bugs. Both Sucanat and Florida Crystals are made from cane sugar, the same stuff that C&H sells.

The difference between refined white sugar and these new products, finding their way into a myriad of health food store items, are traces of vitamins and minerals. Sucanat is an unrefined, granulated sugar-cane juice, containing the nutrients that naturally occur in sugar cane. Raymond Francis, an MIT-trained scientist without credentials in nutrition, bio-chemisty or medicine, claims in an article that Sucanat does not rob your body of B vitamins like refined sugar, or contribute to cancer, vitamin C transport, tooth decay, or other health problems. His article on Sucanat is not documented. A preliminary study at Joslin Diabetes Center in Boston indicated that Sucanat reduced glucose levels in diabetics who were not on insulin. A second study to substantiate this one is planned. What I like about Sucanat is that some of the cane sugar used in it is organic.

Florida Crystals is made from unbleached cane sugar. The growers rotate the sugar cane crop with rice, some of which is organic. This company seems to have a commitment to sustainable agriculture, organic farming, and the environment. Nowhere in their literature are there claims that Florida Crystals are absorbed differently into the body than refined sugar, or that they contain substantially more nutrients.

For now, if you're trying to reduce your sugar intake, that includes reducing foods made with Florida Crystals and Sucanat. If you're going to have some sugar, these forms may be a little healthier for you and a lot healthier for the environment.

blood-sugar regulation and protect you against other illnesses, rather than increase your risk for them.

Basic Dietary Rules

Keep your protein and vegetable intake high, and your carbohydrates reasonably low. A high-carbohydrate diet simply does not work well for many diabetics or people who have trouble losing weight. Be sure a good portion of your diet comes from vegetable protein like beans and soy products so you don't overeat animal fats.

An article in the *New England Journal of Medicine* (vol 319, no 13, 1988) found that a low-fat, high-carbohydrate diet can increase cholesterol, triglycerides, and cause a deterioration in blood-sugar control in people with type II diabetes.

Your best choice would be to reduce all carbs except for beans. An occasional slice of whole wheat bread, half a cup of brown rice, or a single piece of fruit for a snack should be just fine. If beans and soy give you gas, remember to take some Beano with your meals, or find a pancreatic enzyme product at your natural foods store (papaya enzyme simply isn't strong enough for most people).

Don't skip meals. To regulate your blood sugar, you need to eat every five hours or so. By lowering carbohydrates, you'll begin to lose weight without missing meals. And remember, you're combining your dietary changes with increased exercise.

Not all fats are bad, although saturated fats from animal protein and some sugar-free baked goods can increase your risk of heart disease. Essential fatty acids (EFAs) are necessary to good health. Reduce animal fats and increase the fats found in raw nuts and seeds as well as in soy products like tofu or soy milk. EFAs also help increase your metabolism, resulting in ... yes, more weight loss!

Specific foods: Jerusalem artichokes (called sun chokes), burdock root, and dandelion, all contain inulin, a substance that can lower insulin levels after a meal. Jerusalem artichokes are crunchy, slightly sweet roots that can be chopped up and added to salads. Or you can add them to soups or steam/sauté them as a cooked vegetable. When cooked, they taste more like potatoes. Some pastas found in health food stores contain Jerusalem artichokes, as well.

If you're interested in exploring this area more completely, you'll want to pick up Dr. Kathi Head's book, *Your Natural Guide to Diabetes.* It's inexpensive and packed with well-researched information on both nutrient and drug therapy. Here's an overview of some basic nutrients found to be helpful in regulating blood sugar.

Chromium: Found in abundance in brewer's yeast, and to a lesser degree in brown rice, cheese, potatoes, and whole wheat bread, this mineral is needed to help your body use fats and sugars. Interestingly, when you eat a diet high in sugar, your body uses up more chromium. So you may easily be chromium-deficient. Chromium helps your cells become more sensitive to insulin, allowing the hormone to do its job in regulating blood sugar more effectively. A number of scientific studies have shown the effectiveness of chromium in blood-sugar regulation. While 200 mcg is the usual amount found in high potency supplements, you may need much more. For effective control, 600 mcg or more may be required, but don't take more than 600 mcg without talking with an experienced health-care provider. Although chromium is safe, anything in large enough doses can contribute to other imbalances. A skilled health-care partner will help you understand if you need more chromium or need to make other adjustments in your diet, exercise, or nutrient program.

Magnesium: Many diabetics are deficient in magnesium, a mineral that helps insulin work better. In 1992, the American Diabetes Association came out with a statement that "magnesium deficiency may play a role in insulin resistance, carbohydrate intolerance, and hypertension." (*Diabetes Care*, vol 15, no. 8, 1992). Magnesium is necessary for the production and release of insulin, as well as increasing the number of insulin receptors. Low magnesium is also associated with a number of complications of diabetes like heart, nerve, eye, and kidney diseases. Unless you already have kidney disease, magnesium may be taken to bowel tolerance — as much as you can handle without getting too much of a laxative effect. In some women, this amount will vary from 100 mg to 1,000 mg.

Gymnema sylvestre: The leaves of this plant, native to India, have been used for thousands of years to treat diabetes. It is just recently being studied in this country. It is believed that Gymnema helps regenerate pancreas cells responsible for secreting insulin. Because most studies have been conducted on animals, although Gymnema appears to be safe, I advise you use it only under the supervision of a trained health professional (acupuncturist or naturopath, for instance). The typical dose used is 400-600 mg of a standardized extract of 24 percent gymnemic acid.

Other herbs: *Momordica charantia*, known as bitter melon, and the common herb fenugreek (*Trigonella foenum graecum*) have both been used to regulate blood sugar. Many of the studies originated in India, where these herbs are prevalent. Other Indian herbs used traditionally for diabetes include *Coccinia indica* and

All Complex Carbs Are Not Alike

Now that we're becoming familiar with the difference between complex carbohydrates (starchy vegetables and beans, for instance) and simple sugars (white sugar and honey), there's new information that will either confuse us further — or give us more energy. We've been told that complex carbos turn into sugar more slowly than simple sugars, and for that reason provide more constant energy over a longer period of time. By switching from a high-sugar meal to a high-starch meal, we'll be more energetic and healthier. But all complex carbos are not alike.

Some starchy foods raise our blood sugar and insulin levels higher than sugar. And the longer it takes for foods to turn into sugar, the more sustained our energy. Fats slow down the absorption of simple sugars, so an ice cream cone containing fats doesn't cause a sugar rush and sudden energy drop. But a baked potato could! It all depends on the glycemic index, which tells us how fast certain foods turn into sugar. If you're eating a diet high in complex carbohydrates that turn to sugar quickly, you may be having periods of low energy. Even if the foods are healthy foods.

Potatoes, sweet corn, and grains (even whole grains like brown rice) are higher on the glycemic index than beans. Keep plenty of garbanzos, black beans, kidney beans, navy beans, etc. in your diet. Sweet potatoes are lower on the glycemic index than white-fleshed potatoes, so eat more of them for better energy. If you're eating grains, corn, or potatoes, add a little fat to them to slow down their conversion into sugar. Just a half teaspoon of olive oil or butter will give you more sustained energy.

Ref: Blaak, EE, Saris, WHM, "Health aspects of various digestible carbohydrates," *Nutrition Research* 15, 1547-1573 (1995).

Pterocarpus marsupium, but there aren't a lot of studies on these herbs as yet. In Israel, Salt Bush (*Atriplex halimus*) seems to have growing data supporting its use for blood-sugar control. I support the use of herbs for diabetes and other conditions, but without sufficient studies, we suggest you limit your use of herbs to those with more scientific studies, unless you're working with an experienced herbalist. You may want to consult Dr. Head's book on diabetes and share the information with your health-care professional.

Treatment for Diabetic Side Effects

Different nutrients and herbs have been found to be helpful in stopping the progression of such diabetic side effects as heart disease, stroke, nerve damage, and eye problems. Since no two people are exactly alike, the program you need may be different from someone else's. Dr. Head's book can lead you and your doctor to some nutrients that may benefit your blood sugar and give extra protection to whatever areas you both believe may need more support.

Lipoic acid (200 mg three times a day with meals) has been widely used in Germany to reduce symptoms of diabetic neuropathy. So have various essential fatty acids, like three to four grams daily of evening primrose oil, borage seed oil, or black currant oil.

Diabetes and Supplements

Eating correctly and losing weight may not be all you can do for diabetes, especially if you're not on insulin. Nearly 60 diabetic patients who had non-insulin dependent diabetes mellitus took two grams (2,000 mg) of vitamin C each day for three months. Their blood-sugar levels improved. A side benefit was that their cholesterol and triglyceride levels were lowered as well.

The same people had their blood pressure reduced when they were given 600 mg of magnesium a day for three months. Diabetics who were insulin dependent received similar results from the magnesium.

If you are diabetic, you may want to discuss this study with your doctor and consider boosting your supplementation a bit. Neither supplement has any side effects other than, possibly, looser stools.

Eriksson, J. AMagnesium and ascorbic supplementation in diabetes mellitus,@ *Annals of Nutrition Metabolism,* 1995;39:217-223.

However, the oils can take a few months to work. Vitamins E, B$_6$, C, and magnesium are nutrients that may help prevent diabetic complications in the eyes.

We all want a quick fix for our problems, even when they have to do with our health and may have taken years to create. But quick fixes, known by some health practitioners as "silver bullets," are not always the best solution. It may be easier to take a handful of supplements and herbs, but resist this temptation and begin with changing your diet and exercising regularly. Then add one or two nutrients to your program like magnesium and chromium. This way you'll feel the importance of lifestyle changes and won't become dependent on pills. Without diet and exercise, nutrient therapy won't work as well, anyway.

Preventing Diabetes

There's no way around it. Diet and exercise come first. They are the two aspects of your lifestyle that can not only reverse type II diabetes, but help you prevent it. If you're obese, check with your doctor before beginning any exercise program, but don't use this as an excuse to put it off. Start with a five-minute walk every day on a flat surface. Gradually increase your time and speed, but begin slowly. If you haven't exercised regularly before, this can be a challenge. But so is diabetes. And in many cases, when you lose weight, you lose diabetes.

Remember to eat enough protein. If you limit animal protein to once a day, at most, you can have vegetable protein like soy sausage, protein powder, bean soups, humus, veggie burgers, and beans in salads in your other meals. You can eat them with each meal, if you like. Be creative and take charge. The health you save is your own. The quality of life you experience from now on may be based on the changes you make today in your diet. Type II diabetes is both preventable and reversible in most cases. The odds are in your favor if you're willing to make a few important changes.

Modify your diet. Begin by reducing starches, and especially refined grains. An article in the *Journal of the American Medical Association* (February 12, 1997) found that refined grains, low fiber, and foods high on the glycemic index were associated with an increased risk of diabetes in women. Re-design your diet to include more beans as well as plenty of yellow vegetables and fruits. These fruits and vegetables are high in beta carotene. Don't forget tomatoes, if you tolerate them well. They're particularly high in lycopene when they're cooked (as in tomato sauce or tomato paste). Both beta carotene and lycopene have been found to be lower in diabetics than in people whose blood-sugar levels are normal.

Q: How do you suggest I eliminate or diminish the pain in my feet and legs caused by diabetic neuropathy after the diabetes is under control? — *S.B., Oklahoma City, Oklahoma*

A: As you may already know, the pain of diabetic neuropathy is usually caused by damage to the capillaries supplying the peripheral nervous system. If you don't already, include aerobic exercise in your daily routine. Walking is ideal and will help oxygenate and stimulate metabolic function within capillaries and surrounding tissues.

According to Dr. Melvyn Werbach, MD, in his textbook called *Nutritional Influences on Illness* (Third Line Press, 1996), some of the B vitamins have been found in studies to be beneficial. Diabetics with both neuropathy and a vitamin B_6 deficiency improved after taking this nutrient. Vitamin B_{12} deficiency has also been associated with diabetic neuropathy, and both inositol and biotin improved sensory nerve function and improvement. A double-blind study showed that evening primrose oil was also beneficial. You might want to take a vitamin B complex. But if you have type I diabetes, evening primrose oil could increase your cholesterol. Check with your doctor before taking this essential fatty acid.

If you haven't already, now may also be the time to discover the power of Traditional Chinese Medicine (TCM). TCM can improve circulatory problems and the resulting inflammation, swelling, and pain of neuropathy.

Acupuncture can even reverse neuropathy. Dr. William Cargile, CD, LAc, FIACA, Chairman of Research, American Association of Acupuncture and Oriental Medicine, used acupuncture to treat a 90-year-old patient who had been bedridden for years and had no feeling in his feet. After the third session, the patient regained feeling in his feet and resumed walking (eventually increasing his regimen to three miles a day).

Chelation may also provide additional relief, according to Garry F. Gordon, MD and co-founder of the American College of Advancement in Medicine, by improving circulation. To locate TCM and chelation specialists in your area, call the American Holistic Health Association at 714-779-6152.

Using the Glycemic Index

All foods eventually turn into sugar, even fats and proteins. Carbohydrates turn into sugar more quickly, and the rate at which these foods raise blood-sugar levels is the basis for the glycemic index (GI). For people with diabetes (high blood sugar) it's extremely important to eat more foods lower on the glycemic index. For everyone else, eating more foods with a lower GI means having more energy over a longer period of time. When your energy is more even, you feel hungry less frequently and it's easier to exercise more. Even long walks become less tiresome. End result — weight loss.

Now, don't misinterpret this to mean that foods with a high GI should be eliminated. Just mix them with foods lower on the scale. Combining high GI foods with large amounts of fats or protein also lowers the total glucose response. But you probably don't want to eat a meal high in fats. Try eating those foods with a high GI along with a protein meal, like chicken, fish, or beans with a small amount of rice or a potato. Keep your starches low, because when you eat a lot of these high-carbohydrate foods, your blood glucose level goes higher than it would with a smaller amount of the same foods.

Here's an example. Glucose, on the GI, is 100. A baked potato is 85. That's pretty high, considering that pasta is only 33! How, then, can you eat a baked potato without having your blood sugar jump to the ceiling? By first choosing a slightly smaller potato than usual. Then, by adding half a cup or so of chili beans to it. The protein in beans lowers the total GI, the fiber in beans causes them to already have a low GI.

Both the particle size and the gelatinous degree of a starch influence the glycemic index as well. Let's go back to our baked potato and look at particle size. The potato is one unit of starch surrounded by skin. The same amount of lentils or kidney beans would be lots and lots of tiny starch particles surrounded by skin. Less particles, more skin results in a lower glycemic index. That baked potato with a GI of 85 compares with lentils or beans at around 30!

The more gelatinous the grain, the higher the GI. White bread is more gelatinous, or chewy, than pasta. White bread has a GI of

71, while pasta comes in at around 33. And oatmeal, which is certainly good for you, is up at 65. So what do you eat for breakfast? Taking a look at oatmeal as an example, it all depends on how much you eat and what you add to it. By adding foods lower on the GI, you turn a potentially high blood glucose into one that keeps on going over a longer period of time.

A large bowl of oatmeal is 65, plus maybe a few points if you eat a huge bowl of it. Add raisins (64) and honey (73) and you've got a meal with a glycemic index that will upset the blood-sugar level of any diabetic and many of the rest of us. But what if you limit yourself to 1/2 to 2/3 of a cup of oatmeal, rather than a cup and a half? And instead of raisins, you add half an apple (36). Rather than honey, try sprinkling granulated fructose from a health food store on your cereal (21). Better yet, add a small amount of granulated Stevia extract. This herbal substitute is sweeter than sugar with a zero on the GI! (Stevia can be found in health food stores in liquid or granulated form.)

When you opt for a meal of pasta, have a small amount, with lots of vegetables in a marinara or soy sauce. If you have a choice of a little more pasta or a few slices of white bread — choose the pasta.

Choose your foods wisely!

Food	GI	Food	GI
Glucose	100	Soy beans	14
Orange juice	57	Barley	22
Bagel	72	Pasta	33
Orange	43	Corn meal	68
Rye bread	63	Carrots	71
Pear	33	Corn on the cob	60
White bread	71	Baked potato	85
Raisins	64	White rice	56
Whole grain bread	45	Sweet potato	54
Garbanzo beans	33	Brown rice	55
All Bran cereal	30	Honey	73
Kidney beans	27	Apple	36
Cream of wheat	74	Fructose	23
Lentils	30	Banana	53
Oatmeal	65		

Sugar, Cholesterol, and Triglycerides

Cholesterol and triglycerides are fats made in the liver. Most cholesterol is manufactured inside your body; only a little comes from the fats in your diet. Some people have a genetic defect that causes their liver to make more cholesterol than they need. Some of these people, even when they're on an excellent diet, need medications to keep their cholesterol reasonably low. Triglycerides are made from stored sugar — too much sugar in your diet for your body to use at this time.

So eating more foods high in sugars can increase your cholesterol. When your body stores some of the extra sugar in your diet, triglyceride levels go higher. If your blood test shows you have high triglycerides, you're simply eating too many sweets. Even too much fruit and fruit juice can raise triglycerides. Sugars can also contribute to high cholesterol, as can stress, so if your cholesterol is unreasonably high, pay attention to the importance of daily stress reduction and look closely at the total amount of sugars in your diet.

Q: My parents, aunts, and uncles all died of diabetes. My blood sugar is high. I crave sweets all the time. I don't want to use artificial sweeteners and use honey a lot instead of sugar. Can you help me? — *E.G., Robesonia, PA*

A: Yes, I can. First, stop all honey! While it is a natural form of sugar, honey is absorbed quickly into the bloodstream, much like refined sugar. It will cause your blood sugar to rise and your sugar cravings to continue.

One of the best supplements for diabetics seems to be chromium picolinate. A recent study on 180 diabetics showed that after four months, those people who took the highest amount of chromium (500 mg twice daily) had the best results. Chromium acts by helping slow down sugar metabolism. All foods eventually turn into sugar. Chromium also helps take away sugar cravings. So does a diet high in protein (including beans) and vegetables. Reduce your refined carbohydrates in favor of small amounts of brown rice, whole wheat bread, and oatmeal. Concentrate on legumes (all beans), chicken, tofu, and fish. And don't skip meals, ever.

Bradbury, J. "Added chromium may help type 2 diabetics," *The Lancet* 350, 1997.

Anderson, R., et al. main source paper in Diabetes 46, 1997.

To help keep your blood fats, or lipids, lower you can simply eat more foods lower on the GI.

High Glycemic Index Foods

Again, I'm not suggesting you throw out all foods that have a high GI. Some of them, like cornmeal and corn on the cob, have valuable nutrients and fiber. They belong in our diets. And there's nothing wrong with adding a few raisins to your cereal. Just choose your cereal wisely or reduce the amount of raisins and other sugars in that meal. Watch the effect that eating foods with a lower GI has on your blood sugar — if you're a diabetic or pre-diabetic — and pay attention to your energy. After a few weeks eating more foods with a lower GI, do you have less fatigue in the afternoon? Are you no longer tired after you eat some meals? Pay attention to how the foods you select cause you to feel both physically and emotionally.

Whether or not you have a blood-sugar problem, knowing about and using information from the glycemic index can be a valuable tool for energy and weight control. Very few health practitioners teach their patients about this, and I don't think it's smart to wait until you need it. Use the glycemic index for preventive health care today, and feel more energy tomorrow.

Section 3

Easy Ways to Get and Stay Healthy

Chapter 13

Is Your Health a Priority?

Gina was not making progress with her digestive problems. After seeing me for two months, she still hadn't found time to prepare some of the foods we had discussed. She continued to skip breakfast and eat lunch in her car in between appointments, and had not temporarily eliminated dairy to see if it was causing some of her problems. In fact, she hadn't been able to keep away from dairy for more than a few days in all the time we had been working together. "It's just too difficult to do anything right now," she explained. "We're doing a lot of entertaining and eating out two or three times a week. I'm extremely busy and stressed."

Her eating patterns and food choices were adding to Gina's stress. Somehow I needed to find a way to get through to her so she would take the time to make necessary changes. If I failed, Gina was likely to continue having gas, bloating, and constipation. I stopped writing notes in her chart and looked her in the eyes. "Tell me, Gina, what would you say are your three priorities in life right now?"

She thought for a moment. "Why, my work, my family, and my health," she replied.

"I can see that your work and family are priorities. That's where you spend your time and energies," I answered. "But I don't think your health is a priority yet. You may *want* your health to be a priority. That's why you're here. But priorities are what we do, not what we would like them to be. And you're not making enough time to make simple dietary changes to get to the bottom of your digestive problems. To find those answers you have to make your health a priority."

What's a Priority?

Your priorities are not based on the amount of time you spend in any area. For something to be a priority, you need to spend *enough* time doing something to get the results you're looking for. If you're a working woman, you've probably realized for quite a while that work is a priority. It has to be if you want to remain employed or have a successful business. If you're a mother, you may be making your family a priority by shopping for food and seeing that the laundry and other chores are done. If you're in a relationship, you may find that you're spending time talking over problems as they come up or just being together.

The same is true with your health. To make progress with any health concern you need to spend enough time to shop for the foods you need. You have to find time to prepare them and eat sitting down in a relaxed setting. You may need to make notations of what you're eating to see how foods affect the way you feel. And for your health to be a priority, you must remember to take your supplements — every day.

To lose weight or firm up, you have to get regular exercise. Years ago, I read an article about a world-class female runner in a magazine. She was asked, "What is the most difficult part of your training?" Her answer: "Putting on my shoes in the morning." Making exercise a priority can be a challenge, but you won't get results until you exercise regularly. And you won't solve your health problems until you make consistent changes.

It's difficult for many of us to make our health a priority. What mother is going to sit down and eat a healthy breakfast when her children need to be driven to school? How easy is it to prepare the foods we need when our mate or families eat differently? How can we go for a walk after work when someone needs to make dinner?

Making Your Health a Priority

How can you put your health closer to the top of your priority list? If your family is at the top of your list, remember that you're a primary role model for your children. Children don't do what you say, they do what you do. So if you improve your own health, you'll probably improve the health of everyone in your family.

Use whatever tools you need to remind yourself of the steps you want to take. Basically, this means thinking and planning ahead. Creating a new habit takes time and concentration at first. Then it's easy. Here are a few tips:

• Set your supplements out the night before. This will help you remember to take them the next day.

• Prepare some meals ahead. If you're having difficulty eating enough vegetables, make extra veggies for dinner and use the leftovers for lunch.

• Make a shopping list for the foods you need. You're likely to forget the ones you need and remember what everyone else eats.

• Keep a checklist with the most important steps you need to take. Include such things as "15 minute walk," "stretch before bed," and anything else you know you need to do, but never find time for.

• Read your checklist every morning. Put something on the list into action that day and check it off after you do.

It may not be easy at first for you to put your health near the top of your priority list, but it's often the best way for you to reach your goals. Take a look at what you want in your life. Are you investing enough time to get it? Take the time to re-think your priorities. A shift in your actions — making your health a top priority — can make all the difference between what you want and what you have.

That's what this section is about, making your health a priority. It's about taking control of your health, instead of handing it over to a doctor or a drug.

I'm not suggesting you stop taking your medications. That's not smart. Some may be your best option, while others may need to be reduced slowly before they're stopped. Still, you can learn more about your condition and more natural options. Then make a well-informed decision about what solution is truly best for you.

I'm also not saying you shouldn't see a doctor. However, most conventional doctors are trained in the use of medications, so that's usually what they suggest. Had they been trained in nutrition or herbs, they might suggest alternatives to drug therapy.

Start taking control of your health by asking your doctor to explain your condition. Or, if it's a common complaint like menstrual cramps, pregnancy-associated nausea, menopausal symptoms, anxiety, or depression, look them up in reference books that offer nutritional and herbal solutions. Two of the most valuable books I've seen on natural healing and recommend for your personal home reference library were written by doctors. They are *Healing With Foods* by Melvyn Werbach, MD (Harper Collins, 1994) and *The Healing Power of Herbs* by Michael T. Murray, ND (Prima Publishing, 1995). These authors, who have written nutritional and herbal textbooks for doctors as well as lay persons, base their information on good, sound scientific studies, not just personal experience or hearsay.

Let me walk you through this concept of taking more control of your health. Let's say you are anxious and your anxiety has bothered you enough for you to consult with a doctor. Your doctor gave you a prescription that you take and now you're not as anxious — so long as you continue taking your medication.

First, look to the cause of your anxiety. All of us are anxious at times, sometimes appropriately. But if you're frequently anxious and it's interfering with your life, you obviously have to do something. You may understand why you're anxious and feel stuck, even if you're in therapy. But does this mean that medications are the next step? Not necessarily. Most conditions have both emotional and physiological components. When you remove the physiological imbalances it's much easier to deal with your emotions. With this in mind, let's look at what Dr. Werbach and Dr. Murray say about more natural answers to anxiety.

Dr. Werbach explains the association between anxiety and refined sugar, caffeine, and food allergies. If you eat a lot of candy, cookies, or ice cream it would be smart to eliminate sugar entirely from your diet for two weeks. This is all many people need to do to reduce their anxiety or depression. Since natural sugars don't cause the same effect, you can substitute fruit-juice sweetened desserts and not feel deprived. If sugar is not the answer, try eliminating caffeine or look for a source of food sensitivity. Dr. Werbach tells you just how to find out which foods you react to that may be contributing to anxiety.

He continues by explaining the association between anxiety and a number of B vitamins, calcium, and magnesium, and a fatty-acid deficiency. And he tells how much of each nutrient to take as well as when you need medical supervision. If you read his clear analysis and follow his program step-by-step, you will find out how much of your anxiety is caused by nutritional excesses or deficiencies.

Dr. Murray adds to this information by naming two herbs that reduce anxiety: kava and valerian. He suggests beginning with kava for one month and, if you're still feeling anxious, trying valerian. Valerian root is one of a number of relaxing herbs used in Celestial Seasoning's Sleepytime Tea. Other herb tea companies also make relaxing teas with valerian that you can safely drink during the day or before going to sleep.

Here are a few suggestions for drug-free approaches to other common complaints:

For hot flashes associated with menopause: reduce the amount of spicy foods, fats, and sugars in your diet. They create heat. Add more foods that cool you from the inside out like fruits and vegetables. Add lemon to your water and sip it frequently throughout the day. Remember, water puts out fire. If your problem persists, consider a natural substance found in citrus fruits, a flavonoid called hesperidin. I have given many of my menopausal patients two capsules of hesperidin in the morning and evening and find it eliminates their hot flashes within a week or two. Dr. Murray also lists a number of herbs that have been used successfully to eliminate hot flashes including dong quai, licorice root, chaste berry, and black cohosh.

For nausea associated with pregnancy, you want to avoid medications as much as possible since they can affect the fetus as well as you. Begin by trying a light abdominal massage — or increase your intake of vitamin B_6. If these don't work, have some ginger, an herb used for motion sickness and morning sickness. The ginger can be taken in capsules or grated into a cup and made into ginger tea. Traditional Medicinals herb tea company has a delicious tea called

Ginger Aid found in most health food stores and some supermarkets. (Note: Some nutritional supplements and herbs are not recommended during pregnancy, so as always, check with your health-care provider about the safety of any treatment you are considering.)

For menstrual cramps, Dr. Werbach suggests a program of 100 IU of vitamin E three times a day for two weeks beginning 10 days before your menses. He also points out a frequent need to increase your magnesium intake, a mineral that causes muscles to relax. Calcium has the opposite effect and causes muscle contractions, so you may want to reduce your calcium intake, including all dairy products, and eat more whole grains and beans, which are higher in magnesium. Check your vitamins to make sure you're taking more magnesium than calcium if you have menstrual cramps. Bilberry is an herb you may want to try that contains a flavonoid that relaxes smooth muscles. Common over-the-counter drugs like ibuprofen cause the cycle of menstrual cramps to continue by destroying anti-cramping substances called prostaglandins along with the prostaglandins that cause cramping. Although they may take away your pain this month, they will guarantee you have them again next month — a good solution only for the manufacturer, which is interested in selling as many pills as possible.

Get a Second Opinion

If the only doctor you've visited is a conventional doctor, I suggest you find an Doctor of Osteopathic Medicine (DO or osteopath, for short) in your area. They offer everything a medical doctor (MD) does — and a lot more!

Osteopaths are fully trained and licensed physicians, just like an MD. Osteopaths can also specialize in family practice or any other specific field of medicine.

Born in the U.S.A

Osteopathy originated in the United States in the late 1800s, based on the work of registered physician Andrew Taylor Still. He went on to found the first school of osteopathy in Kirksville, Missouri in 1892, and by 1917, over 5,000 osteopaths had been trained and licensed — an impressive rate of growth that reflects osteopathy's early popularity.

Osteopathic philosophy is one that aims to treat the whole person, not just symptoms. Osteopathic medicine is a complete system of medical care that emphasizes the interrelationship of structure and function. Like Traditional Chinese Medicine, osteopathy is very concerned with balance, but the osteopathic approach to balance is more akin to that of chiropractors or physical therapists. Osteopaths believe body structure can be related to a wide range of health disorders. In the course of treatment, osteopaths use various forms of physical manipulation — skeletal and soft tissue — which is aimed at bringing the entire body into better balance, and in turn, allows the body's ability to heal itself to operate more efficiently and effectively.

Osteopathy has been proven effective in treating spinal and joint problems, arthritis, allergies, cardiac diseases, breathing dysfunctions, chronic fatigue syndrome, hiatal hernias, high blood pressure, headaches, sciatica, and other disorders related to inflammation of nerves. And in fact, there are few health disorders that don't respond to osteopathic treatment. "Osteopathy can help or resolve many problems that previously have failed to respond to medicine and surgery," says William Faber, DO, of Milwaukee, Wisconsin, head of the Milwaukee Pain Clinic. Research has also shown that osteopathic treatment is a good choice for children, with faster recovery rates and fewer negative side effects. Osteopathy does this by treating the underlying causes of serious health conditions. For example, osteopaths view coronary heart disease as having a musculoskeletal component and will treat it as such, then consider whether a prescription drug might provide additional benefits.

In this way, osteopaths tend to be conservative about prescribing drugs. That's great for patients since recent estimates are that prescription drug use is now a leading cause of death, claiming roughly 150,000 lives in the U.S. every year. This also reduces the risk of adverse prescription drug interactions for patients. And a person who is presently taking handfuls of, or just one or two, prescription pills each day, but is interested in cutting back on, or getting off of, these medications, is also a good candidate for an osteopath. Since osteopaths are licensed to prescribe drugs, they also understand the intricacies of combining them, cutting back on them, or eliminating their use entirely.

Manipulative healing therapies used by osteopaths include:

Gentle mobilization, moving a joint gently and slowly through its range of motion and gradually freeing the joint from restrictions.

Articulation, a quick thrust.

Functional and positional release, places the patient in a specific position that allows the body to relax and release muscular spasms.

Muscle energy technique, relaxing muscles through gentle tensing and releasing.

Other soft tissue techniques, to release restrictions in various soft tissues of the body.

Cranial manipulation, gentle cranial (head) manipulation to treat headaches, strokes, spinal cord injury, temporomandibular joint syndrome dysfunction; especially beneficial for young children suffering from hyperactivity, mood disorders, dizziness, and dyslexia.

Emphasis on Prevention

By restoring better musculoskeletal balance, osteopathy not only treats health disorders, but can produce exciting secondary effects that restore overall wellness. Many osteopaths further assist patients in preventive health care through the teaching of relaxation techniques, improved breathing methods, postural correction, and individualized nutritional guidance.

"If you consider that the musculoskeletal system makes up the largest body system, using far and away the greatest amount of energy," says Leon Chaitow, ND, DO, of London, England, "and if you reflect on the fact that it is through the musculoskeletal system that you live your life, you will begin to appreciate osteopathy's importance."

Chapter 14

The Best Way to Achieve Optimum Health — A Good Diet

Some people function best on a high-protein diet, such as the one featured in *Enter the Zone*, a popular diet book by Barry Sears, PhD. For many others, however, a high complex-carbohydrate diet is the best one for feeling satisfied after meals and providing a steady stream of maximum energy. But how can you determine which foods will keep you free from illness?

As I've researched various health conditions from digestive problems to osteoporosis, breast disease, and heart disease, I've found that scientific studies are showing that diets lower in animal protein and higher in vegetable protein are healthier. In fact, when I wrote my first book, *The Nutrition Detective* (Tarcher, 1985), I was one of the first authors to explain how diets high in dairy increase premenstrual symptoms (PMS) and actually contribute to osteoporosis — as well as menstrual cramps, fibromyalgia, food sensitivities, and atherosclerosis. I put together an anti-illness diet in my book that talked about eating a diet higher in whole grains, beans, and vegetables, and lower in fats and animal protein.

Today, little has changed in my anti-illness diet. We're now seeing, however, that cultures that eat large amounts of soy products have a reduction in osteoporosis, breast and prostate cancer, and other illnesses. Ditto for green tea. So I've added soy to the diet, as it's one of my main sources of vegetable protein. And I've added three cups of green tea to the diet.

I realize there are some people who are sensitive to soy. A good friend of mine in Los Angeles is a physician, Dr. Cathie-Ann Lippman, who works with people with food sensitivities. We have talked about this subject and agree that people who are sensitive to soy should avoid it, but soy has so many benefits for the rest of us that we should keep it in our diets as a regular protein source. Soy has become quite controversial lately, so I'll discuss it more in a moment.

Flaxseed is another recently discovered nutrient powerhouse that in my opinion is not just a fad but is here to stay. It's rich in essential fatty acids and has strong antioxidant properties. I have a special coffee grinder that I use to grind a tablespoon or two of flaxseed daily, which I then sprinkle on a salad.

The biggest problem I ran into when formulating the diet was how to get enough protein. Complex carbohydrates from whole grains are an essential part of a healthy diet, but they don't replace the need for slow-burning energy in the form of protein. You can slow down the rate at which carbs are burned by adding either protein or fat. This, in fact, is the basis for the Zone diet. From a health standpoint, I believe adding vegetable protein is healthier than adding more fat.

With all that said, let's discuss some of the issues surrounding a healthy diet and how you can easily switch to a diet that will keep you healthy for years to come. What follows is a dietary plan that will give you the most energy and help you attain your proper weight. At the same time, it's probably the best protection against illness for both you and your family.

Protein: Striking a Healthy Balance

The subject of protein can be confusing. In this country, we tend to eat too much of it. Animal protein, that is. And we do know that too much animal protein can contribute to health problems from osteoporosis to heart disease and cancer.

A diet too high in calcium and phosphorous (common in diets high in animal protein) can leach calcium out of your bones. And it tends to be high in the saturated fats that are not health promoting.

Proponents of a high animal protein diet go back to our ancestors, who ate what is called the Paleolithic diet, and suggests we eat the way they did.

Before agriculture, our ancestors lived mostly on wild game, birds, and insects. They did not have the diseases we have today. How could they? Their life expectancy was an average of 35 years!

We know that breast cancer, colon cancer, and heart disease can all be affected by a diet high in animal fats. We also know that it can take 20 to 30 years for these diseases to become detectable. To return to a Paleolithic-style diet seems short sighted, but perhaps looking at the balance in their diet, high in plants and protein, could give us a key we can use today. Perhaps we do need more protein. I suggest you would be healthier with more vegetable protein than with more animal protein. And, of course, by eating more vegetables with your meals.

With the advent of agriculture, the emphasis in diet was switched from animal protein to grains. Since then we have jumped on a seesaw that switches between a high fat, high animal-protein diet to one that is primarily grains. Neither is healthy. We need a balance of protein — not necessarily animal-based — and some grains. But our diets are often too low in vegetables, along with legumes.

While animal protein is high in saturated fat, vegetable proteins contain unsaturated fats, some in the form of essential fatty acids. And essential fatty acids are just that — essential to good health and important in weight-loss programs. Too much of one kind of protein may be harmful, and not enough protein throughout the day could cause you to hold onto the weight you'd like to lose or cause fatigue. So I thought this would be a good time to discuss vegetable proteins and give you some ideas on how to incorporate them into your diet.

For many years it was thought that you had to combine legumes (beans and soy products) with grains at the same meal to make a complete protein. Now we know you can eat these foods throughout the day and your body will combine them.

Too Many Carbohydrates May Keep You From Losing Weight

In an effort to be more health conscious, some women are limiting their animal protein and eating more carbohydrates (fruits, sugars, and grains). Not all, but some of these women, find they have increased fatigue, mental fuzziness or confusion, and difficulty keeping those extra pounds off. The problem is that they are particularly sensitive to carbohydrates. Eating carbohydrates stimulates their pancreas to make more insulin, and insulin is a hormone that helps the body store carbohydrates in fat cells. These women simply can't lose weight if they eat a lot of starches and sugars. And their energy levels and mental clarity fluctuate greatly, as well. If you struggle with extra pounds that threaten to stay on no matter what you do, and if you're feeling more tired than you think you should, consider eating more protein and less starches for a while.

Eat More Vegetable Protein

This means all kinds of beans, including soy with all its cancer-protecting nutrients. While beans are starchy and do contain some carbohydrates, they are a good source of slow-burning energy and are high in protein as well. To feel satisfied and keep from getting hungry an hour or two after breakfast, begin your day with some form of plant protein. Remember, you don't have to eat breakfast food first thing in the morning. You may choose anything from some lentil or split pea soup to a Boca Burger (made from soy protein, and found in the frozen section of many supermarkets) or humus (pureed garbanzo beans with lemon juice and garlic).

This isn't your idea of breakfast food, you say? Then save these ideas for lunch and make a protein shake, add some soy protein powder to your whole grain cereal, or put a little nut butter on a slice of whole grain bread (my favorite is soy butter). While nut butters are high in fat, these fats are the health-promoting kind, and nuts also contain protein. Soy butter, now available in many health food and specialty stores, is higher in protein than peanut butter, and healthier, as well. Because nut products are high in fat, and fat is difficult to digest, limit the quantity you use at any one time.

On days when you have more time to cook, try sautéing crum-
bled tofu in a bit of light olive oil, add mushrooms and any leftover
veggies, and season with soy sauce or herbs to make scrambled tofu.

Increasing protein and decreasing carbohydrates is important
for lunch and dinner, as well, especially if you're trying to lose a few
pounds (or more). Stuff half a whole-wheat pita bread with some fat-
free bean dip or vegetarian refried beans. Add sprouts or lettuce and
plenty of salsa for a high-protein meal. Thicken soups by pureeing a
can of white navy beans, a slab of tofu, or half a cup of cashews or
almonds with a few ladles full of soup out of a full soup pot. Any of
these makes the soup creamier and boosts its protein content.

How Much Protein Is Enough?

There's no need for you to count protein calories or any other
calories. Just try eating more vegetable protein and keep your animal fats low. Have some source of protein at each meal, and limit
your animal protein to one meal per day at most.

Don't go overboard with nuts and seeds, but consider adding
a few (meaning a very small handful) of nuts, pumpkin seeds, or
sunflower seeds to a protein free meal. Sprinkle raw walnuts or
almonds over a salad, or add some to a dish of veggies over a half-
portion of rice. Nuts and seeds are filling, and adding them will
make the meal more satisfying.

Tips:
- Choose any non-dairy protein powder and add it to drinks
  and cereal.
- Eat snacks with a little protein, like bean dip or humus
  and carrots or crackers.
- Experiment with pureeing tofu in sauces and salad
  dressings to boost their protein content.
- Have a little vegetable protein at night to help you sleep
  better and wake refreshed.
- A half cup of lentil, bean, or split-pea soup makes a good
  low-fat snack or side dish to salad.
- If vegetable protein gives you gas, try taking Beano or

other enzymes to help you digest them better.
- Learn to like the foods that contribute to your energy, health, and proper weight (the secret is in seasonings, and in being open to change).

We should learn from our ancestors, both the meat eaters and those who began growing their own foods. Each has something to teach us. But to think that any extreme diet is healthful is to miss the point. A diet high in animal protein will not keep you healthy. Neither, we are finding, will a diet so high in grains that there is very little protein for sustained energy.

How Much Protein? Let Your Energy Be Your Guide

How much protein do you need to consume for maximum energy? The answer depends on who you ask. Different experts will give you different answers. In *Becoming Vegetarian*, author Vesanto Melina, RD, et al, recommends around 49 grams of dietary protein daily for a 135-pound person. I agree with this general recommendation, but also consider it an approximation — different people have different dietary needs. How much protein you actually need

---

Diet and Ovarian Cancer

Although ovarian cancer causes more deaths than any other gynecological cancer, and is the fifth most common cancer that results in mortality, we still don't know very much about what causes it. However, we're getting closer to an answer. A study that appeared in the *American Journal of Epidemiology* (1999) looked at 29,000 women and found that diets high in cholesterol like meats and eggs increased the risk for ovarian cancer. So did a diet high in refined carbohydrates found in candy, cookies, and desserts.

What's protective against this form of cancer? Apparently, lots of veggies. In this study, drinking a little alcohol was more protective than having no alcohol, but previous studies show that alcoholic drinks could increase the risk. If you have one drink a day, or an occasional glass of wine, we don't see any reason to stop. On the other hand, we are not advising you begin drinking if you don't. It may be quite a while before we know for certain whether alcohol's risks outweigh its benefits.

Kushi, L.H., *et al.* "Prospective study of diet and ovarian cancer," *American Journal of Epidemiology,* vol. 149, no. 1, 1999.

to consume may be more or less than Melina's suggestion of 49 grams. In my opinion, it's best to let your energy be your guide.

If you've been experiencing fatigue for no apparent reason, such as lack of sleep or a health condition, you might try increasing your protein intake for 1 month. Do this by decreasing your intake of fast-burning foods, such as refined flour and sugar. Instead of these foods, consume a little more animal protein and/or beans, peas, and tofu. For some, a protein powder might be an easy solution. At the end of one month, if your energy level has increased, you will know a lack of protein was playing a role in your lack of energy.

When Fats Are Fine

Health issues aside, if we could eat whatever foods we wanted in unlimited quantities most of us would eat a high-fat diet. In fact, the majority of people already eat 35 to 40 percent of their energy as fat according to a study published in *Trends in Food Science Technology*. Is this preference for fat our body's way of telling us what it needs? Apparently not. It seems to be more of a learned response connected to our feelings of fullness and satisfaction after eating.

Although we know eating fatty foods isn't good for us, advertisements for high-fat foods bombard our senses daily in newspapers, magazines, television, and even in the movies. Since we are clearly in love with something that's not good for us that the media tells us to keep eating, how can we significantly lower fats in our diet? Perhaps by better understanding why dietary fats are harmful in high amounts, and which are best for us.

Are all fats harmful? In any quantity? John McDougall, a medical doctor in Santa Rosa, California, might answer "yes." He advocates a totally fat-free vegetarian diet to prevent illnesses and to reverse disease. In response to his popular books and radio shows, many restaurants in northern California now offer fat-free vegetarian "McDougall" menus. Still, a fat-free diet is difficult for most people to achieve. Tofu, avocado, nuts, and seeds are high-fat components of vegetarian diets. Are small amounts of fats okay? If so, which ones? Before I answer this we should a take a look at why so many people are saying we should avoid a high-fat diet.

Why Fats Have Gotten a Bad Rap

For the past decade, research linked a high dietary fat intake with numerous diseases: including coronary heart disease, digestive disorders and both colon and breast cancers. A study in *Preventive Medicine* investigated the relationship between animal, vegetable, and fish fats and deaths from breast cancer in 30 countries over a 15-year span of time. The results were impressive. *All fats, with the exception of fish oils, were correlated with increased deaths from breast cancer.* Although small amounts of vegetable oils did not seem to be a problem and could prove to be beneficial for other aspects of health, *high* amounts of previously thought-to-be-safe vegetable oils (polysaturated oils) were found to be harmful.

In an article published in *The Lancet* in 1990, both women and men showed significant reversal of their atteroschlersis after one year on a low-fat vegetarian diet. During this time, the only animal products they ate were egg whites and one cup of non-fat milk or yogurt a day. In addition to these dietary changes they stopped smoking and consuming caffeine, exercised, and used relaxation techniques.

Some Fats Are Just Too Sticky

A recent study published in *The Lancet* reports on the intake of particular group of fats, called *trans-fatty acids*, in women. Trans-fatty acids are the fats, which are formed when vegetable oils are solidified into margarine and vegetable shortening. And they increase the ratio of "bad" cholesterol (low-density-lipoproteins, or LDL) to "good" cholesterol (high-density-lipoproteins, or HDL).

To simplify it for you, think of the HDLs as being the healthy cholesterol. They are slick and keep the sticky LDLs from adhering to the walls of your arteries. You want enough "good" cholesterol to keep the "bad" cholesterol from causing a buildup of sticky fats (or plaque) in your arteries. But as safe as you may have thought them to be, baked goods made without butter are usually made with margarine or vegetable shortening. And this study, conducted on over 85,000 women, says they showed a significantly higher risk for coronary heart disease. *Since heart disease kills more post-menopausal women than all cancers combined, it is important to reduce your dietary intake of margarine and vegetable shortening.*

Animal fats (from meat, poultry, and dairy products) are called *saturated fats*. They are made up of a long chain of atoms. The longer the chain the slower they are to burn up and turn into energy. When you eat a lot of foods high in saturated fats, these fats tend to stick together and become deposited in cells, organs (like the liver), and arteries (often resulting in heart disease).

How Fats Play Havoc With Our Bodies

When fats mix with oxygen in our bodies they produce free radicals. In themselves, free radicals are not a problem. They become a problem when there are too many of them. In his book *Fats and Oils,* Udo Erasmus writes, "...a free radical is a subatomic, free-wheeling, loose-living electron playing the field for a mate to settle down with, and willing to break up other pairs to find that mate." As free radicals increase, they can damage cells and leave us open to many degenerative diseases like heart disease and cancers.

Antioxidants prevent oils from getting rancid in our bodies. Antioxidants include vitamins A, C, E and large number of other chemicals found naturally in fresh fruits and vegetables. No matter how high or low your fat intake is, your diet should include two to four cups a day of fresh fruits and vegetables, high in antioxidants.

This rancidity of fats can lead to other degenerative diseases as well. In one study, animal fats and fried foods were associated with increased incidents of endometrial cancer, a form of cancer found to be particularly high in obese women.

A high fat intake is also linked to increases in hormones like estrogen, and the longer a woman produces estrogen, the greater her risk for cervical, endometrial and breast cancers. Other cancers, like pancreatic, gall bladder, and colon cancers, have also been associated with high estrogen production. The more fats you eat, the more estrogen you tend to produce and store in your fat cells.

In addition, a high-fat diet is difficult to digest, especially as you get older. It takes more digestive juices to break fats down into small, usable particles. The foods you eat along with the fats may not be digested, as well. They join the fats in your intestines, fermenting and causing gas. This is not only embarrassing; when undigested food particles are too large to get into your cells they can't nourish you. They also produce harmful chemicals that can lead to colon cancer.

Finally, some women have a genetic predisposition to obesity no matter what they eat. Others become obese when their calorie intake exceeds the calories they burn. Each gram of fat equals 9 calories. The higher your fat intake, the more calories you're eating from fat.

People who are greatly over weight from overeating tend to eat food high in saturated (animal) and processed polysaturated (vegetable oil) fats. These fats contribute to disease.

A lowered-fat diet with more essential fatty acids and fish oils would lower your risk of disease. In addition, it would reduce your calorie intake...and reduce you.

What are the best fats to eat in a low-fat diet?

Since even vegetables like carrots and celery contain some fats, a non-fat diet does not exist. And some fats like essential fatty acids and fish oils contribute greatly to your health. A low-fat diet is you best choice, accompanied by plenty of fresh fruits and vegetables — that contain antioxidants which protect you from some of the harmful effects of fats.

The Best Fats You Can Eat: Essential Fatty Acids

Essential fatty acids are called "essential" because your body needs and can't manufacture them. They are responsible for the production of hormone-like substances called prostaglandins, which can either cause or eliminate menstrual cramps as well as protect against coronary heart disease. Deficiencies of essential fatty acids are found in people with cancer, multiple sclerosis, heart disease, cystic fibrosis, premenstrual tension and menstrual cramps, arthritis, in men and immune problems.

Linoleic and linolenic acids are essential fatty acids that must get into your body through the foods you eat. Foods highest in essential fatty acids are soybeans (like soy oil or tofu, pumpkin seeds, raw walnuts and walnut oil, and flaxseeds and oil.)

Many people advocate purchasing "cold-pressed" vegetable oils for cooking and salad dressings. However, heat is not the problem. All non-chemical forms of extraction produce heat. Cold-pressed, or expeller-pressed, oils are considered most beneficial primarily because they are not extracted with chemical solvents, and not refined using caustic chemicals which remove the essential fatty acids from the oil. Therefore, *cold-pressed* or *expeller-pressed* oils are best. You can find them in health food stores and some supermarkets.

The oils in fish, especially cold-water fish like halibut and salmon, contain fatty acids that don't break down easily. These fatty acids, EPA (eicosapentaenoic acid) and DHA (docosahexaenoic acid) are less saturated than the fats found in meats (arachadonic acid). The more fish you eat, the more helpful EPAs and DHAs replace arachodonic acid in your body.

Fish oils appear to have anti-inflammatory properties and studies have shown them to be helpful for some people with rheumatoid arthritis and itching skin. They have been used to treat atherosclerosis, reduce hypertension and lower cholesterol, help regulate the immune system and protect against heart disease and cancer. Since all oils can go rancid in your body, causing free radicals, if you increase your intake of fish oils through your diet or supplementation, increase your antioxidants — vitamins A, C, and E — as well.

Vegetable oils were thought to be beneficial in the past, but more recently these polyunsaturated fatty acids, found in corn, sunflower, and safflower oils have been shown to lower the "good" or healthy cholesterol (HDL).

Olive oil, on the other hand, is monounsaturated oil. It has been shown to be effective in reducing cholesterol in both men and women. Because it is not a harmful oil and does not break down at higher temperatures, many people think of it as being beneficial. Mostly, it is not harmful in small quantities.

Canola oil is also monounsaturated oil. It is made from rapeseed and has been used for centuries in the Orient. The name of the rapeseed oil was changed to present a more favorable image to the public. Both canola and olive oils are good choices for cooking — in small quantities.

A Fat That Burns Like a Carbohydrate

Fats are difficult to digest, burn slowly, and collect in tissues and arteries when we consume more than our body can use. This is why we need to limit them in our diet. Now a "new" oil, medium-chain triglycerides to the public. The molecules in this oil, made from vegetable sources, are ⅓ to ½ the size of molecules in other oils. They are more water-soluble (easier to digest) and are burned quickly for energy. In fact, *this fat burns as fast as a carbohydrate!*

Medium-chain triglycerides may be new to the consumer but they have been used for more than 30 years in hospitals to give energy to premature babies and have been given to people with compromised digestion. Now available to the public as ThinOIL, this oil can be used in baking, cooking, salad dressings, and toppings for bread. In fact, ThinOIL can be used in place of any other oil. Because its molecules are so small, it is less viscous than other oils and you can use half the amount you'd usually use. It absorbs other flavors with more intensity than other oils, like garlic, for instance, and actually gets into your taste buds more easily due to its small molecules.

Remember, the longer the chain of molecules in an oil, the more difficult it is to digest and burn. Most oils burn like large moist logs and don't always get completely burned. What isn't burned gets stored and can become rancid in your body. Medium-chain triglycerides burn like dry wood chips and are rapidly used up. Because it is not stored in arteries, it may be the oil of choice for postmenopausal women who are at increased risk for heart disease. ThinOIL is available in four flavors, original, butter garlic and, olive oil, through Sound Nutrition, Inc. (1-800-THIN-OIL).

Medium-chain triglycerides are still considered a fat, although a fast-burning one. That means 9 calories per gram, just like any other fat. The difference is that those fat calories will get burned not stored. Keep all fats in your diet low, even these.

When Are Fats Fine?

An editorial in *The New England Journal of Medicine* suggests that animal fats and trans-fatty acids like palm kernel oil, coconut oil, and margarine should be eliminated or limited to almost none. The authors, two medical doctors from Harvard, Walter Willet and Frank M. Sacks, propose we stop calling fats "good" or "bad." Instead, they suggest we use the terminology "land-mammal fat" to designate fats from red meat, lard, and dairy products.

These doctors believe all trans-fatty acids should be considered suspect until they have been proven safe. They are concerned that margarines have been allowed into our food system without their effects on our health being examined more closely.

Instead of looking for a safe fat, it's becoming clear that a low-fat diet that contains plenty of vegetables, accompanied by a lifestyle that includes regular exercise, is the way to lower your risk for such conditions as coronary heart disease, a major health problem for older women. No fat is safe if it's eaten in large enough quantities, and nobody seems able to come up with a specific amount of how much fat is fine for everyone. Therefore, my best advice is to include a variety of the following fats, *in moderation*, in your diet: essential fatty acids, fish oils (unless you're a vegetarian), and olive oil for high-heat cooking, and medium-chain triglycerides. Remember we're all biochemically different and some of us have a family history of heart disease, while others do not. When it comes to solid, saturated fats (butter, margarine, vegetable shortening, lard), it's best to eat as little as possible. Bread with margarine is no better than bread with butter and may, in fact, be worse. Eat your bread with more moist foods such as soup or salad (or chew bread more thoroughly) and you may discover you don't need butter or margarine. If a topping is necessary for you, mix butter with ThinOIL for a safer spread. Or better yet, use sugar-free jam or another alternative lower-fat spread.

Since liking fats is an acquired taste, eating a low-fat diet for two to four weeks can result in a reduction of craving high-fat foods. Or use the lighter ThinOIL in your salad dressing, sautéd foods, and home baked goods. After two weeks you won't want to go back to the thicker taste of other oils.

How Safe Is Soy?

I don't know about you, but in the past few years, I've gotten very confused about the safety of soy. Both as a food and in supplement form, soy has been sold to women as a miracle food, especially after menopause. It has been found to reduce hot flashes, lower cholesterol and risk of heart disease, prevent breast cancer, relieve vaginal dryness, and strengthen bones. In fact, soy appeared to be so beneficial that last October the Food and Drug Administration (FDA) ruled that food manufacturers could say that soy protein (not its isolated isoflavones that are found in supplements) can help lower cholesterol and protect against heart disease.

But not everything we're hearing about soy is positive. Sixteen years ago, a Canadian mother, Noni Anderson, fed soy milk to her baby girl who had a problem with cow's milk. "She now has all the symptoms of a classic soy baby: menstruated at the age of 10, low thyroid, frequent and intense migraines, learning disabilities, and a skin disease that has been associated with low thyroid called vitilago." Anderson says. While she doesn't blame soy for all her daughter's problems, she does wonder why there was no hint of a possible problem that could come from a diet of soy formula.

Noni's story is not an isolated case. Other people have had bad reactions to soy as well. Several studies linking tofu intake to brain aging and atrophy, thyroid problems, and even the growth of breast tissue have sent out signals of alarm. The media, as usual, ran with the scary headlines. After all, it sells newspapers, magazines, and advertising space on radio and TV. But Elizabeth A. Yeatley, PhD, lead nutrition scientist at the FDA's Center for Food Safety and Applied Nutrition (CFSAN) commented that "every dietary health claim that has ever been published has had controversy."

So what's the real story about soy? I decided to talk with some of the experts on the subject and try to understand what people are saying, why they're saying it, and what's behind their statements alleging that soy causes more problems than it solves.

It's truly difficult to get a clear picture since not all the studies cited to back up any particular point are as good as we'd like them to be. In fact, some are seriously flawed. People and organizations with vested interests often heavily influence the slant of articles both pro and con. Meanwhile some scientists are concerned about soy's safety based on preliminary studies, and it will be years before we get more studies to either back up these opinions or refute them.

I'm convinced that some people don't tolerate soy well, but that doesn't mean soy is harmful to everyone. Let's look at just some of the allegations, and take a peek behind them at the "other" side.

Does Tofu Consumption Cause Brain Atrophy?

Dr. Lon White, MD, senior neuroepidemiologist at Pacific Health Research Institute and Professor at the University of Hawaii School of Nursing, conducted a Hawaiian study that concluded that Japanese men and their wives who ate the most tofu from ages 45-65 had the greatest loss of cognitive function after age 75. In addition, their brains appeared to shrink and atrophy. But Mark Messina, PhD, Chairman of the Third International Symposium on the Role of Soy in Preventing and Treating Chronic Disease, notes that Alzheimer's disease has typically been found to be more prevalent among Japanese men living in Hawaii than those living in Japan. In fact, that dementia is lower in Asia than in Europe.

The study, from which this extrapolation was taken, wasn't designed to show a relationship between brain size and function and its possible cause. Could eating soy be just one factor in a lifestyle that leads to lower cognitive function as Messina asks? Or could the isoflavones in soy have been responsible for the end results?

Other factors may have influenced the outcome of the Hawaiian study as well, such as the aluminum content of tofu. Aluminum is suspected of being implicated in Alzheimer's. Dr. William Harris, MD, of Honolulu had 16 samples of soy products tested for aluminum at the University of Hawaii. Some of the tofu was high in aluminum, and it was found that aluminum content of soy is increased when it is cooked in aluminum pots. We don't

know about the aluminum content of the tofu ingested by the people Dr. White found had decreased brain function. We do know that
a two-year study of Japanese women living in Seattle did not show
an association between tofu intake and cognitive decline.

Vesanto Melina, MS, RD, co-author of *Becoming Vegetarian*
and *Becoming Vegan* (Book Publishing Co., 1995 and 2000 respectively), points out that, "The Hawaii study's research design was
seriously flawed in a number of respects, including not quantifying
the amounts of soy consumed. It is a single study, is not more widely reflected, and clearly factors other than soy could be responsible
for the findings."

I contacted Dr. White, who replied that only one other study
had ever investigated this question, and it was a poor study. His, he
claimed, is about as good a study as it gets so far. "But it is still an
observational study," he said, adding, "Bottom line is that we have
too little information to attach significant importance to such com-
parisons beyond just saying they are interesting."

Is Soy Bad for Your Thyroid?

As far back as the 1930s, studies have suggested that soy produced goiters in laboratory animals. A goiter is an enlargement of the
thyroid caused by an iodine deficiency or hypothyroidism (low thyroid function). A small number of babies who were fed soy formulas
without added iodine also developed goiters. Today's formulas contain iodine, which appears to have eliminated the problem. In addition, when soy is heated, the properties that lead to goiters are reduced.
Dr. Messina points out that there have been no studies that have been
designed to study the effects of soy formula on thyroid function.

Researchers at the National Center for Toxicology Research
(NCTR), looking at laboratory (not human or animal) studies, pro-
posed that isoflavones and other flavonoids may lead to goiters. At
the same time, they said that this is most likely to occur in people
with low iodine intake. It appears that low iodine may be more of a
problem than a high soy diet.

Seafood, seaweed, nutritional yeast, and iodized table salt all
contain good amounts of iodine. So do most multivitamin/mineral

formulas. Dr. Messina points to recent studies examining the effects of soy on thyroid that have failed to show much of a connection.

What about Noni Anderson's daughter? There's so much we don't know. Was she was born with hypothyroidism? Did her soy formula contribute to her problems, or were there other factors involved?

Is Soy Harmful for Women With Breast Cancer?

Soy contains phytoestrogens, plant-based chemicals with a weak estrogenic effect, called isoflavones. One of the isoflavones in soy, genistein, has been found in studies to slightly stimulate estrogen-receptor-positive breast cells. But higher amounts of genistein inhibit both estrogen-receptor-positive and estrogen-receptor-negative cell growth. Let's complicate this by pointing out that these studies were done in vitro (in laboratories) not in vivo (in humans). Animal studies, which are better than in vitro studies, show soy actually *inhibits* chemically induced tumors. And there are no studies I've found that show soy foods increase the risk for breast cancer. Everything I've seen indicates the opposite is true.

The American Dietetic Association has suggested that women who are taking tamoxifen to prevent a recurrence of breast cancer should avoid soy. But Dr. Messina reports an animal study that found the combination of miso with tamoxifen inhibited the development of chemically induced breast tumors by 50 percent. Tamoxifen alone had no inhibitory effect. While some oncologists actually use high amounts of isoflavones to help shrink breast-cancer tumors, it might be wise, if you've had breast cancer, to avoid soy isoflavones in supplement form unless your doctor says otherwise.

Other Studies/Other Allegations

There are other allegations that suggest soy may be harmful, but I think it's important not to jump to this conclusion yet. Until we have more long-range, double-blinded, placebo controlled studies or other well-designed studies with a large number of participants, we don't know the whole picture. This research is many years away from being completed. Meanwhile, we need to consider both sides of the soy picture — the positive and the negative.

It's important to realize that not all foods are good or safe for everyone, and that too much of a good thing may turn it into a harmful substance. A diet heavily weighted in soy will undoubtedly lead to negative side effects in some people, although the same amount may be safe for someone else. Health writer Bill Sardi points out that the companies that grow and distribute soybeans are over-promoting this food. Clearly, there are other forms of protein than soy, even in vegetarian diets.

Some of the negative allegations about soy have come from two scientists at the Food and Drug Administration (FDA). The FDA responded by saying that the benefits of soy outweigh any potential problems, and that soy contains healthy substances and is safe to consume. More information can be found at www.fda.gov.

How Much Soy Is Safe?

Last October, the FDA announced that 25 grams of soy protein a day along with a diet low in saturated fat and cholesterol may reduce the risk of heart disease. In *Becoming Vegan*, Vesanto Melina, RD, points out that one cup of cooked soybeans (like edamame) contains 28 ½ grams of protein, while half a cup of tofu has 17-20 grams. One veggie burger or soy hot dog has 9-13 grams of protein.

How much do some soy experts eat?

James W. Anderson, MD, does soy research on people at the University of Kentucky. He believes that soy is more beneficial to our health than any other food we could eat. He eats two or more servings of soy a day, beginning with 20-25 grams of soy protein for breakfast.

He also eats soybean chili, soy nut snacks, and includes tofu in stir-fry twice a week.

Mark Messina, PhD, has about 10 servings of soy a week, and estimates he's eating from 10-40 mg a day.

My Personal Recommendations Are:

• Everyone is different. Soy may be fine for you, but not for someone else.

• Don't overdo soy or any other "miracle" food or supplement. More of something good isn't always better. One or two servings a day appear to be safe for most people.

• Use the most natural form of soy you can find. Boiled green soybeans (edamame) are less processed than tofu. Tofu and tempeh are less processed than soy dogs, soy burgers, soy cheese, and soy protein powder.

• Use isoflavone supplements judiciously and let your health practitioner know what you're taking in case he or she feels you should be monitored for any possible estrogenic side effects.

• Add other legumes to your diet both for variety in taste and ingredients. People who emphasize soy frequently de-emphasize lentils and other legumes.

As for me, I add one scoop of soy protein powder to my non-soy cereal in the morning. That's about 12 grams of soy protein. Then I choose from edamame, tofu, and an occasional veggie burger or soy dog for another meal on most days. I do eat many other legumes, as well, and that's what I recommend you do, too.

No Time to Eat Well? No Problem!

Many women know which foods are healthier than others but not how to put them together into an acceptable meal everyone in the family will eat. Besides, cooking healthy meals that taste good takes time, doesn't it? Not necessarily.

Over the years, I've found a simple formula that has helped hundreds of my patients eat the way they want and need to. It's based on one of my favorite eating out experiences as a child when I was taken to a Chinese restaurant and could choose one item from column A and one from column B. The excitement of creating my own taste sensations is one I've always remembered.

The formula I've given to my patients begins with the first question: Which ethnic foods do you like to eat and what sauces or condiments give foods that flavor? Begin with tomato sauce if you like Italian. For Chinese-flavored foods, you want soy sauce with perhaps a little grated fresh ginger (it's easy to keep a small piece of ginger root in your vegetable bin). Curry turns a meal into an Indian one, and curry powder can be mixed with a can of lentil soup, then pureed together for a curried lentil sauce to pour over vegetables. For Mexican-style meals, think of salsa and corn tortillas.

Think of any other ethnic food you like— perhaps from the country where your grandparents are from — and the flavors that could turn a starch, vegetable, and protein into a meal that has a taste you enjoy. Your list of sauces and condiments, then, might look something like this:

> tomato sauce with garlic
> soy sauce with ginger or oyster sauce
> curried lentil sauce
> salsa

Next, begin a column of starches — those low-fat, filling foods that add bulk to our meals. This column might include any or all of the following:

> brown rice
> pasta (any kind)
> potatoes
> corn or whole wheat tortillas
> couscous (cracked wheat) or millet

Your next column is for vegetables. We all have our favorites and not-so-favorites. But add some of these for quick, easy meals:

> mixed Chinese vegetables (frozen or prepackaged)
> green beans
> broccoli
> mixed vegetables (fresh or frozen)

Then there's the protein column. Protein may or may not include animal protein. When it does, you can keep this protein to a small amount. Here are some ideas for protein: beans (black beans for chili, fat-free refried beans for Mexican food, pureed garbanzo beans for hummus, white beans to add to pasta sauce, pureed lentils with curry powder)

> chicken, turkey, fish, meat
> eggs
> tofu (soy bean curd)

Now you're ready to mix and match. Let me give you a few ideas and you can see how easy this is.

Italian: Toss steamed broccoli or asparagus with tomato sauce and pasta. Serve with salad (add garbanzo beans or white beans for protein) and garlic bread (use a little olive oil instead of butter). If you like, put a little ground turkey or chicken in the sauce.

Indian: Combine mixed sautéd vegetables with diced potatoes, winter squash or yams, or eggplant (whichever you prefer) and a good helping of frozen peas. Add small chunks of chicken if you want and pour over rice or millet. Add curried lentil sauce. Serve with mango chutney. If you like Indian food, but your children don't, serve their vegetables with tomato or soy sauce for a flavor they may prefer.

Chinese: Combine mixed sautéd Chinese vegetables (or add bean sprouts to frozen mixed veggies) with a little diced tofu, which adds texture but not much taste. If you want to buy just a small amount, Mori-Nu brand comes in small boxes and does not have to be refrigerated until after it's opened. Keep some in your pantry. Add a little soy sauce and fresh grated ginger if you like and serve over rice (white or brown) with oyster-flavored sauce (ready-made sauces are available in many markets, and some are vegetarian).

Mexican: Corn or whole wheat tortillas with fat-free refried beans (either pinto or black), a little leftover rice, shredded chicken if you like, and topped with salsa and romaine lettuce. Serve with a salad or put out various raw vegetables that can be added to these tostadas (tomatoes, cucumbers, sprouts, chopped carrots, avocado).

Mediterranean: If you like this taste, try pureeing a can or two of garbanzo beans and adding fresh garlic (one or two cloves) and lemon juice. Now you have fat-free hummus. The hummus sold in stores has a lot of olive oil and sesame seed paste (tahini), so it's fairly high in fat.

Next, make some couscous (cracked wheat) or millet (cooks like rice, but takes less time) and add lemon juice and a bunch of finely chopped parsley. Finely chop two or three tomatoes and add. Now you have tabouli.

Serve with a salad that has a lot of cucumbers, tomatoes, and onions with a dressing of olive oil and lemon juice. Add some whole wheat pita bread and you have a Middle-Eastern meal.

High-Energy Meal Ideas

Breakfast: Don't skip this meal! Your body needs fuel in the morning. Contrary to popular diets, fruit and fruit juice is not sufficient for most people. It's high in fruit sugars and gets digested too quickly to give you lasting energy. You may want to begin with a little fruit or diluted juice, but follow it with a whole-grain cereal. Cream of brown rice and oatmeal are two good hot cereals. Fat-free granola, Nature's Path Millet Rice flakes, or New Morning Oatios are good-tasting cold cereals that will keep your energy up. Van's International makes both organic whole wheat frozen waffles and some that are wheat-free. Look for them in health food stores and top them with a little fruit, or fruit jam.

Lunch: If wheat doesn't make you sleepy, you could have a sandwich and salad. Otherwise, look for soups like lentil, split pea, black bean — either canned, dried or homemade. Add a grain to it (throw in a little leftover brown rice or have rye crackers or rice cakes) to give you a complete protein for longer-lasting energy. Remember, mixing grains and legumes makes a complete protein, which also provides slow-burning energy.

Dinner: Keep your portion of animal protein low. About the equivalent of a half a chicken breast is sufficient when you're eating plenty of grains and beans. Make sure you add brown rice, millet, rice noodles or pasta to your protein and vegetables. Or skip the animal protein for a high-energy vegetarian meal like stir-fried vegetables over brown rice, leftover vegetables with rice and beans in a corn or whole wheat tortilla, or a veggie burger like Boca Burgers with oven-baked potato slices and cole slaw.

Snacks: Baked corn chips with or without bean dip, popcorn, whole grain crackers, fruit-juice sweetened muffins or cookies like Nana's (made with organic grains, raisins and maple syrup). Avoid snack foods made with evaporated cane juice or unrefined sugar like Sucanat. The minerals they contain may not be sufficient to keep your energy from spiking and dipping.

Give this kind of a program a few weeks, and see how your energy improves. Animal protein can take several hours from the time you eat it until it becomes energy. Complex carbohydrates turn to energy in a fraction of that time. Sustain your energy throughout the day with good quality whole foods rather than sugar and caffeine. You'll love the difference good foods make in your energy level! And if you prepare meals for other family members, too, they'll appreciate the difference as well.

Easy to Be Prepared

These meals do not have to take a lot of preparation. Some foods can be made ahead of time, others can be bought frozen, like vegetables and boneless chicken breasts. Some, like beans, can be canned.

Rice, millet, couscous, and even pasta may be made in large quantities some evening after dinner when you are going to be home. After they've been cooked and cooled down a bit, put them in plastic containers or Ziplock bags and store in the freezer. When you come home tired and rushed, simply take out a bag or two of your starch and heat it in the microwave. Sauté a package or two of frozen vegetables in a wok with a little olive oil, add your seasoning and present your family — or yourself — with a delicious, healthy, low-fat meal.

Perhaps the best way to eat well without doing much cooking is to take advantage of the many quick and healthy foods found in the health food section of supermarkets and in health food stores. I've talked before about the Polenta meals made by San Genarro and Food Merchants. Both brands need no refrigeration and come in 13 oz servings. The polenta (corn meal) is organic, and each container has some kind of topping, like marinara sauce or black bean sauce. If you want to have a fast, healthy meal, add a package of frozen broccoli and a little more sauce (dried curried lentil soup from Taste Adventures can be make into a sauce by adding boiling water). By adding some kind of beans, you've turned the instant polenta meal into one high in protein. Each serving really does serve two people. Percentage of calories from fat — 20 percent.

Casbah brand has come out with a line of Teapot Soups — dried soup mixes in individual pouches. The cup-of-soup containers get crushed easily, are difficult to pack if you're traveling, and often come apart if they're mishandled (mine get a pretty rough treatment at times). These pouches take up less space and won't rip open by accident.

Want a soup ready to heat and eat, but something healthy? Try Imagine Foods creamy soups made without dairy like creamy butternut squash or creamy broccoli. To keep from eating sugars in the afternoon, or for an after-work snack on days when dinner may be a bit late, carry a piece of fruit with you. Pick up an apple or bag of baby carrots on the way to or from work. This gives you a serving of a fruit or vegetable as well, something that's likely to be missing from a busy person's food plan.

Healthy meals do not need to be boring or take a lot of time when you have a few easy formulas to follow.

My Favorite Recipes

Like many of you, I used to cook two or three meals a day for my family. Often I cooked what other people wanted just to avoid making more than one entrée. I have always been a good cook, thanks to all I learned from my mother, and it was not uncommon for me to make elaborate dishes that took hours of preparation. Cooking was one of my hobbies.

Now I live alone and have other interests in addition to food. So while I enjoy tasty meals, I'm not willing to spend a lot of time making them. And I often cook in advance, preparing a dish that will last two, three, even four meals. Sometimes I freeze them for days when I'm busy or not in the mood to cook at all. Life is simpler, but the food I eat is still healthy and delicious. To help you get a jump-start on preparing healthy food, I'd like to share some of my favorite recipes.

Lemon-Baked Chicken

Yes, I'm a vegetarian, but years ago I wasn't. This simple chicken dish takes almost no preparation and the chicken is tenderized by its flavoring — slices of lemon.

Thin lemon slices
Boneless, skinless chicken breasts
Seasonings

Cover the bottom of a baking dish with slices of lemon. Season the chicken with salt and pepper to taste. Place the chicken breasts down on the lemon and cover with another layer of lemon. Cover and bake in a pre-heated oven at 350° for half an hour.

Two-Minute Brown Rice or Millet

If you like brown rice and/or millet (try this mild-flavored, nutty grain if you haven't), but don't want to spend a lot of time preparing it, cook it ahead and freeze it. This allows you to eat whole grains even if your family won't. Yes, it takes more than two minutes to make these grains initially, but only two minutes to re-heat them. I think they taste just as good as if you made them right before a meal.

For most grains, take one cup of the grain to two cups of water. Bring to a boil and simmer, covered, for 20 minutes. Then, without looking in the pot, turn off the heat and walk away. Half an hour later, your grains are done. I start with two to four cups of grains, which gives me four to eight cups of cooked grains. Then I let them cool down and put them in individual portions in Ziplock baggies and freeze them. When I'm ready to fix a meal, I take one or more packages out of the freezer, remove the baggie (microwaving plastic can be harmful to the food), and microwave on high for two minutes per serving. It couldn't be simpler.

Lasagna Al Forno

This lasagna is made with tofu, rather than cheese, making it lower in fat and healthier than the familiar dairy-soaked recipes. But let me begin with a confession. I'm a vegetarian who's not particularly fond of tofu. It's bland and I don't like its texture. Never have. Still, tofu is an extremely healthful food that takes on other flavors well and can easily be disguised. Filled with essential fatty acids (so you don't need to buy the low-fat variety) and isoflavones (protective against breast and prostate cancer), tofu is an important food to add to our diets regularly. In addition to blending it into soups to increase their health quotient and make soups creamy, I have found some tofu dishes I really like. This one is from a book called *Cooking Vegetarian,* by Vesanto Melina, RD, and Joseph Forest (Chronimed Publishing, Minneapolis, MN, 1998), and it's worth making. Some soy recipes are simple and some take a little more time to make, but are well worth the extra effort. For now, start with a take-off of a familiar favorite — lasagna.

> 12-oz extra-firm tofu, crumbled
> 1/2 tsp. salt
> 2 bunches spinach, washed,
> cooked, drained, chopped
> One 28-oz can tomato sauce
> 1 cup grated soy cheese or Parmesan cheese
> 6 cooked lasagna noodles
> 1 tsp. onion powder
> 8-oz grated soy cheese or low-fat
> 1 tsp. oregano
> 1 tsp. basil

Preheat oven to 350°. Combine tofu with spinach, two-thirds of the soy or Parmesan cheese, and onion powder, oregano, basil, and salt. Spread 1/4 cup of tomato sauce in 9x13-inch baking dish. Cover with three noodles, followed by one-half tofu mixture, half of grated cheese, and 1 1/2 cups tomato sauce. Repeat layers with three noodles, remaining tofu, tomato sauce, and soy cheese. Sprinkle top with remaining Parmesan. Bake uncovered for 30 to 40 minutes or until the moisture bubbles on the sides of the pan. Makes eight servings. Per serving: protein 15 gm, fat 28 percent.

Swiss Chard With Capers

I've made this vegetable dish for guests and put it over pasta, and I use it as a side dish often with lentil soup or a bean entrée. If you don't like capers, you can omit them.

Wash, chop, and sauté one bunch of Swiss chard in lemon juice (I like the red chard best, but any will do, as will beet tops or spinach). When the chard is tender, add two tablespoons of capers, more lemon juice to taste, and serve.

Breakfast Shakes: Fast, Easy, Tasty Ideas

I just finished drinking my breakfast. It took less than five minutes to make and it was delicious. What's more, it will give me energy from 7:30 until noon.

Yesterday I ate a high-carbohydrate, organic breakfast cereal at 7:00 a.m. and I was hungry at 10:00. What's the difference? Today's breakfast drink was high in protein and contained essential fats, and I feel best with a breakfast that includes protein.

When the weather gets hot, I don't feel like eating much. That's when I make a protein drink, or smoothie. With all the excellent products available in health food stores and supermarkets, your drinks are only limited by your imagination.

The ones I'm sharing with you today are not only nutritious, they are not too high in carbohydrates and contain good quantities of vegetable protein. This means your energy will be sustained, instead of peaking and dropping. Too many carbohydrates in the form of grains, fruits, juices, or other sugars — natural or refined — can cause a low-blood sugar slump in some people.

The components of a protein drink are: liquid, protein, essential fats, and flavoring. Let's look at each category to find the best-tasting choices that are low in carbohydrates and high in protein.

Liquids: Many people begin with fruit juice, but ounce-by-ounce, fruit juice is much sweeter than soy milk, rice milk, and oat or almond beverages. In fact, a cup of apple juice (21 grams of carbohydrates) or apricot nectar (36 grams of carbohydrates) is three to five times as full of sugars as soy milk (from three to seven grams, depending on whether or not it's sweetened). Even ProSoya's So Nice Chocolate soy milk has less — 17 grams of carbohydrates per cup. I suggest you choose 1/2 to 1/3 cup of one of the following:

Rice milk (low in carbs)
Almond beverage (low in carbs)
Soy milk (check brands for one you like;
low in carb calories)

All soy milk is rich in isoflavones, those cancer-protecting chemicals found in soy. Since these chemicals are found in the essential fats, don't reach for a low-fat or no-fat soy beverage. The regular formulas are the ones that are high in isoflavones, and high in essential fatty acids (see below).

Protein: This will help keep your blood-sugar level. In the past, it was popular to put a raw egg in breakfast drinks, but raw egg

Some Great Tastes for Breakfast

Breakfast shake ideas can run the gamut from something simple (all vanilla), fruity, or chocolate. Here are a few we like to get you started.

Cherry Vanilla Smoothie
1/2 -1/3 cup of vanilla soy or rice milk
1/2 cup fresh or frozen pitted cherries
1-2 scoops vanilla protein powder
1 tsp flaxseed oil

Chocolate Almond Protein Drink
1/2-1/3 cup of chocolate soy or rice milk
1/2 tsp almond extract
1-2 scoops chocolate protein powder
1-3 tbsp ground flaxseeds

Banana Nut Smoothie
1/2-1/3 cup of liquid of your choice
1-2 scoops plain protein powder
Half fresh or frozen banana
1/4 cup raw walnuts

Mango Delight
1/2-1/3 cup of liquid of your choice
1-2 scoops vanilla protein powder
1/2 cup fresh or frozen mango
1 tsp flax oil

white robs the body of biotin, an important B vitamin. With all the talk of salmonella, I don't think it's a particularly safe choice, either. Also, the yolks are high in saturated fat. We prefer vegetable protein powders.

I searched through health food stores for brands of protein powder that were high in protein and low in total calories. The ones that best met my criteria were GeniSoy Fat Free All Soy Protein powder (24 grams of protein/100 calories per serving) and Naturade Vegetable Protein Powder without soy, made from peas, rice, potato, and sesame proteins (23 grams of protein/100 calories per serving). By comparison, Schiff Women's Natural Replacement (I was drawn to it by its name) is made from soy and rice proteins, and contains a fair amount of sugar in the form of fructose (just 15 grams of protein/120 calories per serving).

What about putting some tofu in with the liquid if you're out of protein powder? That will work. MoriNu tofu, which comes in 12-oz boxes and doesn't have to be refrigerated until it's been opened, contains about 12 grams of protein and 70 calories for six ounces (half a box).

Why not use milk or a dairy-based protein powder? Many women are lactose-intolerant and already are taking too much calcium and not enough magnesium. Soy contains plenty of calcium and magnesium, making the calcium better absorbed. If you prefer a dairy-based liquid or protein for your drink, like milk or yogurt, you may want to take extra magnesium to assure that the calcium in your foods is absorbed.

Another plus for soy milk: Many soy beverages are now made from organic soybeans, free from pesticides. And if a soybean crop gets "sick" it's not given antibiotics. So soy milk can be a cleaner, safer alternative to dairy.

Essential Fatty Acids: Some fats slow down your metabolism, like saturated fats found in animal products. Others speed it up. These are the essential fatty acids (EFAs) found in flaxseed, walnuts, sunflower, and pumpkin seeds — and soy. You can also find EFAs in cold-water fish like salmon and mackerel — but they don't taste good in breakfast drinks!

According to Udo Erasmus, author of *Fats That Heal, Fats That Kill,* essential fatty acids increase your metabolism, helping you burn calories faster, while saturated fats slow it down. I suggest you add some EFAs to your breakfast drink.

I grind up one scoop (3 tablespoons) of organic flaxseeds in a coffee grinder and add it to my soy milk. It has a nutty taste and thickens the drink. You can add the equivalent of flaxseed oil (1 tsp) or throw in a small amount of raw walnuts, sunflower seeds, or pumpkin seeds, if you prefer. A friend of mine likes to use a Vita-Mix machine (which retails for $399, but she found for $10 at a yard sale), because it grinds nuts and seeds, and blends the rest of the ingredients at the same time. Heat destroys essential fats, however, so don't use roasted nuts or seeds. EFAs not only help speed up your metabolism, all fats keep you feeling satisfied longer.

If you prefer using flax oil, I suggest Spectrum or Barlean's. Both are good quality and are found in the refrigerator section of health food stores. Use 1/2 to 1 tsp a day, at least, and don't heat it. Heat destroys the EFAs, remember? Flax oil can be put into breakfast shakes or used on salads or cooked foods. For more information on recipes, get the excellent book, *Flax for Life,* by Jade Beutler (Progressive Health Publishing, Encinitas, CA, 1996). It's only $5.95 and has over a hundred recipes using flaxseed and flax oil. For more flax information (with a free newsletter they'll send you), or if you have difficulty finding this book, call the Barleans hotline at 800-445-3529.

Flavoring: Here's where you can go wild. Your liquids can be plain, mixed with fruits, or flavored-chocolate, vanilla, and even cappuccino (ProSoya So Nice soy milk). Mix plain or vanilla drinks with a cup of frozen berries, half a cup of frozen or fresh mangos, pitted cherries, or half a banana.

For a coffee-like flavoring without the caffeine, use either some decaf coffee or one of the following beverages found in most health food stores: Inka, Roma, Pero, or Caffix. One coffee substitute, Teeccino, has to be brewed like coffee. Make some ahead of time and add it to your morning drink. Teeccino comes in a variety of flavors including chocolate mint, almond amaretto, and vanilla nut. Let your imagination take you to new tastes. If you use fruit juices, keep the amount low — 1/2 cup or less.

Enjoy a quick breakfast even when you're hot or rushed. Your body needs the nutrients, and your taste buds will thank you.

Healthy Fast Foods

What do you do when you're too rushed to fix a meal and there's nothing in the house? Or when you don't feel like cooking? While women are thought of as the homemakers and cooks of the world, many of us reach a time in our lives when we just don't want to be bothered. It takes time and preparation to shop for fresh foods, then put aside the time to clean, chop, cook them into a meal that's gone in a short period of time, then clean up. When faced with this dilemma, many women turn to fast foods.

Originally, fast-food restaurants were designed to provide an occasional meal for people, but they've become the source of daily food for too many. Since *The Fast-Food Guide* by Michael Jacobsen, PhD, of the Center for Science in the Public Interest (CSPI) was published in 1986, health writers have sought to separate the worst foods from the least-worst. If you choose carefully, you can still buy an occasional fast-food meal that at least won't hurt you too much. Two more recent publications may help you make your decisions.

Eating on the Run, by Evelyn Tribole, MS, RD, (Leisure Press, Champaign, IL, 1992) covers the gamut from frozen foods (there are many more available in health food stores than she knew about in the early 1990s) to making better choices in restaurants. She also gives advice on how to handle the junk foods that are present in offices and at meetings. "If you can, find out who orders the doughnuts where you work and suggest bagels and fresh fruit instead of, or at least in addition to, the sweets." I suggest you bring something with you that you can munch on, like a Clif Luna bar or Barbara's Natural Choice fruit bar. These bars are individually wrapped, sweet, and have little or no refined sugars. They're easy to pack in your purse and have for any emergency, anywhere.

Perhaps the most valuable section of this book is the chapter on One-Minute Information. Tribole lists everything from the nutritional power of beans to high-fiber foods, and foods high in hidden fat (coleslaw, for instance, is 80-87 percent fat!). There's also a chapter on the nutritional information in fast foods that includes calories, grams of fat, percentage of fat calories, sodium, and cholesterol. All in all, a valuable book with lots of good tips to make your eating choices easier and healthier.

A smaller book you can take with you in your purse or at least keep in your car is *The Fat-Gram Guide to Restaurant Food* by Joseph C. Piscatella (Workman Publishing, NY, 1997). This book breaks down foods by categories, and then lists those found at specific fast food restaurants across the country. While it's important to look at the fat content in a food, it would be more helpful if the fat were broken down into cholesterol and essential fatty acids (dare we ask for something as important as this?). If you're just looking at percentage of fat calories, this book would lead you away from broiled halibut (40 percent calories from good essential fats) and right into the arms of a turkey club sandwich with bacon, tomato, and mayonnaise (25 percent calories from more harmful saturated fats). Piscatella's book can be helpful if you know something about foods, first. Like understanding that essential fatty acids found in fish oils, walnuts, soy, and other vegetables help increase the metabolism and are necessary to good health.

I'm also a little concerned that people are just looking at the fat content of foods. There are entire lines of foods in supermarkets that are fat-free but made from white flour and sugar. Cookies, cakes, puddings, etc. can be made to be tasty without fats, but the empty calories they contain in the form of carbohydrates just means you have more to burn off and less nutritional value to support your health. Many are also packed with negative nutritional value — chemical additives, preservatives, food dyes, etc. — that can adversely affect your heath. So use *The Fat-Gram Guide* wisely, or you can still end up eating foods that are not particularly good for you.

Chapter 15

Using Herbs to Supplement Your Diet

Until recently, herbs were used for centuries by a majority of people for most health problems. Then came pharmaceuticals, and everything changed. People forgot that most pharmaceuticals originated in the plant kingdom. Herbs were our first drugs, but because they grow abundantly in the wild, herbs were not profitable products.

Also, since the active ingredients in herbs can vary greatly, pharmaceutical companies offered a way of insuring the same quality and activity. Standardized herbs, where all capsules or tinctures contain the same amount of active ingredients, became more widely used. With standardized extracts, we've come full circle, back to herbs.

So How Good Are Herbal Products?

The media bombards us with information about herbs like St. John's wort (for depression), kava (for anxiety), and echinachea (to support the immune system). Today, people are taking herbal products more than ever. Suddenly, suppliers of herbs have been asked to double, triple, and even quadruple the quantities they are shipping of these and other herbs. People trained in how and when to pick a specific plant, how to store it, and how to get it to the manufacturer when it's still potent, have been joined by people looking to make a quick profit at any cost. Unfortunately, that cost is being passed on to the consumer in the form of herbal products that don't deliver what they promise. The problem is not with the herbs themselves, but with the quality of herbs.

Obviously, with a greater demand, the supplies of many of the more popular herbs have become limited, although many growers now are moving into the lucrative field of planting and farming herbs. But some take years before they can be harvested, and while we're waiting for plants to grow to maturity, even pharmaceutical companies are jumping into the herbal arena and coming out with products containing the more popular herbs.

To meet the demands for more raw materials, some herbs are being harvested before their ingredients are most potent. The result is that the quantity of active ingredients may vary considerably from batch to batch, and from company to company. If the herbs you buy are not potent, you may not get the results you expect. The two sides on the issue of herbal potency revolve around standardization.

To Standardize or Not to Standardize?

When an herb is standardized, it means its active ingredient remains the same from batch to batch. There's no doubt that all herb products don't start out the same. Depending on the source of the herb, when and how it was picked, how it was handled and stored, you may be buying something that is high in potency or pretty much worthless. Jane E. Brody, health writer for the *New York Times,* cites a study of 64 ginseng products that were sold as being pure, although 60 of them were so diluted with cheaper herbs that there was little activity from the ginseng itself. Most of the products that were tested proved to be worthless.

In an effort to help us know what we're buying, the FDA (along with many supplement companies) is suggesting that all herbs and herbal extracts should be standardized. After all, they say, most research on herbs has been done using standardized products. This makes for better science and helps to validate the results of the studies. It also allows supplement and pharmaceutical companies to make claims as to the effectiveness of an herbal product.

In a way, this makes a lot of sense. Standardized herbs should be researched thoroughly. They're like over-the-counter medications. When you separate one or two chemicals from the whole plant and standardize it to a particular potency, you've created an enhanced product that may have originated in nature but does not have the same properties. At this time, herbs are considered to be a food, not a drug. Standardizing herbs puts these plant products closer to the category of over-the-counter drugs than food.

But there's a serious flaw to the subject of standardization. The standardized ingredient, considered to be the "active" part of the plant, is not the only part of the herb that causes it to be effective. A capsule containing vitamin A doesn't work the same way as a food containing vitamin A, all the carotenoids, and other vitamins and minerals.

If whole foods are better than extracts made from whole foods, aren't whole herbs better than those that have been manipulated?

The therapeutic uses of herbs have been observed for hundreds of years using non-standardized herbs. Many of today's most talented herbalists have relied heavily on observations on the effectiveness of whole — not standardized — herbal products. They say standardization is not necessary, and they prefer to use what is known to have worked in the past.

They also like to monitor their clients carefully for the necessary dosage since they realize everyone's body is a little different. This watchfulness is part of the treatment in herbal medicine now being practiced by medical doctors, naturopaths, herbalists, and nurse practitioners across the country. With standardized herbs there's a tendency to use the amount found to be effective in scientific studies. While this puts the use of herbs more in the hands of the consumer, the benefits of a qualified herbalist cannot be minimized.

Health practitioners familiar with herbs understand that when knowledgeable people picked these, they were picked and handled in such a way as to ensure their potency. With the public's demand for herbal products growing daily, it's clear that some herbs are harvested just to meet industry needs.

Which Should You Use?

To be fair, both standardized and non-standardized herbs have their place, but I consider standardized herbs to be in a similar category as over-the-counter drugs. While still relatively inexpensive, standardized herbs may act more quickly than the whole herb. If you're among the majority of the population impatient for an answer to your health problem, you may opt for standardized herbs. At least you know the amount of the known active ingredient of what you're buying. But if you're willing to wait a bit longer and perhaps end up with a more positive outcome, remember that the co-factors, not just the known active ingredients, in a plant are found in the whole herb and herbal tincture. You can't out-do Mother Nature.

Which Should I Buy?

Janet Zand, founder of Zand Herbals, reminds us that herbal tinctures are more stabile than dried, encapsulated herbs. Light and air destroy active ingredients, while alcohol preserves them. Unless you can't take any alcohol, opt for a tincture. One way to avoid ingesting alcohol and still get a product that survives time is to put the drops of herbal alcohol tincture in a glass of boiling water. The water will destroy the alcohol.

Here's another usage tip. Some homeopaths prescribe herbal extracts in homeopathic doses. In practice, this generally means taking one or two drops of an extract (often diluted in a little water) in place of an entire dropperful. If you discover this works for you, it can help you save some money.

Buy products from companies that have been in business for a long period of time and are headed by herbalists. Two of my favorites are Zand Herbal and Herb Pharm. Both companies sell to health food stores throughout the country, and both use organic herbs whenever possible. Herb Pharm supports the use of wild-crafted herbs, which means herbs that are gathered in the wild responsibly, allowing for new growth for future years. Wildcrafted herbs are usually gathered by people who have been trained in respecting both the herbs they're picking and the environment in which they grow.

If you decide to try a different company's products, make sure their products are quality controlled and each batch of herbs is tested. Call the company and ask for Customer Service, to get your questions answered. Then try the product for two or three months. If you don't get the results you're looking for, try another company. I believe in starting at the top and using the best quality herbs I can find. Then, after three months, you're more likely to be able to tell if a different herbal product works as well. Meanwhile, you will have benefited by getting the best. If an herbal product doesn't work, it most likely either isn't the most appropriate one for you to take for your particular condition, or it's not of a high enough quality. Herbs work. Some herbal products work better than others.

Finding the Best

Some foods and nutritional products seem to work better than others, even when they appear to be the same. With all the media hype, it's easy to get confused and not know which products to buy. The reason results may differ is simple: Both the content of the product and the form it's in are factors in how a product works. Let's take a closer look at this phenomenon with foods, vitamin/mineral supplements, and herbs — and begin to de-mystify the subject so you can get the products that best suit your needs.

Food Differences

Tomatoes are high in lycopene, a valuable carotenoid in the vitamin A family that protects the heart and eyes. So tomatoes are important for people with a family history of macular degeneration or heart disease. But scientists have found the lycopene in tomato paste is absorbed two-and-a-half times more than lycopene in fresh tomatoes. If you're looking to boost your diet with lycopene, adding tomato paste to soup or spaghetti sauce will give you more lycopene than adding tomato to your salad.

Supplement manufacturers know that fresh tomatoes don't have enough lycopene for preventive purposes and have begun marketing lycopene supplements. It's too early to know if our bodies use the lycopene in a supplement in the same way as lycopene in tomato paste, which contains other co-factors that may enhance the properties of this substance.

The form of a food determines how slowly or quickly it is digested. For example, a fresh apple is digested more slowly than applesauce. Applesauce is digested more slowly than apple juice. Since apples are a form of carbohydrate that give quick energy, an apple can give you a little lift if you're not yet exhausted. But if you already feel faint, go for the apple juice.

Cooking affects nutrient values and not always negatively. The vitamin A in a cooked carrot is more bioavailable than the vitamin A in a raw carrot. If you're looking for additional vitamin A to ward off a cold or infection, a plate of steamed carrots will give you more beta carotene than a glass of carrot juice.

To maximize your nutrient intake and reduce confusion, eat plenty of fresh fruits and vegetables and be aware of the form your foods are in. You can eat them cooked or raw, depending on your preference. Some people digest cooked foods more easily than raw. Avoid deep fried veggies like potatoes and tempura. Eat foods that are as unrefined as possible, and chew your food well so their beneficial nutrients can get into your cells and support your health.

Supplement Quality

Vitamin and mineral supplements that appear to be alike may not be. Studies show that natural vitamin E (d-alpha tocopherol) is absorbed twice as well as synthetic vitamin E (dl-alpha tocopherol). The carrier to which it is attached, or bound, determines the absorption of some minerals. Calcium carbonate, for instance, is less well absorbed than calcium citrate, calcium malate, or calcium aspartate because calcium — along with iron and magnesium — are best absorbed in the presence of acid. Citrate, malate, and aspartate are all acidic.

The Confusing World of Herbs

Some herbs are "standardized" to contain a certain amount of a particular chemical known through scientific studies to produce a certain result while the co-factors contained in whole plants may give different results. Herbal products are filling the shelves of natural food stores, drugstores, and even some supermarkets, and not all are equally effective. Herbal tinctures remain potent longer than dried herbs in capsules because the alcohol acts to preserve the oils that often contain medicinal activity.

Aloe vera, a plant that soothes burns and the intestinal tract, is an excellent example of varying potency. The gel of a mature aloe vera plant placed directly on a burn soothes and heals quickly. Aloe vera products have a reputation for healing based on properties in the raw aloe vera gel, which are greatly diminished when the plant is heated. Most aloe vera products on the market have been heated.

The only unheated aloe vera products I've found are by Herbal Answers, Inc. (phone: 888-256-3367). Its Herbal Aloe Force Skin Gel is being used in nursing homes. I have used it on poison oak and it removes the itch almost immediately and lasts hours longer than any other product I've tried. It also keeps the rash from blossoming and spreading. Author and naturopath John Finnegan, ND, has used it on his patients with great success for psoriasis, ulcers, rosacea, fungus, and warts. You can expect similar results with the gel from fresh cut aloe leaves from your own plant.

Friendly Bacteria

Probiotics, friendly bacteria like acidophilus and bifidus, are important because their populations decline with diarrhea, a high-sugar diet, and antibiotics. But not all probiotics are the same. When several varieties are mixed together, they compete with one another and become less potent more quickly than individually packaged bacteria. Begin by using a bottle of acidophilus (for the small intestines) and follow it with a bottle of bifidus (for the large intestines). This approach is no more expensive than several bottles of mixed probiotics, but it's more effective.

Probiotics are patented strains of particular bacteria. Many acidophilus products on the market use the same low-potency acidophilus that is added to yogurt. DDS-1 is a stronger strain of acidophilus developed by a Dr. Shahani that you can find in natural food stores in the refrigerator.

Selecting the Best

First, you need to know what you're looking for. This means doing your homework. You could search the Internet, ask your health-care practitioners (especially if they don't sell the product), and talk with knowledgeable friends.

Beware of Multi-Level Marketing companies whose products are frequently either inferior in quality or overpriced. Their sales force usually consists of untrained non-professionals who are trying to make money and don't understand who should and should not use specific products.

Check libraries and bookstores for additional information on both the form and content of a product. Don't be swayed by persuasive arguments from people with a vested interest in selling any product.

Finally, if you try something that you think should work for you, and it doesn't, look at the form it's in. You may only need to make a slight adjustment to get the results you're looking for.

Smart Herb Use

I like using herbs a lot. Many natural plant products have advantages over traditional pharmaceuticals. You've heard me say many times that just because something is natural doesn't mean it's safe. This is especially true in the area of herbs. We have an abundance of folklore available on how and when to use specific herbs, but we're just beginning to understand how they affect our contemporary lifestyle. And what we're seeing leads me to these suggestions for smarter herb use.

When herbs were first used, they were taken for specific health problems over a relatively short duration. They were not taken everyday. So we are not certain of side effects from long-term use. More studies are needed. But herbal medicine began with observation and was built upon the perceptions of skilled herbalists who looked closely at their patients. Now, doctors are beginning to take a closer look at certain popular herbs.

Before Surgery

At a recent meeting of the American Society of Anesthesiologists, physicians were urged to speak with patients about possible allergic reactions to herbs and adverse drug-herb reactions. The drug-herb interactions are particularly worrisome, because some herbs, like the popular kava kava and St. John's wort, may prolong the effects of some narcotics and anesthetics. Kava can also increase the effects of some antiseizure medications.

A number of herbs interfere with blood clotting. This means that even simple surgical procedures can result in profuse bleeding. Some of the herbs that reduce platelets, needed for your blood to clot, include: ginkgo biloba (used for memory), feverfew (used for migraine headaches), garlic (used to lower cholesterol and blood pressure and fight infection), and ginger (used for nausea and digestion). Other substances, like aspirin and vitamin E, also thin the blood. If you are taking several of these on a daily basis, you might consider cutting back. One elderly woman I know was taking an aspirin each day along with ginkgo. When she began bleeding from a cut on her leg, the cut wouldn't stop bleeding and she ended up being hospitalized. Now she skips the aspirin.

Ephedra, or Ma Huang, is an herb used in many weight-loss products. It may interact with pharmaceutical antidepressants and blood-pressure medication, causing high blood pressure or an increased heart rate. Ginseng, which is used to increase energy, can also increase hypertension, cause rapid heart beat (tachycardia), and blood thinning.

Taking Responsibility for the Herbs You Take

We suggest that you speak with your doctor about any and all supplements, medications, and herbs you're taking to make certain that you will benefit as intended. If your doctor is not familiar with herbs, you need to do your homework, present it to your doctor, and sit down and discuss what is and is not advisable for you to take.

Stop taking any herbs two or three weeks before any surgical procedure, especially, but not only, if you will be given any anesthesia. This includes dental surgery. By stopping the herbs prior to surgery, you give your body time to clear them out of your system. If you can't do this, bring your herbs in their original bottles, to the hospital so your surgeon and anesthesiologist can know which herbs and in what quantities you've been taking.

Play It Smart

Add up all the supplements you're taking that have any particular action, like thinning the blood. Then speak with your health practitioner about reducing or eliminating any unnecessary products. Often, there are other non-herbal products that do not cause negative interactions with medications. To take the best care of yourself, take herbal products only when there is a real need for them, not on a whim.

Treating Illness With Herbs and Food

Let's start with the "big" illnesses and work our way down to the common cold. Most people don't realize that herbs can be used to treat and prevent some of the worst health problems you might experience. I definitely wouldn't be one to say that herbs will cure everything. In fact, most herbs aren't strong enough to cure such things as cancer or heart disease. But if you use herbs wisely, in conjunction with a good diet, you'd be surprised at how effective herbs can be. We don't have room here to go into all the herbs and how they can be used, but I do want to give you a few of my favorites. You'll notice that many of these herbs could also be classified as foods. I'm not as concerned about defining the blurry line that exists between the two. I'm just interested in what works.

Resveratrol: A Cancer Preventive That Works

Back in the 1920s, a doctor named Johanna Brandt wrote a book claiming that grapes cured her cancer. In the book, called *The Grape Cure,* Dr. Brandt explains that a grape fast, eating only grapes, is the method she used to treat her disease. At one point, she was eating as many as *four pounds* of grapes a day!

Obviously, Dr. Brandt's cure hasn't hit the mainstream, but the principles of the grape cure are now shaking the medical community.

It started when *Science* magazine published an article from the University of Illinois, Chicago that stated, "resveratrol can inhibit all three stages of chemical carcinogenesis — tumor initiation, promotion, and progression" (quoted from the *The Lancet*).

Grape plants produce resveratrol as a natural defense mechanism against fungus infection. But not all grape plants will produce the protective substance. It's only when the plant comes under the attack of a fungus that resveratrol is produced to fight off or kill the fungus. And it's this protective mechanism that has proved to be so beneficial in fighting off cancer.

This specific class of bioflavonoids that has such powerful anti-cancer effects is also found in pine bark, lemon tree bark, hazel nut tree leaves, blueberries, cherries, cranberries, and others. But the most concentrated quantity is found in the skins of certain purple grapes (resveratrol is also found in the grape seeds, but in lower concentrations).

To find resveratrol, suppliers must travel throughout the world testing grape skins and seeds for their resveratrol content. Once they find a vineyard with a high content of resveratrol, they purchase the entire lot. The grapes are then transported to a facility where they undergo a natural process using water to make a high potency extract, which is then used in the supplements.

While the therapeutic value of resveratrol is quite broad due to its antioxidant activity, results of some very sophisticated tests provide a strong rationale for its use in vascular disease as well. Resveratrol and quercetin, both found in the seeds and skins of grapes, block human platelet aggregation, i.e., they prevent the tiny poker-chip-like cells in the blood from clumping together causing clots, which cause heart attacks and strokes.

Another cardiovascular effect of resveratrol is vasorelaxation, a relaxation of the walls of the arteries that may prevent angina attacks, heart attacks, and strokes.

Resveratrol has also been found to be an effective combatant against the latest cancer dragon called COX — cyclooxygenase. This enzyme stimulates tumor cell growth and suppresses "immune surveillance," the early warning system that signals your body to attack the dangerous cells that are going cancerous. COX can also activate some carcinogens. So we need "COX inhibitors" to fight this new-found enemy within.

Work done at the University of Illinois, Chicago, has proven resveratrol in grape skins to be a powerful COX inhibitor. And it's worth repeating that resveratrol can inhibit *all three stages of chemical carcinogenesis,* an unusual phenomenon and highly significant in the treatment of cancer.

We've all had many disappointments in the treatment of cancer, so let's not assume the battle is anywhere close to being over. However, resveratrol is the most significant molecule to challenge cancer, at least in the laboratory, in many decades and perhaps ever.

Resveratrol interferes with the development of cancer on several levels, such as growth inhibition of cancer cells and reversal of pre-cancer cells to normal. As *The Lancet* put it: "Grapes are good for you, but leave the skins on." But you'd have to drink a lot of wine to get an effective dose of resveratrol — and you wouldn't want to do that. The leader of the study even went so far as to remind us that "eternal health is not to be found in the bottom of a wine bottle."

So, although not a perfect answer to the problem, grape skins and grape seeds are what we have to work with for the present.

What to Do

I don't suggest you go on a grape fast like Dr. Brandt. But I can heartily recommend taking resveratrol — especially if cancer runs in your family. If you can't find a good brand at your local health food store, our friends at Women's Preferred have a high-quality product. Please call 800-728-2288 for ordering information.

Resveratrol is nontoxic and there is essentially no known toxic dose. As with anything, you probably could overdose, but it wouldn't be easy. In an experiment with dogs, they were given *132 mg per 20 pounds of body weight per day for 12 months with no deleterious effects.* During tests on pregnant women, there was no toxicity found in the women or their babies. Nutritionists have found that a dose of 20 mg per 20 pounds of body weight for humans gives the best results. But for general prevention, stick to the recommended dosage on the label.

Some of you may be taking a product called Pycnogenol, which contains pine bark extract, and may be wondering if you need to take resveratrol. The answer is yes. Remember, the grape skin extract is far superior to any of the other types of extracts, so I recommend Resveratrol Plus or other quality grape-skin products over any of the other extracts.

Herbs (and Other Nutrients) for the Eyes

Eye health is one area where herbs can have an amazing impact. Not only can they prevent serious eye conditions, but in many cases, they can actually reverse the problems. Let's take a look at three major eye problems that afflict the elderly: cataracts, glaucoma, and macular degeneration.

Cataracts

The human eye has a compound focusing system similar to that found in a camera. This system consists of the cornea, or curved clear window of the eye, an iris diaphragm to control the light entering the eye, and a crystalline or transparent lens located just behind the iris. A cataract is a clouding of the normally clear and transparent lens of the eye. It's not a tumor or a new growth of skin or tissue over the eye, but a fogging of the lens itself. When a cataract develops, the lens becomes cloudy like a frosted window and may cause a painless blurring of vision.

The lens, located behind the pupil, focuses light on the retina at the back of the eye to produce a sharp image. When a cataract forms, the lens can become so opaque and unclear that light cannot easily be transmitted to the retina. Often, however, a cataract covers only a small part of the lens and if sight is not greatly impaired, there is no need to remove the cataract. If a large portion of the lens becomes cloudy, sight can be partially or completely lost until the cataract is removed. When this blurring of vision becomes severe enough to interfere with the individual's daily activities, then cataract surgery may be necessary to restore visual function.

Various conditions may cause cataracts to form: heredity is the determining factor in congenital and juvenile cataracts; toxic substances, certain eye injuries, chronic systemic disease (such as diabetes), or other specific eye diseases may cause cataracts. But, by far, the most common cause is simply the aging process. As we grow older, the lens gradually loses its water content and increases in density. The lens becomes hard in its center, and the ability to focus on near objects is diminished (usually requiring bifocals by age 45). As the lens ages it also becomes less clear.

Can Cataracts Be Prevented or Cured?

Depending on how far along your cataracts have progressed, you may or may not be able to avoid surgery. While surgery is rarely the best course of action, cataract surgery is a relatively safe surgi-

---

Rosemary and Breast Cancer

We know that the results from animal studies do not always translate into similar results for humans, but an interesting study published in the *Journal of Nutrition* showed that the herb rosemary kept normal cells from mutating into cancer cells in the breast tissue of rats. One reason for this, the authors of the study believe, could be an antioxidant found in rosemary called rosmanol.

Rosemary contains a number of other chemicals that may contribute to this anti-tumor protection. But don't think you can sprinkle a little rosemary on your chicken or add it to your vinegar and eat whatever you like. Rats who were on a low-fat diet with rosemary had fewer tumors than rats on a high-fat diet. And for now, we don't know how much rosemary would be helpful to add to your diet. But using it a little more freely in your cooking sounds like a good idea for added antioxidant protection if you like its flavor.

cal procedure and, coupled with appropriate corrective lenses, has preserved or restored sight for millions.

When cataracts cause enough loss of sight to interfere with your work, hobbies, or lifestyle, it's time to remove them. Depending on individual needs, you and your ophthalmologist decide together when removal is necessary.

Surgery, which can be performed under general or local anesthesia, and often on an out-patient basis, is the only effective way to remove the cloudy lens from the eye.

Before Submitting to Surgery

But before your cataracts get that far along, I suggest you try a few things at home that may prevent the cataract from getting worse and may even help in some cases.

The most important fighters of cataracts are antioxidants, including vitamins A, C, and E. These are absolutely vital! Vitamin C alone has demonstrated the ability to halt the progression of cataracts.

If you have a cataract forming, I suggest you take as much as 25,000 IU of vitamin A (unless you're pregnant); 1,000 mg of vitamin C, three times a day; and 800-1,200 IU of vitamin E.

In addition to these antioxidants, I heartily recommend you take either Pycnogenol (which is available in most health food stores) or Healthy Resolve's Herbal Antioxidants (call 800-728-2288 to order), especially if you're a diabetic. These antioxidants, coupled with those mentioned above, can reverse early cataracts and halt more developed ones.

Many alternative doctors and researchers also believe that it's important to take at least 200 mcg of selenium in order to prevent or halt the development of cataracts. Researchers have found that many cataract sufferers are selenium deficient. This doesn't prove cause and effect, but taking extra selenium can't hurt.

And let's not forget diet. Get rid of the sugars and starches and eat plenty of soy, spinach, garlic, carrots, yams, and any other dark green or yellow vegetables.

Glaucoma

Although it is a relatively rare condition, glaucoma — a leading cause of blindness in the United States — receives a lot of attention in the media. This is because most of the cases of blindness due to glaucoma are thought to be preventable.

If your doctor tells you you're suffering from glaucoma or that the blood pressure in your eyes is high, he may prescribe drugs or encourage you to undergo laser surgery. While these approaches may help some, the side effects and risks are high enough that there are things you need to do before submitting to them.

The first thing you need to do is find out if the higher pressure in your eye is being caused by allergies. Avoiding known allergens has been shown to lower the eye pressure by as much as 20 millimeters. This may not solve your problem entirely, but it's the best place to begin.

Once you've identified and avoided the things you're allergic to, it's time to add additional supplements to your diet, specifically

Will Zinc Help Your MD?

Can vitamins and minerals help to alleviate macular degeneration? Even the conservative American Academy of Ophthalmology (AAO) agrees that zinc can help. Zinc is highly concentrated in the eye, particularly in the retina and tissues surrounding the macula. Zinc is necessary for the action of over 100 enzymes, including chemical reactions in the retina. Studies have shown that some older people have low levels of zinc in their blood, either because of poor diet or poor absorption of zinc from food.

In February 1996, researchers at the Department of Veteran Affairs announced the results of a study related to macular degeneration in the elderly. A study of U.S. veterans, published in the *Journal of the American Optometric Association,* found that taking a natural combination of nutrients, which includes zinc and vitamins C and E appeared to prevent the progression of age related macular degeneration.

This is great news and offers hope to thousands of older Americans with early symptoms of macular degeneration. Finally, there is scientific evidence that proves antioxidant therapy, led by zinc, can perhaps slow the progression of this leading cause of blindness. I suggest 25-100 mg of zinc picolinate daily (picolinate is more easily absorbed by the body).

bioflavonoids and magnesium. The bioflavonoids are absolutely crucial to your health, including the health of your eye. A healthy person needs only about 100 mg a day, but for glaucoma sufferers, 1,000 mgs a day is more appropriate.

As for magnesium, a report in the journal *Ophthalmologica* indicates that 122 mg of magnesium daily can improve visual-field defects by increasing the blood flow to the eye. I suggest you take as much magnesium as your body can handle. Start with 500 mg and work your way up to 1000 mg. If you begin to experience diarrhea, cut back until it goes away.

And, finally, make sure you're taking at least 100 mg of Coenzyme Q10 (CoQ10). This nutrient does wonders for the circulatory system and should be part of your daily supplement regimen anyway. The best product on the market is produced by Vitaline and can be purchased direct by calling 800-648-4755 (www.vitaline.com) or through Healthy Resolve (800-728-2288).

Macular Degeneration

In macular degeneration, the macula, or central area of the retina deteriorates, resulting in the loss of sharp vision. It is the leading cause of severe vision loss in the United States as well as Europe for persons 55 and older, affecting men and women about equally.

Protection against macular degeneration should start with a well-balanced, nutrient-dense diet, backed up with the extra protection of a top-quality daily multiple vitamin/mineral supplement. Also include extra amounts of dark berries and dark leafy green vegetables, such as spinach and kale in your diet. These foods respectively provide extra flavonoids and carotenoids, nutrients that are especially beneficial to eye health. In addition to a daily multiple, taking a lutein and zeaxanthin supplement will give eye tissue extra support, in view of strong research to date on the special role of these two carotenoids in eye health. Finally, your digestive system needs to be kept in good working order as well or vital nutrients will not be properly absorbed and assimilated.

For even more protection against macular degeneration, reach for the herbs *ginkgo biloba* and *bilberry.*

Ginkgo Biloba: Although generally referred to as an herb, this extract actually comes from the leaves of the deciduous ginkgo biloba tree.

In double-blind studies, this herb has consistently demonstrated significant improvement in long-distance visual acuity associated with macular degeneration as well as diabetic retinopathy. In other studies, ginkgo biloba has been shown to help protect against free-radical damage to the retina. In two studies, it has even been shown to prevent diabetic retinopathy in diabetic rats, which suggests a similar effect on humans with diabetes.

The effects are explained in large part by ginkgo biloba extract's primary use, which is to treat vascular insufficiency, including cerebral vascular insufficiency, by exerting beneficial effects on the circulatory system, including microcirculation throughout the brain, (which includes the eyes). More than 50 double-blind clinical trials have confirmed gingko's ability to enhance vascular function.

Ginkgo appears to help prevent and reverse symptoms of macular degeneration through its antioxidant action, ability to

---

Vitamin and Mineral Program May Help Macular Degeneration

Here's why: Chemical reactions from light in the eye activate oxygen that may cause macular damage. Therefore, antioxidants may help to limit these unwanted chemical reactions that can lead to macular degeneration. The best known antioxidants are vitamins E, C, and A, along with selenium, zinc (of course), taurine (an amino acid), and beta-carotene. The new herbal antioxidants are also important.

All of these nutrients are very important for the eye to function properly, especially zinc and taurine. Some people have been helped by simply adding vitamin E and selenium supplements. And still others have needed zinc and selenium administered intravenously before their eyesight improved.

Researchers at the University of Illinois found that failing to get enough vitamin A in your diet makes you twice as likely to develop macular degeneration. If you are noticing MD symptoms, bump your intake of vitamin A up to 25,000 IU.

improve cellular-fluid regulation, and enhance circulation, all within the eye itself. Most studies on ginkgo have used standardized extract containing 24 percent ginkgo heterosides, 40 milligrams, three times daily. Some studies have used up to 80 milligrams, three times daily. This extract is considered extremely safe.

Bilberry: The name bilberry is another name for European blueberry. Unlike American blueberries, the fruit of the European species is blue inside and out. The active compounds in bilberries are flavonoids called anthocyanosides. Bilberry extracts are included in conventional medical treatment in Europe for many vision disorders including cataracts, diabetic retinopathy, night blindness, and macular degeneration. Bilberry appears to improve these conditions, mainly, by improving blood flow and delivery of oxygen to the eye, as well as through antioxidant activity. Many eye diseases have been linked to free-radical damage, including cataracts and macular degeneration.

In one small study, bilberry extract combined with vitamin E halted cataract formation in 97 percent of the patients, all of whom had been diagnosed with senile cortical cataracts. Bilberry's effectiveness in preventing and treating glaucoma is believed to result from its beneficial effect on the eye's collagen structures, which in turn enhances cellular and tissue integrity. This effect may explain the results of another small study in which 31 patients with retinopathy all showed improved membrane permeability and less hemorrhaging when treated with bilberry. Another study showed that bilberry reduced capillary leakage in persons with varicose veins, suggesting bilberry extract may improve capillary strength and decrease leakage in the eyes as well.

In Europe, bilberry preparations are usually standardized to contain 25 percent anthocyanidins. The usual dosage for this type of preparation is 20 to 40 milligrams, three times daily. The usual dosage for bilberry extract, with 25 percent anthocyanidin content, is 80 to 160 milligrams, three times daily. Extensive testing shows no toxicity.

While I prefer liquid extracts for their superior quality, they are also less convenient to use. So if your eye health is good, and

you want to use ginkgo biloba and bilberry for long-term prevention, powdered extracts in capsules may be a better choice —one
you're more likely to continue on a long-term basis. Others needing
more immediate results are advised to use liquid extracts, under the
supervision of an experienced herbalist or other knowledgeable
health practitioner. Your vision is too important to entrust to anything less than the best professional support and care available.

More Information

If you suffer from one of these eye problems, I strongly recommend that you do a lot of research before submitting to any drug
or surgery. The best place to start is your local bookstore. Here are
a couple of books I recommend: *Healing the Eye the Natural Way*
by Edward Kondrot, MD (call 1-877-341-2703 to order, $19.95)
and *Save Your Sight* by Marc R. Rose, MD and Michael R. Rose,
MD (Warner Books, 1998, $13.99). The latter is primarily about
macular degeneration, but also has information about other forms of
eye disease.

Antibiotic Resistance:
The Herbal Solution

Just when the Food and Drug Administration (FDA)
announced that feeding antibiotics to chickens and turkeys was
causing antibiotic resistance in humans, they turned around and recommended approval for still another antibiotic, Zyvox. Zyvox, they
say, is more effective against staph infections than our most potent
antibiotics. But how long will it take before we become resistant to
Zyvox? Not long at all, I predict.

Have you noticed that antibiotics are not working as well as
they once did? When you understand bacteria, you may marvel, as
I do, that any of them still work at all! I constantly see patients with
chronic bacterial infections and suppressed immune systems from
overusing or misusing antibiotics. Unless we can find an alternative to conventional antibiotics — one that won't result in resistance

— our health is in real jeopardy.

Antibiotics are effective only against bacteria, not viruses, and they work by interrupting bacterial growth, says Cindy L.A. Jones, PhD, author of *The Antibiotic Alternative*. About one-third of the 150 million prescriptions written annually for antibiotics are unnecessary, announced researchers at the Centers for Disease Control and Prevention. Repeated exposure to antibiotics results in only more resistance.

Each year, drug-resistant bacteria kill 100,000 people because antibiotics aren't working. According to Stephen Harrod Buhner, author of *Herbal Antibiotics,* one reason is that bacteria are ganging up on us.

Buhner calls bacteria the biggest gossips on earth. They communicate silently from one organism to another and even from one species to the next! When bacteria are exposed to antibiotics, they create solutions that are antagonistic to antibiotics. In fact, they secrete chemicals called pheramones that attract other bacteria and help them communicate with one another. What do they "talk" about? How to stay alive by resisting antibiotics.

Spreading the Word

Resistance to bacteria spreads quickly through a species and even crosses the species boundary from animals to humans. Bruner tells a chilling story about chickens fed small amounts of antibiotics in their feed. One to one-and-a-half days afterward, their feces contained bacteria resistant to E. coli drugs. Three days later, chickens in adjacent cages were resistant to E. coli drugs *and* other antibiotics they had not been exposed to. Three months later, chickens never fed antibiotics that lived outside the barn containing the antibiotic-fed chickens became resistant. Six months later, people living in a nearby house who had no contact with these chickens became resistant to multiple antibiotics.

Synthetic vs. Natural — Does It Matter?

We can't escape bacteria or some resistance to them. Bacteria live in us and on all living things. Right now, about one to two pounds of your weight come from bacteria. Some are good guys (like acidophilus and bifidus), some are pathogenic and may, if their colonies become overgrown, require some kind of treatment.

Pharmaceutical antibiotics are usually made from one chemical that fights bacteria, says Buhner. Herbs contain hundreds of compounds. Since it's easier to develop a resistance to one chemical than many, I prefer herbal antibiotics, whenever possible. Prescription antibiotics have their place. They save lives. But there are times when herbs may be a safer answer that works just as well — or better.

Ingredients in plants may interact adversely with medications, so check with your doctor or pharmacist before using any herbs if you take drugs, including hormones. Herbal antibiotics may be appropriate for uncomfortable, non-life-threatening conditions, suggests Dr. Jones, such as bladder, skin, or sinus infections. They can be useful at the first sign of a cold, since bacterial infections may be present with viruses. Always get a medical diagnosis before you treat your condition. If you have a fungal infection, use an anti-fungal. If you have a bacterial infection, use antibiotic herbs. If it's a virus, choose a plant with antiviral properties.

Plant-Based Antibiotics That Work

Grapefruit seed extract (*GSE*) — This is a powerful broad-spectrum antibiotic used throughout the world. In very small doses, it fights bacteria, yeasts, and fungi. GSE can be used to kill off intestinal or skin bacteria. If you take too much, you'll kill off some good bacteria as well. Buhner suggests taking three to 15 drops of GSE in citrus juice two to three times a day, but I find that one or two drops twice daily is often sufficient.

Garlic (*Allium sativum*) — Second in usefulness to GSE, and the most studied herb in the world, garlic has been found to be antimicrobial against bacteria, fungi, viruses, and protozoa, as well as skin infections, including athlete's foot. Garlic is effective against both gram-positive and gram-negative bacteria, and most major infectious bacteria, notes Buhner. It can be used in food or found in capsules. If you're on any blood thinner, don't use more than one clove a day. Garlic is an anticoagulant, and high amounts could thin your blood too much. Other than that, garlic is very safe.

Aloe vera juice — You can use aloe vera juice externally, as an antibacterial, antimicrobial, or antiviral. It's effective against staph infections and burns. The best quality I've found is Herbal Aloe Force (518-581-1968), which is unheated, untreated, and extremely potent. I use it on any cuts to avoid infection.

Goldenseal (*Hydrastis canadensis*) — This herb contains berberine, an ingredient with antibiotic properties. Goldenseal has been used for tuberculosis, H. pylori, and diarrhea resulting from E. coli. It's also used for skin, vaginal, and eye infections. Goldenseal can be found in tinctures, capsules, salves, or tablets. All work well. You can use it at the beginning of a cold or infection and take it for a week or two at a time. Avoid using it every day, since there are not enough long-term studies on its safety and effectiveness when it's used constantly. Goldenseal works on smooth muscles, so Dr. Jones cautions against using it if you're pregnant.

Lemon balm (*Melissa officinalis*) — As it's an excellent antiviral and antibacterial, lemon balm is used in some ointments for cold sores. I've found it works beautifully, often preventing a sore from occurring. The product I've used for years is Herpilyn by Enzymatic Therapy (800-783-2286), found in many natural food stores.

Ginger (*Zingiber officinale*) — Effective against food-borne illnesses caused by Shigella dysenteria, E. coli, and salmonella, the root of the ginger plant has both antibacterial and antiviral properties. Because it also acts as an expectorant and antihistamine, it works well for upper respiratory infections. You can use it as a tea, in capsules, or in food in any amounts due to its low toxicity.

What You Can Do

Use antibiotics appropriately. They don't work for viruses, so make sure your doctor has found a bacterial overgrowth and that any prescribed antibiotic is both necessary and appropriate against that particular bacterium.

Take friendly bacteria (probiotics) like acidophilus and bifidus for several weeks. They fight pathogenic (disease-producing) bacteria and keep them under control.

Use antibacterial soaps and cleaners appropriately. They kill good bacteria as well as pathogens. Keep your kitchen and bathroom low in bacteria, but don't scrub your hands with them throughout the day — just when you've been exposed to something nasty.

If your infection is not serious, try using herbs with antibiotic properties, or ask your doctor if you can try them for a few days. With a little trial and error, you'll find which herbs work best for you. And by having them on hand, you can begin treating yourself at the first sign of discomfort — when it's easiest to control.

Medicinal Mushrooms: Strong Immune Boosters

Colds always makes me nervous — or at least they used to.

You see, ever since I was a child exposed daily to second-hand smoke, colds would settle in my chest. As an adult, they often became full-blown pneumonia. I couldn't remember the last time a cold had remained a simple head cold with a runny nose. In spite of being healthy most of the time, I had to be extra careful during the fall and winter to avoid getting sick. Seasonal weather changes were typically when I, and thousands of other people, were most vulnerable to viruses. Over the years, I tried many dietary plans and supplements to enhance my immune system, but none really worked all that well.

One year, during a serious bout of pneumonia, I realized that I simply had to solve this lifelong lung weakness. I was determined to find an answer — and I did, but it wasn't anything I thought it would be.

I was at a health convention, coughing away, when I asked Janet Zand, who started the McZand Herbal company, what she'd suggest. Janet is an experienced acupuncturist and herbalist with an encyclopedia of herbal information. She immediately replied, "Cordyceps and Shiitake mushrooms. They stimulate the immune system and strengthen the lungs."

Not only did the mushrooms work then, but they have continued to work ever since. Her advice started me on a search for more information on medicinal mushrooms that led me to David Law, co-owner of the northern California company, Gourmet Mushrooms, Inc, which grows medicinal mushrooms for the supplement industry. David introduced me to the realm of medicinal mushrooms, a realm based on thousands of years of usage and dozens of scientific studies.

Why Medicinal Mushrooms Are Important

Out of more than 100,000 species of fungus, over a dozen varieties have been used in China for more than 3,000 years to increase immunity, strengthen the lungs and other organs, and as part of cancer therapy. They are included in traditional Chinese medicine and used extensively by acupuncturists under their Latin names.

With my history of lung problems, they appeared to have been made for me. And because respiratory illness is one of the leading causes of death in seniors, especially those with congestive heart failure, mushrooms can be valuable in boosting our immunity as well as giving specific lung support.

Mushrooms appear to be particularly valuable because of their various-sized molecules. The smaller ones contain nutrients, while the larger ones are used by the immune system to make antigens. Antigens, in turn, produce antibodies to fight disease-producing substances. David explained to me that these large mushroom molecules have a unique shape that your immune system remembers. When you are exposed to bacteria or viruses that have similar shaped molecules, your body remembers that mushrooms can produce the antibodies you need to fight these harmful invaders. As long as you have mushroom molecules circulating in your body, your immune system is on alert, ready to take action at a moment's notice. This is why David believes it is best to take medicinal mushrooms more than once a day — so those molecules are always present.

The part of your immune system that remembers the size and shape of these large mushroom molecules are your T-cells, a group of cells living in the thymus gland. Your thymus gland protects you against harmful bacteria, viruses, and parasites, but it shrinks as we age, reducing our army of T-cells. This is why it's so important to boost your immune system as you get older, especially before winter weather changes increase our susceptibility to cold and flu viruses. Various medicinal mushrooms may be your answer to a cold- and flu-free winter.

Shiitake (*Lentinus elodes*)

If you've ever cooked with dried Chinese mushrooms, you've used shiitake mushrooms. The use of shiitakes goes back to the Ming Dynasty in China where they were used for lung problems and to increase stamina. Shiitakes contain a chemical called lentinan which has been shown to reduce tumors. They are currently under investigation as a potential cancer-fighting drug. Studies are indicating, however, that there are substances in shiitakes other than lentinan that fight cancer, which is why using the whole mushroom may be best.

Donald R. Yance, Jr., CN, MH, AHG, author of *Herbal Medicine, Healing & Cancer* (Keats Publishing, 1999) points out that shiitakes help the body make interferon, a powerful antiviral substance. He found these mushrooms have been used for an over- growth of Candida albicans, for bronchial inflammation including asthma, environmental allergies, and frequent colds and flu.

Reishi (*Ganoderma lucidum*)

Reishi mushrooms strengthen the immune system by increasing white blood cells and cells that fight tumors. Herbalist, mushroom expert, and acupuncturist Christopher Hobbs, LAc, found studies indicating they specifically helps the lungs by regenerating lung tissue. Reishis also appear to prevent bronchitis, strengthen the adrenal glands (the glands that handle all types of stress), and have antiviral effects through their production of interferon, says Hobbs. In his practice, he has found reishis to be particularly effective for nervous or anxious people with adrenal exhaustion and even prefers to use them in these cases instead of the herb Valerian.

The Japanese government has formally listed reishis as a supplement to be used for people with cancer. They have studies showing that reishis protect against radiation, so anyone who has had radiation treatments should consider taking the supplement. I would also recommend it for cancer protection or remission.

Maitake (*Grifola frondosa*)

Maitakes are becoming quite popular for one isolated substance they contain called D-Fraction. D-Fraction has been shown to have anti-tumor activity and also supports the immune system in general. But so does the complete mushroom, says Christopher Hobbs, who found a study showing maitakes blocked the growth of tumors in 86 percent of mice. People and mice are different, of course. But the history of medicinal mushrooms indicates that once again, the whole mushroom may contain co-factors that either enhance the absorption of D-Fraction or add to its usefulness as an immune supporter. One Japanese study using rats showed that powdered maitakes lowered cholesterol and increased the excretion of bile, a substance we need to digest fats. This means that maitakes could help with fat digestion. Nutritionist Shari Lieberman, PhD, and Ken Babal, CN, note that maitakes were used in ancient China for respiratory problems, poor circulation, liver support, weakness, exhaustion, and to strengthen the life force (Chi).

It appears that using D-Fraction may be more like using an over-the-counter medication, while taking the complete mushroom is more like eating a food that enhances immunity and helps the body function more effectively. Each has its place in your immune-boosting program.

Cordyceps (*Cordyceps sinensis*)

Cordyceps sinensis is one of the most interesting species of medicinal mushrooms. It is a small, finger-shaped fungus that, in its natural habitat, takes over caterpillar and insect larvae with its spores. The spores germinate, emerging from the parasitized larva. This fungus has been reported to have anti-tumor activity and strong immune properties. In this country, Cordyceps are grown in sterilized mediums without the insect larvae, and appear to have the same kind of protective effects as those found in the wild.

Cordyceps seem to be a lung and kidney tonic, according to

Hobbs. He also notes that they help relax smooth muscles, making them the nutrient of choice for people with asthma and respiratory problems. Like the other medicinal mushrooms, Cordyceps has been used as an anti-cancer agent. In the Orient, one study showed that they strengthened legs in frail older people and reduced their dizziness. For people like me with a history of coughs accompanying chest colds, Cordyceps may be ideal.

Using Medicinal Mushrooms

While different medicinal mushrooms have slightly different properties, all contain beta glucan, a form of sugar called a polysaccharide that supports immunity by communicating with your immune system, telling it to defend you against harmful viruses and bacterium. Some mushroom products contain concentrated quantities of beta glucan, while others contain the whole mushroom with beta glucan and all the co-factors that help beta glucan and other substances work. Just remember that the complete mushroom powder or extract is a supportive food, while products that emphasize one ingredient are similar to over-the-counter medications.

Mushroom grower David Law suggests taking the whole mushroom in powdered form several times a day in small quantities. Over time, the mushroom's strengthening abilities may be seen if you pay close attention. Let me give you an example from my own experience. One day I over-exercised (I was kayaking against the wind and had no choice). My muscles were exhausted when I finished and I could hardly drive home. The next morning my arms were still very fatigued and I didn't know when they would feel strong and rested. But that afternoon, barely 24 hours later, I was ready to go paddling again. My muscles had recovered much more quickly than they had before — when I was years younger.

Some medicinal mushrooms can be found alone, while some, like cordyceps, are usually found in a mushroom combination. In either case, you may want to choose the powder over a tincture. If you do use a mushroom tincture, and some are very good, just make certain you shake the bottle well before taking it to get the little particles into the dropper that have the activity you're seeking.

High quantities of mushrooms, or herbs for that matter, tend to stimulate the system. If you're in a crisis, like a persistent cough or asthmatic attack, you may want to take some every hour for a few days. Janet Zand suggested I take a dropperful of an extract with cordyceps and reishi every hour for three days to knock out my cough. Now that I'm well, I hope to stave off the colds that lead to coughs by taking a smaller amount daily. In my private practice, and with my own health, I've found that taking less is better — and much less expensive.

Finally, consider buying a pound of dried shiitake mushrooms at an Oriental market — if one is nearby. Soak a handful of them in warm water, and add slices of them to a stir-fried dish or soup. Don't throw away the water they soaked in, since it contains beta glucans and other immune-stimulating substances. If you like, you can freeze this mushroom-water in ice cube trays and add some to soups and sauces. Let food become your medicine, as Hippocrates suggested centuries ago, by adding medicinal mushrooms to your diet and supplement program, especially if your immune system needs support, or you tend to suffer from chronic respiratory problems.

Unless you have an allergy to yeasts, molds, and fungi (having an overgrowth of the yeast candida albicans is not the same as having a yeast allergy), taking mushrooms is not only safe, it may be one of the most protective substances for winter illnesses.

Look for mushroom combinations in your local natural food store. If you can't find them, you can call Gourmet Mushrooms at 707-823-1743 and ask for the TriMyco-Gen capsules. A bottle of 100 capsules is $24 including shipping, but if you get two or more bottles, it's only $19/bottle. I take two capsules morning and night, but you may want to start with more if your immune system is suffering.

Usnea — A Mushroom That's Not a Mushroom

Another fungi you need to know about is Usnea, an especially valuable herb for people with chronic lung problems. It's also the perfect herb for anyone who wants to stop a cold or flu from taking hold. Even people who previously resorted to antibiotics have not gotten sick when they took Usnea early.

Usnea is not a plant, but two plants that live together off one another in a symbiotic relationship. It's a form of lichen, and lichens are a combination of an algae (a one-celled plant) and a fungus that live off one another so closely they look and act like a single plant.

Usnea's Properties

Usnea is commonly called "Old Man's Beard"; the native Americans called it "The Lungs of The Earth." Its main properties are antibiotic, antifungal, antiviral, and antibacterial against gram positive bacteria like Streptococcus, Staph, Pneumo-nococcus, and Mycobacterium tuberculosis. This rare combination of properties may be one reason why Hippocrates suggested using usnea for uterine problems centuries ago, and why it has been used extensively in China for numerous conditions.

Some of the most common antibiotic acids found in lichens are Usnic and Barbatic acids, substances not extracted in water. So don't drink usnea tea. It needs to be extracted in alcohol, and here's where it gets tricky. Some usnea tinctures are extracted in a hot alcohol process and some in a cold alcohol base.

To find out which was best, I went to two herbalists: Christopher Hobbs, who has written a booklet called *Usnea: The Herbal Antibiotic* and *Richo Cech*. They were a wealth of information.

The Best Form of Usnea

Either process has its place, but Richo is in favor of a hot alcohol extraction. He says this gives the tincture more usnic and barbatic acids, for more antibiotic and antiviral activity. A cold alcohol extraction, he says, results in fewer beneficial acids, and more polysaccharides, chemicals that are primarily immune-enhancing. But polysaccharides are easily added by taking some dried marshmallow root (found in herb and health food stores) and putting it into a jar of room temperature water for a day. Add some of this liquid to your usnea tincture and you have the best of both worlds.

Christopher Hobbs agrees, and said that for the hot alcohol

extraction of usnea to be potent, the bottles it is sold in must be filled while the tincture is still hot. If not, the active ingredients can fall to the bottom of the container. Herb Pharm does just that, so their product is quite strong. If you find another brand in your favorite health food store, call the company to find out whether they use a hot or cold alcohol extraction before buying it. Or call Herb Pharm and they'll send you a bottle (around $9/1 ounce).

How to Take Usnea

On the advice of Janet Zand, president of McZand Herbal, a company that used to make usnea extract, we suggest you take one dropperful of the tincture every hour at the first sign of a cold or cough. Stop taking it when you feel better (usually within one to two days). Just take it when you need it, not prophylactically. The one exception is when you're in an airplane for many hours, or around people who are sick. In this case, take one dropperful either before or right after exposure. I carry a bottle of usnea as my all-in-one first aid kit whenever I travel, from flights across the country to a week camping in the Grand Canyon.

Other Uses

Usnea is most valuable for lung problems, since usnic acid relaxes the bronchial tubes as well as fights bacteria and viruses that contribute to pneumonia and other lung problems. There are times when you get a bacterial infection and have a slight touch of a virus. Or vice versa. Taking an antibiotic without an antiviral may help a little, but you still get sick. By taking usnea, you get a combination that can prevent illness and shorten the healing time if you're already sick.

Ready for more? The Chinese found usnea to be effective in inhibiting Candida albicans and Trichomonis, making it a valuable herb for women both orally and in a douche. They used it as a disinfectant for infections and to promote the healing of second- and third-degree burns. In laboratory studies it was found to inhibit cancer growth, as well as the Epstein-Barr virus. Usnea also is anti-inflammatory, has analgesic properties and is antifungal. You can even use the tincture topically on such external fungus conditions as athlete's foot. It has been used extensively for urinary tract and bladder infections as well. Since it's non-toxic, you can safely try it for many conditions.

In time, I suspect you'll hear more about usnea. It's a plant that has been used for centuries and overlooked too long. Over the past 18 months, I've used it with dozens of people for numerous lung and urinary tract problems. It has always proved beneficial. A miracle herb? Nothing's a miracle. But I think usnea comes close!

Ginger: Help for Nausea

Ginger, or *Zingiber officinale*, is one of the most valuable commonly found herbs. It has been used in China for 25 centuries, both as a spice and as a medication. Its most popular use is to aid digestion and eliminate nausea — both in pregnancy and for motion sickness, but it also warms the body nicely.

Thought of as a root, ginger is actually a rhizome, grown in various parts of the world. Its oil and resin give it its medicinal properties, so the best ginger is fresh, found in grocery stores.

If you take dried ginger that's been in your cupboards for years, or buy a powdered ginger that sat around in a store or herb supplier's warehouse, you may not get the results you're looking for. Still, powdered ginger can be effective when it's fresh and is the form that's been used in most scientific studies.

There's a lot of myth and folklore mixed with facts about herbs. It's easy to accept anecdotal evidence as fact, but sometimes this is wishful thinking. For the sound information you've come to expect from us, I turned to *Tyler's Herbs of Choice,* a recently published herb book that looks at scientific studies and the pharmacology of herbs, not just how they've been used traditionally. Two professors emeritus of pharmacognosy at Purdue University, James E. Robbers, PhD, and Varro E. Tyler, PhD, ScD, wrote this excellent book which separates fact from fiction.

These authors point out that while ginger has been alleged to be helpful for everything from migraines, high cholesterol, ulcers, depression, and impotence, there is not enough scientific support to use it for these reasons. As a digestive aid, and for motion sickness, however, ginger has an important place in our lives.

Daniel B. Mowrey, PhD, considered to be an expert on herbs, concurs. With a PhD in psychopharmacology, he talks, in his book *The Scientific Validation of Herbal Medicine,* about his personal experiences with ginger, and reports on the success he has had using it. Dr. Mowrey first used ginger successfully to prevent vomiting when he had the flu. In his studies over many years, he has found ginger to be effective for motion sickness in over 90 percent of people, for morning sickness in 75 percent of women, and for dizziness and vertigo in 40-50 percent of people. When he used it on people who were coming down with the flu, he recommended that his subjects took eight to 10 capsules initially, then two to four capsules every half hour until they began feeling better.

In scientific studies using ginger for motion sickness, half showed it was effective and half showed it was not. Drs. Robbers and Tyler believe this may be due to the use of non-standardized ginger in some studies, or because there are emotional factors with motion sickness that ginger simply can't help. Drs. Robbers and Tyler suggest that the anti-nausea chemicals in ginger, shogaols, and gingerols should be in a standardized form for the best results.

Some herb companies offer standardized ginger tinctures and capsules. Enzymatic Therapy sells 100 mg capsules of standardized ginger in natural food stores in a product called GingerAll. Traditional Medicinal tea company has a standardized tea called Ginger Aid, found in natural food stores and many pharmacies.

Ginger capsules contain about 500 mg of powdered rhizome. Try taking two capsules half an hour before you leave on a plane, boat, or in a car. Then you can take one or two additional capsules every four hours. If you prefer crystallized ginger, as I do, the authors point out that a one-inch square, a quarter of an inch thick, seems to be equivalent to one ginger capsule.

According to Oriental medicine, ginger warms the body. Try a cup of the tea or chew on a piece of root, and you'll find out for yourself. Consider taking a thermos of Ginger Aid tea with you on a trip where you may become chilled or expect motion sickness, or pack a few slices of crystallized ginger.

Remember, fresh ginger is an excellent condiment in salads and sautéd vegetables, and most recipes that use it contain small enough quantities to safely consume as part of a balanced meal plan. Some individuals, may want to avoid ginger because of its blood-thinning effect, such as persons already taking baby aspirin or a prescription medication such as Coumadin to thin blood. Also for this reason you would not want to take ginger for nausea following any surgery.

How safe is ginger? Very safe if it's used appropriately.

Great News About Echinacea

The cold and flu season is over. Now it's time to put away your bottle of Echinacea. Then wait until fall when everyone around you starts getting sick, or you feel a little fluish. Right? Not necessarily.

I know that most health-care practitioners, including herbalists, think of Echinacea, a plant used widely throughout Europe and the United States, as an herb that acts as an immune system booster. They say its use should be limited to those times when our immune system needs support. But a widely-respected Australian herbalist, Kerry Bone, BSc, says there is quite a bit of evidence that Echinacea is an immune regulator, and can be used for long periods of time to strengthen the immune system.

His research shows that early American practitioners, who were called the Eclectics, used it extensively. They first heard about it from Native American tribes who supplied them with their initial information on the herb and its uses. Native Americans used Echinacea against more diseases than any other of their hundreds of plants. They even used it for snake bites, although they had no way of knowing it stopped the venom from penetrating into the body by inhibiting one of its most destructive chemicals. The Eclectics used Echinacea with their patients for up to nine months for dozens of ailments with excellent results.

Modern research shows no reason to limit Echinacea's use.

Dr. Bone believes the reason some people have restricted their use of Echinacea is because they have misinterpreted data from some studies. When Bone examined one of these studies carefully it indicated that when Echinacea was taken for 10 weeks it had a considerably greater effect on the immune system than when it was taken for two weeks — the amount of time many people take it during cold and flu season.

How Does It Work?

The action of Echinacea is, in part, to increase phagocyte activity. Some phagocytic cells called macrophages are the watchdogs of your immune system. By increasing phagocytic cells, Echinacea works best by preventing infections or by signaling your immune system to respond quickly when a pathogen comes along. In other words, it makes it easier for your body to deal with a problem in its early stages by making your immune system aware that there's a problem before that problem becomes a big one. But Echinacea works on a wide variety of conditions.

The active ingredients in Echinacea include polysaccharides (which have immune enhancing properties), flavonoids (as quercetin), caffeic acid (which is antibacterial), and essential oils. The herb appears to have both direct and indirect effects on supporting the immune system, and has both antiviral and antibacterial properties as well. The form of Echinacea determines how effective it is and against which conditions, but all forms appear to work well. Dr. Michael Murray, an herbalist and naturopath, suggests you take any of the following forms of Echinacea three times a day:

Dried root (or as tea): 500 mg-1 gram

Freeze-dried plant (in tablet or capsule form): 325-650 mg

Tincture (1:5): 1-2 tsp

I suggest you try various brands and forms of Echinacea to see which works best for you. If you're coming down with a cold, an effective Echinacea will give you results within 12-24 hours. If you have little or no results, try another brand.

Several varieties of the herb are used for its medicinal properties: E. purpurea, E. angustifolia, and E. pallida. And various parts of the plant are made into tablets, capsules and tinctures, including the juice of E. purpurea tops (sold as "Echinacin"), the roots, and the whole plant. Studies of Echinacin injections for people with cancer showed positive results with no side effects. Extracts of Echinacea root show it has antiviral activity against flu, herpes, and other viruses.

Dr. Michael Murray suggests that for the most active ingredients in a tincture, you might want one made with both water and alcohol extraction. Pure alcohol extraction alone leaves behind some of the immune support of polysaccharides. To get more polysaccharides, you can simply put a few ounces of marshmallow root in several cups of water and let the mixture sit for two or three hours. Pour off the marshmallow root and you have a liquid filled with polysaccharides to take along with your tincture of Echinacea.

What I Discovered

Several years ago a New York based nutritionist with a strong interest in the science behind nutrition called me to say that she had gotten hold of some viruses and was testing them in a lab against various brands of Echinacea. "Have you ever heard of a company called McZand?" she asked. I had. In fact, I had shared patients with Dr. Janet Zand, founder and head of the company, when she was in private practice in Southern California and found her to be exceptionally knowledgeable. "Well," the nutritionist said, "that brand out-performed all others." So I went to Janet Zand and asked her of her experience with people who took Echinacea over long periods of time. She knew of many. One person in particular took the herb daily for 16 years. He only got sick twice, when he stopped taking it. "I think that may be a little excessive, however," commented Dr. Zand.

Dr. Bone agrees with Dr. Zand that there is no reason to suspect Echinacea is harmful when taken over a long period of time. Dr. Murray concurs. Based on its effects as a regulator of the immune system, we would like to suggest you consider taking Echinacea at the end of the summer for a number of months if you tend to get frequent fall or winter colds and flus. By building up your immune system now, you could break your cycle of illness around the holiday season. Don't take the herb for more than six to nine months. Then give your body a rest and see what results you get. Conditions that seem to respond well to Echinacea include wound healing, infections, viruses, candidiasis, rheumatoid arthritis, and immunodepression (including from chemotherapy and radiation).

Chicken Soup for Colds and Flu?

My mother knew it worked, but not why. Whenever my brother or I was sick, she would come into our rooms with bowls of hot chicken soup. "Eat it," she would say. "It will make you feel better." And it did. Maybe it was the rest and fluids — or simply time — that cured us. But decades later, scientists are finding that chicken soup fights colds. Who, besides my mother and possibly yours, would have thought it?

Chicken soup is known in Jewish tradition as Jewish penicillin. It's been used for upper respiratory-tract infections as far back as the 12th century when the Egyptian Jewish physician and philosopher Maimonides wrote about its effectiveness. He took the information from the Greeks, so in truth, chicken soup is Greek penicillin.

How Does It Work?

There are a few ways chicken soup may help fight colds and respiratory infections. The most obvious one is by re-hydrating the body and keeping it nourished. Eating warm soup can clear your nasal passages and help remove mucus from your lungs. Another way it can work is to inhibit the inflammation that occurs with respiratory infections and viruses. This new information comes from a study conducted by researchers who prepared a traditional homemade chicken soup with lots of vegetables (carrots, parsnips, sweet potatoes, celery, etc.) and tested it against blood samples in a laboratory setting.

When chicken soup was tested on blood samples, it had an anti-inflammatory effect by allowing beneficial neutrophils, white blood cells that protect against infection, to remain in inflamed areas where they could reduce inflammation.

A Close Second to Chicken Soup

Oscillococcinum is a long name for a homeopathic product that is very similar to chicken soup in fighting colds and flu. Made by a French company, Boiron, for more than 60 years, from an extract of duck liver and heart, oscillococcinum is the primary over-the-counter cold and flu medication in France.

A study published in the *British Homeopathic Journal* in April 1998 reported that when oscillococcinum worked, it was more than twice as effective as a placebo in eliminating flu symptoms in just one day. In another study (*British Journal of Clinical Pharmacology,* March 1989), one-fourth of the people who used it felt better in two days.

Oscillococcinum can take the place of chicken soup if you think you're coming down with a cold. I suggest you get a few vials of these tiny pellets at your natural food store and keep them on hand. Use it at the first sign of a cold or flu if you're not in the mood to cook up a batch of chicken soup. Like many natural remedies, it works best when taken early on.

Chapter 16

Vitamins vs. a Good Diet

We've heard in the past about studies that showed smokers with lung cancer got worse or developed coronary heart disease when they took a lot of beta-carotene, one of a family of carotenoids found in vitamin A. We've also seen studies that show that beta-carotene levels are low in many people who have lung cancer. So what's going on? Who should we believe? Do we take extra beta-carotene or shun it?

The problem with many of these studies is that they tend to be flawed. They often leave out more information than they contain. What kind of diet were these patients on? How long did they have lung cancer before they began taking beta-carotene? What about people who took the entire spectrum of carotenoids through a diet high in fresh fruits and vegetables, rather than taking just one in a pill form? Does an imbalance of nutrients contribute to health problems? Probably the greatest mistake we're making about taking vitamins and minerals is that we're treating them like drugs.

Many people, on the advice of their health practitioners, or after hearing a media blitz on the benefits of a particular vitamin, mineral, or amino acid, begin to take huge amounts of one or two nutrients. In fact, in some of these studies, vitamins are being both tested and treated as though they were drugs. But they're not.

While a drug may have a specific action or actions on its own, nutrients work in balance with one another. Co-factors (nutrients that enable a vitamin or mineral to work) are as important as the vitamin or mineral itself. Take calcium, for instance. It's an over-prescribed mineral that just won't make it into your bones unless it's accompanied by sufficient amounts of vitamin D, magnesium, hydrochloric acid, and other nutrients. Rather than look at these interactions, we are asking supplements to work like drugs — on their own.

A letter in the British medical journal, *The Lancet*, talks about early studies done by two research scientists, Pauling and Robinson (yes, that's Linus Pauling, winner of two Nobel prizes). Apparently, these two scientists had major feuds, so some of their studies were never published — including animal studies that showed that a normal diet with high doses of vitamin C promoted cancer in mice exposed to carcinogens. But mice whose diet consisted of large amounts of raw fruits and vegetables — with the same amount of vitamin C and the same exposure to carcinogens — had much fewer cancers. In one case, vitamin C promoted cancer; in another, it inhibited it. Diet, not supplementation, made the difference.

Why They're Called *Supplements*

We at *WHL* have always taken the position that supplements are just that: *supplements* to a good diet. There's a reason they're called supplements, not *instead-of's*. Other studies have confirmed Pauling and Robinson's initial findings. A good, healthy eating program is essential. Diets rich in fresh produce are high in fiber, antioxidants, and other immune-building nutrients. They protect us against cancers and other serious diseases.

If you think you can take supplements and make only a few changes in your diet, and still eat mostly low quality, nutrient-sparse foods — high in fats, animal protein, and sugar; low in fresh produce, whole grains, and legumes — you're fooling yourself and playing Russian roulette with your health. It's just not going to give you the results you want.

And by all means, don't take large amounts of single nutrients that are part of a nutrient family. Take beta-carotene, for example. It's just one of around 600 fat-soluble carotenoids that are part of the vitamin A family. And all the nutrients in a food can't be put into pill form. After hearing so much about the benefits of the complete carotenoids, I recently spoke with the president of a large natural-supplement company and asked her when they would be coming out with a carotenoid product.

"Never," she told us. "Some of them are very unstable. And there are too many of them. If we came out with a product that contained a dozen or so carotenoids, we might well be missing just the ones that make a difference in someone's health. It just won't happen." You can't fool Mother Nature, and you can't duplicate her, either. The basis for a healthy diet needs to begin with food, not vitamins used as drugs. High potency supplements may have their place in your health-care program. Indeed, numerous studies have shown them to be beneficial at times. But not at the expense of a good diet.

Antioxidants — like vitamins C, E, and A — protect us by destroying oxidants. Iron oxidizes, which is why if you're not menstruating or otherwise losing blood, you may not want to take extra iron in your supplements. In the past, many women have reached for iron when they felt tired. They believed they had "iron poor blood." Why? Because that's what one of the manufacturers of a synthetic

---

Blood Sugar and Magnesium

Here it comes again. Another reason to re-evaluate your magnesium intake. A study published in the *American Journal of Hypertension* (vol. 12, no. 8, 1999) found that low levels of dietary magnesium are correlated with insulin resistance. And insulin resistance means low blood sugar, with possible symptoms of fatigue, confusion, and headaches. This study indicated that its participants consumed about 200 mg of magnesium a day, rather than the recommended 410 mg.

That's easy to understand. Magnesium is found in moderate amounts in legumes, nuts, and seeds, and whole grains. But unless you're eating good quantities of magnesium-rich foods, you may be under-consuming this mineral. So you may want to take an additional magnesium supplement, especially if your multivitamin contains more calcium than magnesium. High calcium intake lowers magnesium stores, and magnesium is needed to get calcium into the bones.

Bottom line: if you have low blood-sugar symptoms, boost your dietary and supplemental magnesium to bowel tolerance.

Humphries, S., et al. "Low dietary magnesium is associated with insulin resistance in sample of young non-diabetic black Americans," *Am J Hypertension,* 12(8), 1999. From *Int'l Clinical Nutr Rev,* July 2000.

vitamin product bombarded the airwaves and print ads with. Taking extra iron when you don't need it can be dangerous. New labeling laws will make this more obvious on vitamin products in the future.

Fats oxidize, which is one good reason to keep fats low in your diet. The more oxidants in your diet, the more antioxidants you need. Some foods contain natural antioxidants: grape juice and wine, green tea, and just about all fruits and vegetables. Increasing antioxidants and decreasing oxidants through dietary modification is the smartest way of getting or staying healthy. Use supplements to supplement your diet, not to take instead of eating properly. Take balanced formulas, not huge amounts of any one nutrient. It may cause an imbalance, and chances are it won't be as well absorbed as if you took a lower amount more frequently throughout the day. Don't mess with Mother Nature by trying to use vitamin pills like drugs. Ultimately, you won't win.

The Complexities of Vitamins

I'm not arguing against using vitamins. I think, however, you should be aware of some of their limitations. For instance, older blue-eyed adults are more prone to retinal disease than brown-eyed people, because their retinas contain half as much lutein, one of over a hundred carotenoids. Beta-carotene needs lutein to be absorbed. By taking extra beta-carotene without extra lutein, blue-eyed adults may be at more risk for eye problems as they age. Most vitamin pills

Thiamine and Your Brain

Thiamine (vitamin B_1) is one of the B vitamins with antioxidant properties. It's found in whole grains, brewer's yeast, molasses, and meats. While blood tests may not show a thiamine deficiency, a study with 120 women college students indicates a deficiency may not even be necessary for thiamine supplementation to be beneficial.

The women in this study, who were around 20 years of age, were given either 50 mg of thiamine a day for two months or a placebo. The women who took thiamine noticed significant improvements in their mood, as well as in their mental acuity. Multivitamins contain from five to 100 mg of thiamine. If you're taking a low-potency vitamin, you may want to boost it.

have plenty of beta-carotene and no lutein. To get enough lutein to use the beta-carotene in your vitamins, you would need three to five servings of spinach or kale a week. Easy in the summer when spinach salads taste good, but hard other times of the year.

Bill Sardi, a health writer I respect, has spoken about these nutrient imbalances as something the supplement manufacturers need to address. He points out that too much riboflavin (known as vitamin B$_2$), could lead to cataracts and retinal diseases. As author of a now out-of-print, excellent series of books on *Nutrition and the Eyes,* Sardi knows the subject of eye diseases and nutrients well. He points out that the B-complex vitamins that contain 50-100 mg of each B vitamin have too much riboflavin.

Still, Sardi agrees with the position of *WIIL* that when you're getting older, are an athlete, smoke, are pregnant or lactating, or under a lot of stress, vitamins can be an important addition to a good diet. The bottom line is that we don't know as much about the amount of nutrients we need as the media and advertising agencies would have us believe. This is still a relatively young industry with a lot of information still to come.

I suggest you learn as much about your body and its needs as possible. Eat a diet that's the most healthful for you. Then, add the supplements you and your health practitioner believe would boost your nutrient levels to the needed amounts. Use the best-quality, natural (not synthetic) supplements you can find. Take nutrients with any needed co-factors (like lutein with beta-carotene or vitamin C with bioflavonoids). Take a little less rather than a little more. Err on the side of caution. Be careful. Be well. Be happy.

What You Need to Know About Vitamins

Vitamins and minerals are nutrients that feed all the cells in your body. Without them your cells would starve and you would die. When you have too few of one or more nutrients, you run the risk of not feeling completely well and energetic or eventually of having a nutrient deficiency disease. Many of these diseases, like scurvy from a vitamin C deficiency, are no longer a health problem in developed countries. Others, like anemia, which can be caused by iron or B_{12} deficiencies, may result in fatigue. Sometimes nutrient deficiencies result in such discomfort as PMS (often caused by a lack of sufficient B_6 or magnesium) or skin problems and never lead to serious illness.

Your body uses extra amounts of nutrients when you're under stress, exercising, fighting off a cold or flu, smoking, exposed to

Does Zinc Help Colds?

Various studies have looked at using zinc lozenges to shorten the length of colds. Some say it helps, while others say it doesn't. Why is there so much variation in results? The answer may be in the form of zinc, what it's taken with, and how soon you begin using it.

Four dozen people were given 12.8 mg of zinc acetate every two to three hours within 24 hours of experiencing cold symptoms. The symptoms lasted half as long in those on the zinc lozenges as for those on a placebo (4.5 days compared with 8.1 days). Coughs were reduced significantly (three days for zinc; six days for placebo). Dry mouth and constipation in some were the only side effects, and drinking sufficient water could help resolve those problems.

Other studies showed little or no results, but it may have been due to the form of zinc. Zinc gluconate lozenges are proving to be effective in shortening the length of colds and reducing symptoms quickly, according to a study published in *Canadian Family Physician*. In my clinical practice, I have used zinc gluconate lozenges for years with excellent results, so they are the ones I would suggest. They can be found in any health food store.

Be sure to begin taking them within a day or two of your symptoms, and suck on them every two to three hours. Studies suggest you use a zinc gluconate lozenge with a minimum of 13.3 mg of elemental zinc per lozenge (it will say this on the label) and get about 80 mg of elemental zinc a day.

Also, some substances attach themselves to zinc making it less available to your body. One of these is citric acid — commonly found in orange juice and grapefruit juice. So switch to other juices like apple juice or black cherry juice (great for the liver). The sweeteners sorbitol and mannitol also bind to zinc and should be avoided at this time.

Ann Int Med 2000;133: 245-252

Can Fam Physician, 1998;44:1037-42

environmental pollutants, or using medications. Can you get enough of the vitamins and minerals you need from your diet? And when you take vitamin or mineral supplements, how do you know they are getting into your cells and doing their job?

How Much Is Enough?

Many people believe that a healthy diet provides all the nutrients we need. At one time that may have been true. However, environmental toxins from smog, foods containing residues of antibiotics, pesticides and herbicides, and the additional stresses that come from living in the 21st century, all impact on our nutrient needs. A diet that once was enough may now be deficient. And many people are too busy to prepare and eat three balanced meals a day. They get their energy boosts from caffeine, alcohol, or sugar, all of which deplete the body of one or more nutrients. Sugar, for example, requires more B vitamins to be digested than you'll get in your regular diet. Whenever you eat foods high in sugar, you need extra B vitamins.

Supplements, Not Replacements

To evaluate your body's nutrient needs, first recognize that vitamins and minerals are supplements, not instead of's. They do not replace a healthy diet or a good night's sleep. If you want to be healthy, stay healthy, and be free from discomfort as well as disease, begin eating a diet low in fats (and very low in animal fats), low in refined sugar and high in whole grains, beans, and vegetables. Add a little fruit and small amounts of raw nuts and seeds. After you've been eating well for several months, consider taking vitamins and minerals.

Taking a multivitamin/mineral may be the least expensive health insurance you can find — or it may be a complete waste of money. You may be surprised to know that all vitamins and minerals do not necessarily have the ingredients their labels say they contain. Nor are these nutrients necessarily in a form your body can break down and use. There is no agency that monitors the content and bioavailability of vitamins, so you have to do a little of the research yourself.

Look for High Quality

Some vitamins and minerals are made from petroleum byproducts. They are synthetic. Numerous doctors and scientists argue that these are as well absorbed as the "natural" ones and that more expensive vitamins are a waste of money. You may choose to believe them. At one time, I did, too. Then, as a nutritionist, I started looking closely at my patients and their health concerns. I noticed over a period of 14 years that patients who used inexpensive vitamins and minerals from drugstores, discount stores, and even health food stores appeared to be taking sufficient amounts of vitamins and minerals, but still had signs of nutrient deficiencies. I had them take natural vitamins and their deficiencies and symptoms disappeared.

For more than 20 years, I have noticed the relationship between good quality, well-absorbed nutrients and those that do not appear to do anything. My patients often decide to continue taking multivita-

The Link Between CoQ10 and Cancer

Coenzyme Q10 (CoQ10) is a vitamin (vitamin Q10) that, along with vitamin B_6, has been found to be low in people with cancer. CoQ10 is made from tyrosine, an amino acid found in proteins like meats and beans. But to make CoQ10, the body needs a number of vitamins, and without the coenzyme form of vitamin B_6 — one of the necessary vitamins — there can be dysfunctions to the DNA, which lead to mutations and cancer. Most vitamin formulas with B_6 contain pyridoxine HCL. The coenzyme form of B_6 is called Pyridoxyl-5-phosphate (P-5-P).

One more fact about CoQ10: it requires fatty acids to be taken along with it or it can't be absorbed well. Some CoQ10 products have no fatty acids added to them. If they don't, you need to take them with a meal that contains some fats. Other products have fatty acids added, and are well absorbed at any time.

Folkers, K. "Relevance of the biosynthesis of coenzyme Q10 and of the four bases of DNA as a rationale for the molecular causes of cancer and a therapy," *Biochem Biophys Res,* 224(2), 358-361(1996); *Intl Clin Nutr Rev,* July 1997.

min/ minerals because they notice a difference when they stop taking them.

Match Your Needs With a Formula

Look for a complete formula rather than buying bottle after bottle and making your own mixture. Some formulas are put together in such a way that they break down and are absorbed without competing with one another.

Most multivitamin/mineral formulas are based on old information stating that women need twice as much calcium as magnesium. The truth is, excessive calcium without sufficient magnesium is not absorbed into the cells, but rather collects in the joints where it becomes arthritis or in the arteries where it contributes to atherosclerosis. No wonder so many women suffer from heart attacks and painful arthritis as they age!

If you have PMS or are postmenopausal and concerned about osteoporosis, contact Optimox, Inc. They are the only company that has done controlled double-blind studies showing the effectiveness of their ratio of calcium to magnesium on eliminating PMS (Optivite formula) and reversing osteoporosis (Gynovite formula). Their formulas contain more magnesium than calcium and are extremely well absorbed. You can call them at 800-223-1601. Other similar formulas are based on Optimox research. They may or may not break down in your body as well.

One More Thing ...

Most companies put together formulas based on research on individual nutrients. They do not run expensive studies based on their finished product. Therefore, since each of us is unique and requires more or less of a specific nutrient, and our bodies differ in their abilities to utilize them, a formula that works for one person may not work as well for another.

You may want to try a particular formula for three months, and then stop for a week or two to see if you notice any difference. If not, perhaps there is a better formula for you. Is a less than ideal formula better than nothing? If you're stressed, have less energy than you think you should, and if you're living in the same polluted world as the rest of us, you'll probably benefit from a good multivitamin/mineral whether you experience the benefits now or in the future.

What to Look for in Supplements

Vitamins A & E: Studies have shown that water-soluble vitamins A and E are better absorbed than the more commonly found oil-soluble ones. Look for dry or water-soluble forms.

Calcium: The most easily absorbed calcium is calcium citrate. But calcium needs acid in order to be absorbed, so calcium in an antacid is poorly absorbed.

Minerals: Minerals in citrate form usually are not irritating and are well absorbed. If the name of a mineral is followed by the word "picolinate" such as chromium, iron, and zinc, the absorption rate into your body is very high. You get more of these nutrients into your cells than minerals in other forms.

Hearing Loss in the Elderly

A study of 55 women in their 60s, published in the *American Journal of Clinical Nutrition,* found that those with lower levels of vitamin B_{12} and folic acid had more hearing loss than women with normal levels of these nutrients. Mary Ann Johnson, PhD, from the American Society of Clinical Nutrition, one of the authors of the study conducted at the University of Georgia, announced that this is the first study that associates hearing loss with vitamin status.

Older adults may not eat enough dark green leafy vegetables, a source of folic acids. And vitamin B_{12}, found primarily in animal protein, is absorbed in the large intestines. If you have digestive problems and either constipation or diarrhea, you may not be absorbing the vitamin B_{12} you need.

A simple blood test can measure folate (folic acid) and vitamin B_{12}. If your level of either of these vitamins is low, you may want to take a look at the B_{12} and folic acid in your diet. Next, make sure you are not adding to a vitamin B_{12} malabsorption problem by having unresolved intestinal dysfunction. Future studies will give us more information about whether or not adding these vitamins can reduce hearing loss as we age. For now, a healthy diet, good digestion, and good quality nutritional supplements may provide you with some protection in this area.

Calcium and Magnesium: Choose a formula that has at least as much magnesium as calcium. Numerous recent studies indicate that 400 to 600 mg of calcium a day is sufficient, and you get more from the foods you eat. A formula with more than 600 mg of calcium may lead to more problems than solutions.

Iron: If you have had cancer, or if there is a high incidence of cancer in your family, you may want to take a formula without added iron. High iron has been found in women with cancer.

Selenium: Low selenium levels are associated with cancer, AIDS, and other immune problems. A protective amount is 200 mcg.

Chromium: Chromium helps the body utilize carbohydrates and is helpful in stabilizing blood sugar levels and reducing excess weight. You need at least 200 mcg of chromium — often more for weight control and excessive sugar cravings.

Vitamins: Getting Your Money's Worth

All vitamins are not created equal. Some are higher potency than others, some have better ratios of particular nutrients, and some are better absorbed. You usually get what you pay for, so the least expensive supplements are often not the best.

First, they tend to be lower in potency. Frequently, their formulas are based on older research and are not the balance that current scientific research suggests your body needs. Most important, they are not particularly well absorbed. This means that the amount of a nutrient on the label is much less than the amount that gets into your cells. In other words, you're not getting the amount you think you are.

No supplements are 100 percent absorbed, but the cheaper ones tend to be much less absorbable than more expensive ones. Let me give you one example: calcium. According to Dr. Tori Hudson, ND, author of *Women's Encyclopedia of Natural Medicine* (Keats Publishing, 1999), calcium citrate is 45 percent absorbed, while calcium carbonate is only four percent absorbed! If you don't buy supplements that break down and get used by your body, you're wasting your money and fooling yourself about how much you body is actually getting.

What Potency Do I Need?

I believe you need more than the Recommended Daily Allowances (RDAs) suggest. RDAs are the amounts of nutrients you need to maintain health, not the amount you need to get healthy if you have any common deficiencies. RDAs are not high enough to overcome any inherited genetic weaknesses that affect your body's nutritional needs. And they are definitely not enough to make up the nutrients your body loses through stress or dietary indiscretions. (Example: To digest sugar, you need B vitamins, which are usually lacking in sugary foods.) The RDAs indicate the amount of nutrients most people need to not be obviously sick. That's not good enough for anyone who wants to support and improve their health.

What Balance of Nutrients Do I Need?

Women looking to prevent bone loss often need at least as

L-arginine for Bladder Infections

Interstitial cystitis is a persistent bladder irritation that is not caused by any infection. It is painful and can cause an urgency to urinate. Researchers have found that L-arginine, a common amino acid, found in most natural food stores, can reduce both pain and urgency in patients with cystitis.

The patients were given either a placebo or 1,500 mg of L-arginine for three months. Improvements were found in those who took the amino acid. In addition to taking this supplement, we'd like to echo the suggestions made by naturopaths Michael Murray, ND and Joseph Pizzorno, ND. Eat a diet very low in simple sugars, refined carbohydrates, and full-strength fruit juices; drink at least two quarts of water throughout the day every day; and drink cranberry juice or cranberry concentrate (without refined sugar).

Note: L-arginine, used for wound healing, should not be taken by people with viral infections like herpes. Its antagonist, L-lysine, is used for this purpose.

Korting, G.E., et al. "A randomised, double-blind trial of roal L-arginine for treatment of interstitial cystitis," *Journal of Urology,* 161(2), 1999. From *Int'l Clin Nutr Rev,* July 2000.

Murray, Michael, ND and Joseph Pizzorno, ND. *Encyclopedia of Natural Medicine,* Prima Publishing, 1998.

much magnesium as calcium. Old formulas stress high calcium and half as much magnesium, but without sufficient magnesium, calcium just doesn't get into your bones. Since the excess is not simply excreted, it can cause health problems like arthritis and heart disease. How much is needed? Around 500 mg of each, added to a diet containing whole grains, legumes, nuts, and seeds — foods that contain both calcium and magnesium.

If you're menstruating, you may need extra supplemental iron; if you're not, leave it out, since many doctors now consider excess iron to be a risk factor for cancer and heart disease. Iron is an oxidizer and can damage tissues. Antioxidants prevent aging-related health problems like heart disease, eye disease, etc. There is no need to take supplementary iron when sufficient quantities for most people are found in foods.

Vitamin E is a powerful antioxidant that numerous studies have found to be beneficial when other antioxidants just don't seem to work. When very low amounts of vitamin E are added to a supplement (2-5 IU), it is added as a preservative. Low amounts of E (20-50 IU) are added so you will buy the supplement. From 200-400 IU of vitamin E is needed to provide therapeutic doses. Some people need even more, but I'd suggest a supplement with 400 IU of natural vitamin E, the form that's most highly absorbed. Geritol Complete, Theragram-M, and One-A-Day Maximum each contain 30 IU of synthetic vitamin E.

B vitamins are needed for stress, the nervous system, and numerous other body functions. Depressed people need sufficient vitamin B_6 to help the brain make a feel-good chemical, seratonin. A good amount of B vitamins, including B_6, would be 30-50 mg. More could put a burden on the liver, since these vitamins need to be synthesized in the liver to be absorbed.

Chromium and selenium are minerals needed for blood sugar regulation and the immune system. To help your body utilize sugars more slowly, or to help you regain your nutritional balance if you ever drank a lot of alcohol or have diabetes, you need at least 200 mcg of chromium a day. Some people require much more, under the supervision of a health-care provider.

The same amount, 200 mcg a day, applies to selenium. This mineral has been found to be low in people with cancer and other immune-related problems. Theragram-M contains 15 mcg of selenium, and Centrum Silver has 25 mcg.

All women who are concerned about bone loss should have enough boron in their diet and supplement. How much is enough? Studies indicate that the amount found in a healthy vegetarian diet (two to three mg) could help prevent osteoporosis. One mg of boron won't give you the protection you want unless your diet is high in leafy vegetables, nuts, and whole grains, natural sources of boron.

What Forms of Nutrients Are Best Absorbed?

The form of vitamin or mineral you take is even more important than how much you take. The higher the quality, the more it gets absorbed. Each vitamin and mineral has specific forms that are better absorbed than others. Here are a few of them.

Calcium, magnesium, and many other minerals are best absorbed when they are bound to citrate, aspartate, picolinate, or amino acid chelate. Minerals need an acidic base to break down and get used. If your stomach does not produce enough stomach acid (hydrochloric acid) to help the absorption of these nutrients, the form the minerals take will give you the acidity you need to utilize them.

Opponents of natural foods and natural supplements have argued that synthetic vitamin E is just as well absorbed as natural vitamin E. Scientific studies show that natural E is much better absorbed than the synthetic. How can you tell the difference? Simple. Your vitamin supplement will either say d-alpha-tocopherol or dl-alpha tocopherol. You can remember which is natural and which is synthetic by thinking, the extra "l" is for limited absorption. Dl-alpha forms of vitamin E are synthetic.

Most B vitamins will break down in your body, but some forms don't need to go through your liver to be utilized. If you have hepatitis, are a recovering alcoholic, or suspect a clinical or subclinical liver problem, you may want your supplement to contain an easy-to-absorb form of the B vitamins.

Vitamin B_6 is called pyridoxine. It is metabolized through the liver. Pyridoxyl-5-phosphate, or P-5-P, is a co-enzyme form of vitamin B6. That is, it turns into B_6 in your body, and does so without going through your liver. So it's easy to absorb and well tolerated. Co-enzyme B vitamins are best absorbed. If you think you want co-enzyme Bs, look for Pyridoxyl-5-phosphate on the label as an indicator of the form of the B vitamins it contains.

Are capsules or tablets best? It depends on the quality of the supplement. Cheaper tablets may not disintegrate properly, while good quality ones do. Because some nutrients are best utilized in the stomach and some in the small intestines, the better brands are formulated so that the ones that need to be released first, in the stomach, are. Capsules are released in the stomach. Bottom line? Don't shop by price; buy a good quality supplement.

What Do You Think of the Popular One-A-Day Vitamin Formulas?

Not much.

They're all low in potency, and most, if not all, are in the "less well absorbed" category. I qualify this statement because the form of nutrient used is not even listed in numerous popular one-a-day

How Natural Is Cholestin?

Cholestin is a dietary supplement made from red yeast rice, designed to lower cholesterol. But is this product a pharmaceutical or a natural supplement? The FDA called it a drug, even though its manufacturer, Pharmanex, insists it has been used for centuries in China. Is the FDA being unnecessarily hard on Pharmanex? Consumers interested in protecting our right to use alternative or complementary medicine might argue this call. But they might not, perhaps, if they looked a little deeper.

Pharmanex is not fermenting the yeast on rice in the traditional Chinese manner. Instead, they've altered it to produce a product much higher in lovastatin, the active ingredient in Mevacor (made by Merck Pharmaceuticals). Red yeast rice made the old-fashioned way contains little or no lovastatin, but a daily dose of Cholestin has 5 mg of lovastatin. Mevacor, when used to lower cholesterol, is usually taken in doses of 20-80 mg of lovastatin. Does this make Cholestin a drug?

supplements like Theragram-M, Geritol, and Centrum. They frequently contain synthetic coloring, waxes, and other ingredients that bind the tablet together. You could be sensitive to these ingredients. No one needs them for better health.

One-a-day formulas can't give you high potencies of nutrients, either. There just isn't room to put a lot of nutrients into a single tablet or capsule. Supplements with therapeutic amounts need to be taken in larger quantities — from four to six tablets or capsules daily.

This may seem like a lot, but it's not. These formulas usually contain plenty of vitamin C, so you don't need any extra. They also have 200-400 IU of vitamin E. The antioxidants are in higher amounts, so you don't need an extra formula to protect your eyes or heart. You've just saved yourself from taking your one-a-day plus three other supplements. With a good quality higher-dose supple-

When You're Traveling

Whether or not there's a doctor nearby, you may save yourself a great deal of discomfort by packing a few extra items for your next vacation. Even on an adventure travel trip where there will be plenty of Band-Aids and disinfectant. But to prevent shock from injury, nothing beats Rescue Remedy, a combination of flower essences originating with English physician Edward Bach, MD. You can find Rescue Remedy in health food stores. A few drops under the tongue take people and animals out of shock within a few minutes.

Some forms of Acidophilus, friendly bacteria, can prevent the discomfort of diarrhea or an upset stomach. Take it preventively or at the first sign of symptoms. The strongest forms of Acidophilus supplements are those that require refrigeration. Even if you can't keep it cold, it should stay more potent longer than those that do not need to be refrigerated. One variety, lactobacillus GG, or Culturelle, has been used extensively in Europe to counteract the effects of food poisoning, viruses, and antibiotics. Yogurt can also relieve digestive upset.

For sore muscles, use a lotion or ointment with Arnica Montana, a homeopathic, to reduce pain and swelling. Arnica tablets can be taken orally, as well. One effective ointment is Traumed, found in health food stores or wherever homeopathics can be found in your area. By adding these natural substances to your travel first-aid kit, you may save yourself unnecessary health problems on your vacation.

ment, you're getting even more.

Good quality vitamins and minerals can be found in health food stores and through many health-care practitioners. Don't waste your money on low potency, poor quality supplements. Take a better supplement for three to six months. You'll feel the difference.

Vitamin Buyers Beware

I cannot check out every product on the market, but we would like to take this time to caution you about health claims made about nutritional supplements and herbal products. They may be excellent products at a good value. Then again, they may be highly overpriced and overrated.

An example is a product I was told about that is advertised on the Internet, called Inholtra Natural Pain Relief Formula, sold by Discount Natural Foods, a store in Syracuse, New York. Brand names of the many supplements they sell on-line are not given, nor is the breakdown of what form these nutrients take, nor their potency. The company's name, Discount Natural Foods, also implies that this outfit offers good deals.

Inholtra Natural Pain Relief Formula consists of 90 softgel capsules containing glucosamine sulfate (a highly absorbable anti-inflammatory), chondroitan sulfate (a poorly absorbed anti-inflammatory), essential fatty acids, vitamins E and C, and manganese. One bottle costs $35.95. The literature from the Internet says that the "softgel delivery allows for greater absorption and utilization, especially for those with weak digestion (often older individuals with pain)." This suggests that if you were older, you'd want the softgel form over any other form available. However, gelatin or vegetarian capsules are very well digested. There's no digestive advantage to softgels. (They are generally used for products that are more liquid.) If you have impaired digestion, you probably don't have enough hydrochloric acid (HCl) in your stomach to digest the protein (gelatin) that makes up the softgel capsules.

Inholtra's literature goes on to say that the "glucosamine is bound with potassium vs. sodium for those concerned with salt in their diet (i.e. high blood pressure, etc)." However, the amount of sodium in some forms of glucosamine sulfate is so small it has not been found to affect sodium levels. The reason some glucosamine is made without sodium is simply the public's perception of the product.

Since the folks who make Inholtra mention that their product contains vitamin E, I was surprised to find that three capsules contain just 10 IU — an amount that is normally used as a preservative to keep other oils a product contains from going rancid. Therapeutic doses of vitamin E, however, begin at 200 IU, so you need a much higher dosage than you'll find in a day's supply of this product.

The literature claims this Pain Relief Formula is "cost effective," yet studies indicate that to reduce inflammation you need 500 mg of glucosamine sulfate three times a day. Since three of Inholtra's softgels equals 500 mg, if you take the amount of nutrients found to be helpful in pain control, a $35.95 bottle will last you only 10 days. A one-month supply is $108 plus any shipping and handling. I've seen studies showing that 500 mg of glucosamine sulfate alone taken three times a day can significantly reduce pain from inflammation. One company I contacted sells a one-month supply of glucosamine sulfate for $27.95. If you wanted to add essential fatty acids to make a similar product, it would set you back another $21.95/month. Now you're up to $49.90 for a similar product, half of what Inholtra is charging.

Vitamin E and Sun Damage

I've seen studies that showed vitamin E taken internally is a protective antioxidant, but what about using it externally? A preliminary animal study published in the *British Journal of Dermatology* (vol. 138, 1998) indicates that when vitamin E is applied topically it increases levels of other protective nutrients, glutathione, and vitamin C. After exposure to ultraviolet (UV) rays, vitamin E slowed down the harmful effects of skin oxidation. Simply speaking, if you find sunscreens with added vitamin E, they may protect you even more than those without it. Especially if the amounts are high. You can also add vitamin E to your sunscreen or everyday moisturizer yourself. Just cut open a vitamin E capsule and mix around 200 IU of vitamin E oil for each teaspoon of lotion. (This makes a great eye cream, too.)

I called the 800 number I was given for the Inholtra product and spoke with a personable young man at Discount Natural Foods, the store that sells this product by mail. He read off the ingredients of the Pain Relief Formula to me along with their amounts. When I mentioned to him that chondroitan sulfate was poorly absorbed orally, he said, as other manufacturers have told me, that some people prefer a formula with chondroitan sulfate and claim it works better than glucosamine sulfate alone. Good enough. That's what makes horse racing. But glucosamine and chondroitan sulfate are much less expensive than this formula, I pointed out. "We have glucosamine sulfate a lot cheaper than this formula," the young man told me. "So," I replied, "you like this product because it contains essential fatty acids?" "We like this formula because people buy it," he answered without a pause. His honesty was refreshing, but the ethics stunk.

The bottom line is that some companies are looking for formulas that work well at a fair price. Others are looking for formulas you'll buy, regardless of whether they give you results or are fairly priced. Glucosamine sulfate as an anti-inflammatory supplement can take up to three months before it works, so offering it at double what it should cost can be extra profitable for the seller.

What You Can Do

Choose companies with a good reputation. Do some price-comparison shopping. The least expensive product you find may or may not be as good in quality as the most expensive, but you can usually find one in the mid- to upper-range that is well absorbed and high enough in potency to give you the results you're looking for.

If a company is making claims about an exciting new formula that no one else has, it might be true. Some business people, however, are selling formulas that people will buy, whether or not they work. When possible, get input from your health-care provider who may have experience with patients using various brands, and know which ones have a consistent pattern of working. If you're in doubt and have no one to ask, buy the best quality supplement you can afford and try it for three to four months. If it works but cost is a significant issue, try one that's less expensive. Continue with the less expensive brand as long as it works for you. Remember that there's a 30-day placebo effect. This means that anything, even a sugar pill, could appear to work for you as long as one month. If a supplement appears to work for more than a month, it probably is working for you. Finally, if you're confused, you're in good company. We are at times, too, and must investigate further.

All new products are not scams or high-priced versions of other formulas that work just as well. For example, I heard about a product that was said to be protective against breast cancer — calcium-d-glucarate. It sounded too good to be true. I pursued the information and found that a reputable medical doctor at a cancer center in Denver had discovered this nutrient and patented it, and was selling it through Wieder Nutrition and Schiff supplement company. I spoke with a medical doctor associated with Wieder who I have known for decades by reputation as being a good scientist knowledgeable in nutrition. After a lengthy conversation, I was convinced that the science behind this product, NuStart Women's Breast Health Formula, is sound. It's also not expensive ($15-$18/month). Some supplements are worth taking, while others are better ignored. But remember that none take the place of a sound nutritional program.

Vitamin Supplements for Younger Women?

Consumption of some nutrients before conception is important in preventing serious complications during and after pregnancy. For example, not enough folic acid can cause neural tube defects. It is also thought that insufficient nutrition before and during pregnancy increases the risk for infertility, spontaneous abortion, and retarded growth. A recent study suggests that small amounts of vitamin and mineral supplements, prior to conception, could help avoid many of these problems without containing toxic quantities of any nutrients.

Women of childbearing age, many of whom are on constant

weight-loss programs, should be aware that these programs often contribute to nutrient deficiencies. Eating sensibly, with plenty of whole grains and fresh fruits and vegetables, may take a little effort at first. But it provides excellent, inexpensive insurance against future problems during pregnancy and childhood.

Antioxidants are nutrients that counteract the harmful effects that occur when fats in our body break down and "spoil" and produce chemicals called free radicals. We are now seeing that these free radicals may negatively affect embryos and even contribute to spontaneous abortion. Since emotional stress increases the production of hormones that make more free radicals, stress reduction during pregnancy is important. But so are antioxidants that are found in fresh fruits and vegetables. Women who want additional nutritional insurance may also want to take an antioxidant supplement consisting of vitamins E, C, and beta-carotene.

How Harmful Is Vitamin C?

The media is quick to jump on anything they think will make headlines, whether or not it is true or will confuse the public. Take this recent story about the harmful effects of vitamin C, which alleged that it could cause genetic damage in doses over the RDA.

I took a closer look, and what I found was astounding:
First, the story was not based on any scientific study submitted for peer review in any medical journal. It was based on a commentary, or opinion, of some British researchers who completed a small, short study that has neither been duplicated, nor published in a reputable journal or submitted to one.

This study was conducted over a period of only six weeks with 30 healthy people given 500 mg of vitamin C a day. Its conclusion was far from conclusive. The commentary on this study, published in the journal *Nature*, said that if you take more than 60 mg of vitamin C a day, it might cause genetic damage that could lead to such diseases as cancer or rheumatoid arthritis.

One of the research team members, Joseph Lunec, from the University of Leicester in England where this study was conducted, said that vitamin C has both a protective antioxidant effect and the ability to cause damage by producing free radicals. This is not new information. Many substances contain within themselves the ability to both heal and harm. The balance of the two cancels out the harmful effects. Lunec then theorized that the balance between protection and destruction could cause more oxidative stress and lead to disease.

However, the reverse is true as well. It is just as possible that the balance would be tipped in favor of vitamin C's protective abilities, and that it is more protective and less damaging. We think this is the most probable conclusion that will be reached.

This story warning consumers about the potential dangers of vitamin C was reported by the news service Reuters on the same day that nutrition writer Jane Brody had a similar story printed in the *New York Times*. Both stories, based only on this opinion, appeared on the same day.

Jane Brody's article included an interview with Victor Herbert, a doctor known to be vehemently opposed to any vitamin

---

RDA vs. DRI

The Recommended Daily Allowances for nutrients were designed to inform the public about the amount of vitamins and minerals necessary to prevent illnesses, like scurvy and kwashiorkor (uncommon to begin with in this country). They were not to give optimal levels for people to recover from illnesses, or to keep people healthy.

Now, the National Academy of Sciences, which helps set nutrient levels, has asked a nonprofit organization, the Institute of Medicine (IOM), to re-do nutrient levels for specific conditions. The first condition being addressed is osteoporosis. Sound good? Read further.

I believe there is a great deal of confusion about how much calcium a woman needs for healthy, strong bones. The ideal amount, 1,000-1,500 mg, suggested by most doctors will, unfortunately, not get into women's bones. Calcium absorption after age 25 (except during pregnancy) deteriorates. Unabsorbed calcium can lead to arthritis and heart disease. And heart disease is the number one killer of post-menopausal women.

I think the impartial IOM may not be so impartial after all. The current study was funded by the FDA, Health Canada, the National Institutes of Health, and the United States Dairy Association (USDA). With the USDA in the picture, how can we expect impartial information, which must include our body's ability to use various nutrients?

therapy and complementary medicine, who supported this negative theory. I can't help but wonder about the connection between the two. Was Jane Brody fed this opinion and did she examine only one side of the story in order to come up with an article that would make the nightly news? I hope not, but I don't see any other way this timing could have occurred.

I believe that stories that are potentially alarming or signal a danger from either foods or supplements should be based on scientific studies that have appeared in peer-reviewed journals. This means that a number of other doctors have read the report and find it contains conclusions that have merit and make sense. If you want to read some horror stories about the harmful effects of common substances, pick up a copy of the *Physician's Desk Reference* and look at the known side effects of over-the-counter and prescription drugs.

I am concerned about the truth in Jane Brody's article and any anxiety it may have caused in the public. Vitamin C has been used in large doses for many, many years with no side effects in healthy people except for occasional diarrhea. Blowing an opinion, such as this one, out of proportion only serves the press, not the public. And, as for the researcher in England, I can't help but wonder what makes Lunec tick?

Supplement Alert

I am used to seeing pharmaceutical companies launching strong ad campaigns touting their drug as being superior to other similar drugs, but we haven't seen too much of this with supplement companies. Some, but not a lot. Now there appears to be a war waging about the superiority of one kind of glucosamine sulfate over another. Why so much noise about a supplement? Could the answer be money?

I've talked about glucosamine sulfate before. It's a simple substance that has been found to reduce inflammation in numerous studies on osteoarthritis. And with the vast number of people — mostly women — in pain from osteoarthritis, there's a huge potential market out there.

Recently, PhytoPharmica, an excellent supplement company

that markets supplements to health food stores under the brand name of Enzymatic Therapy, has been saying that the patented glucosamine sulfate they carry (manufactured by a European company, Rotta Research) is the only glucosamine sulfate that has been clinically studied in the world. This is true. They suggest that because of this, others may be inferior. This may not be so. Here's why:

Glucosamine sulfate is a single compound that's relatively easy to make, and one, I have been told, where there's no room for variation. One glucosamine sulfate is the same as the other — with one exception: the stabilizing agents used. On its own, glucosamine sulfate is unstable if it comes into contact with moisture, like the

---

Nutritional Discovery for Hot Flashes

Q: I have hot flashes three to eight times a day and am taking soy pills with isoflavones, vitamin E, essential fats, and use progesterone cream twice a day. I'm getting a saliva test to check hormone levels. What else can you suggest? — *B.L.M, Fergus Falls, MN*

A: First, while I understand that many practitioners believe that saliva tests for hormone levels are accurate, the head of one of the largest natural compounding pharmacies has found their results do not correspond with symptoms in many, many people. I have been hearing from numerous doctors who are finding this out for themselves and are no longer using them. Blood levels of hormones appear to be the best "snapshot" of your hormones.

Be sure that if you're using isoflavones in high quantities, you are not at a particularly high risk for breast cancer, or have not had it. There is concern that a lot of isoflavones (more than what you'd find in a serving or two of soy) could stimulate breast cell growth.

Finally, for an answer to your hot flashes, I have found that hesperidin, one of the flavonoids found in vitamin C, works for many, many women to turn off the signal in the hypothalamus that causes hot flashes. Hesperidin is not easy to find in large enough quantities to work, but some years ago I asked AMNI, a supplement company, to consider selling it and they now do.

I have successfully used 1,000 mg (two capsules) of Hesperidin Methyl Chalcone by AMNI morning and night on an empty stomach for women with hot flashes. If it's going to work, you'll have at least some results within a month. A month's supply is two bottles (about $32), and AMNI's phone number is 800-356-4791. Hopefully, in time, other companies will also sell 500 mg capsules of hesperidin.

moisture in the air. It becomes gummy, and you're left with sticky capsules or tablets. So stabilizing agents are used to prevent this from happening: sodium chloride and potassium chloride are two. The PhytoPharmica/Rotta glucosamine sulfate apparently is stabilized with both sodium chloride and potassium chloride. But Rotta is not the only European lab that makes glucosamine sulfate with these stabilizers. They are the lab that holds a patent on a product that has been used in scientific studies.

Some other companies have argued that there's too much sodium in PhytoPharmica's supplement, but unless you're a sodium-sensitive person with hypertension, 150 mg of sodium a day (the equivalent of one capsule three times daily) is not going to harm you at all. This issue aside, it's important to note that the patent on this particular product is on the method of manufacturing, not on the finished product. Besides, what's the real difference between glucosamine sulfates that are stabilized with sodium chloride vs. potassium chloride vs. both?

I can't see any difference in the finished product, because when the hydrochloric acid (HCl) in your stomach comes into contact with these supplements, the sodium chlorides or potassium chlorides are ionized into free glucosamine sulfate and you're left with the same substance.

I understand that by entering into a licensing agreement with Rotta, PhytoPharmica may be adding a licensing fee to the cost of its product that it would like to recoup by selling a lot of its product. I have no reason to believe its product is not excellent. I have always found PhytoPharmica/ Enzymatic Therapy products to be of the highest quality. But so are some others.

What is the consumer to do? Through our nutrition grapevine I've heard there are manufacturers of glucosamine sulfates that may not be as high a quality as the one sold by PhytoPharmica and some other companies. I suggest if you are going to try this supplement for arthritis or other chronic pain that you begin with one of the more expensive brands for the first three or four months. That's how long it takes for glucosamine sulfate to work. Then, after you have results, if you want to try a less expensive brand, you'll know if it's one that works just as well.

You can find Enzymatic Therapy glucosamine sulfate in most health food stores. If your insurance will pay for it if it's ordered through your doctor, have your physician call PhytoPharmica at 800-553-2370, or Thorne Research at 800-228-1966. Both companies sell only to health practitioners and have excellent products.

Colloidal Minerals:
A Marketing Scam That Could Hurt You

Millions of dollars of nutritional supplements are sold each year by pharmaceutical companies and companies that manufacture or package vitamins, minerals, and herbs. The competition is fierce and we have become the victims of numerous unsubstantiated claims.

Take a look at a new form of supplement — colloidal minerals. There is not a single study to support the claims being made about them that Alexander Schauss, PhD could find after searching through 40 years of databases containing almost 30 million papers.

Many claims about the benefits of nutritional supplements are based on scientific studies published in peer-reviewed medical and nutritional journals. Some studies are conducted on laboratory animals, others on people. While studies on people are best, we should at least be able to find some to back up the statements shouting the benefits of a supplement.

What Are Colloidal Minerals?

Simply put, colloidal minerals are minerals found in clay, and then are freed from the clay when it's mixed with water. The kind and amount of minerals depends on what is in the type of clay it comes from. Montmorillonite, bentonite, kaolinite, and vermiculite (used by gardeners as a growing medium) are forms of clay from which colloidal minerals are taken. These clays also contain aluminum silicates, and large amounts of aluminum have been linked to Alzheimer's disease in numerous scientific studies.

Some colloidal minerals have from 1,800 to 4,400 parts per

million of aluminum. Foods usually have less than 10. Can taking colloidal minerals over a long period of time contribute to Alzheimer's? No one knows. There are no studies showing it's safe to use them. If the claims about colloidal minerals being very highly absorbed are true, they could flood the body with toxic levels of aluminum! Magnesium protects the brain from getting too much aluminum, but colloidal minerals high in aluminum are low in magnesium.

Unsubstantiated Claims Can Be Harmful

Higher absorption? According to Dr. Schauss, "When an element is soluble, it is usually more absorbable than when it is insoluble. Calling the product colloidal makes the product insoluble by definition. If it were a soluble solution, it could not be colloidal."

Still, vendors of colloidal minerals are saying they have superior absorption to other mineral forms — 10 to 12 times greater than minerals in tablets or capsules. Some claim their colloidal minerals are 95 percent absorbed. But there is not one study to back up these claims. If colloidal minerals really were absorbed as well as the people who sell them say, you could be getting toxic amounts of them into your body.

Colloidal minerals are also said to be better absorbed because they are negatively charged. This is physically impossible, as doctors and physiologists well know, because the small intestine walls through which nutrients are absorbed are negatively charged. Try this experiment with two magnets. Put the negative side of one against the negative side of another. The two sides are repelled. If, indeed, colloidal minerals were negatively charged, the walls of the small intestines would keep them from being absorbed.

Colloidal Minerals Are "Organic"

Some companies even claim their colloidal minerals are superior to others because they are organic. But minerals, by definition, are inorganic. Can your body absorb them? Sure. Especially if you're low on that particular mineral. Your body comes equipped with a sophisticated process in your intestines that allows you to absorb inorganic minerals from the foods you eat and the water you drink.

All that "organic" colloidal minerals means is that the clay from which they come may contain some humus, which is organic material. This is another marketing ploy to fool you into thinking this product is superior.

What About the Dangers of Iodine?

If these claims weren't enough, colloidal minerals may also cause radiation contamination. Clay is highly absorptive, which is why montmorillonite is used in some intestinal cleansers. It is especially good in absorbing all forms of iodine. We know from studies in the 1960s that clay-humus soils absorb high levels of radioactive iodine from nuclear fallout. And nuclear testing is being done throughout the world. Some clays are old enough to have absorbed radioactive iodine-131 from decades past. Are the colloidal minerals being sold high in radioactive iodine-131? There are no labora-

---

Quick Fix or Hard Work?

Baseball has an important metaphor to offer us. Recently, Mark McGwire and Sammy Sosa beat the previous all-time record for the most home runs set 30 years ago by Roger Maris. So what, you say? Well, if you're not interested in baseball, maybe you'll be interested in the fuss behind the home run king—Mark McGwire, who was first to top Maris.

McGwire is a strong, muscular man, and some people think his muscles and strength don't just come from training. They're supported with androstenedione, a nutritional supplement that may increase testosterone. This supplement, called "andro," is outlawed by the Olympics committee and by other sports, but not baseball. Now andro is flying off the shelves, and some people fear the wrong folks will take it. Like teenage boys whose bodies don't need extra hormones. And women who could end up with hairy faces (hirsuitism).

McGwire may have been first to break the record, but nobody is talking about what Sammy Sosa has been taking to bulk up and stay strong. Sosa takes Flintstones vitamins. Bam-Bam! Another Sosa home run!! We'd like to suggest that maybe these two baseball players are tops in their profession because they have talent and work hard. The public doesn't want to hear this. They want a better pill.

tory analyses we know of that tell us. If they are, how long would it take before any long-term negative effects occurred? No one knows.

How Can These Claims Be Made?

You are probably not a doctor, scientist, or physiologist. Neither are the health food store personnel or sales people in multi-level marketing companies who sell colloidal minerals. And many doctors and health practitioners are too busy or lax to look for the substantiation behind claims of various products. Besides, some people swear by them.

Anecdotal stories boost the sales of products like colloidal minerals. Some people feel terrific after they take them. Why? There are several possible reasons. The first is called "the placebo effect." This is a phenomena — backed up with scientific studies — that says you can get positive results from a food, drug, nutritional supplement, hands-on healing, etc. for up to 30 days if you believe it will work. The placebo effect doesn't last forever.

But many stories told to health practitioners and passed along from person to person are due to this phenomena. If anything you're doing is working for you for one month, but not after that time, it may be due to the placebo effect, not the effectiveness of the substance or course of treatment you're taking.

Another reason some people may feel good after taking colloidal minerals is that people who need minerals will get some absorbed from this source. They will also get them from mineral-rich foods. When your body needs minerals you will absorb more of them from your foods and supplements than if your mineral levels are not low. This doesn't mean that colloidal minerals are either superior or safe, however.

How to Know if Colloidal Minerals Are Superior?

In time, many statements we find to be true today may be found false tomorrow. Or vice versa. Perhaps we will discover that colloidal minerals have something in them that makes them better than other forms of minerals.

For now, a manufacturer or distributor of colloidal minerals would need to show you and me a certificate of analysis from an independent laboratory stating that the product they're selling contains the minerals they say it has, along with the amounts of aluminum and radioactive iodine-131. Anecdotes and testimonials are not enough in an area where there is so little known, and where a product could be much more dangerous to take than beneficial.

Consulting Clinical & Microbiological Laboratory (CCML) is an independent lab in Portland, Oregon that tests the ability of colloidal minerals to inhibit the growth of various microorganisms. In one study, they tested five colloidal silver products. One showed no ability to stop the growth of microorganisms and, in fact, *was contaminated itself.* Other products varied greatly in their effectiveness. If you're going to take mineral supplements, take those that are citrates, chelates, or picolinates. At least they're safe.

CoQ10: An Amazing Cancer Treatment and Heart Disease Preventive

Coenzyme Q10, also known as CoQ10, is one of the hottest selling nutrients on the market these days, but is it possible that one vitamin-like nutrient could treat cancer and prevent heart disease all by itself?

Obviously, I believe that a good diet is the starting point for any health-related problem. However, science is proving over and over again that CoQ10 can have a dramatic impact on both of these illnesses, as well as many others.

In fact, its broad base application is so evident that the National Institutes of Health has launched a $2-million study of CoQ10 in 80 people with early-stage Parkinson's disease and a second $6.5-million study of 347 people with Huntington's disease.

CoQ10 is produced by the mitochondria, which is the furnace or power plant of the cells in your body, and is the only known antioxidant that your body produces on its own. Frederick Crane, who was trying to figure out how heart cells convert sugar into energy, discovered it back in 1957.

It Works to Protect Health in Two Ways

What Dr. Crane discovered was an enzyme, a substance that sparks a chemical reaction in the body, that has at least two important functions in the body: *First, it works in the cells to produce energy, which gives your cells the ability to perform their specific functions.*

You can quickly see why this would be important for the cells in your heart. When your heart cells cease to operate at optimal levels, you experience heart failure.

Richard Delany, MD, FACC, a board-certified cardiologist from Massachusetts, had a patient nine years ago who was suffering from congestive heart failure so severe he couldn't drive his own car. None of the conventional methods of treatment were working, so the patient suggested CoQ10. Dr. Delany was familiar with the nutrient and knew it couldn't hurt to try, so he agreed.

Forty-five days later, the patient not only drove himself to his appointment, but his complexion and composure had changed so dramatically he was hardly recognized by the clinic staff.

Since then, Dr. Delany has used CoQ10 in his practice on a regular basis with great success. Where possible, he has heart surgery patients take CoQ10 for a couple of weeks before the operation. In open-heart surgery, the surgeon will isolate and chill the heart before operating. Once the operation is completed, the heart must be "awakened" from the chill. If the patient was able to take CoQ10 for a couple of weeks before the operation, the heart recovers more quickly from the chilling process, giving the patient a much smoother recovery.

This protective effect was proven in a 1982 Japanese study that was reported in the *Annals of Thoracic Surgery*. The study found that CoQ10 is highly protective of the heart during surgery, even during surgery on the heart itself.

The second function of CoQ10 in the body is that of an antioxidant.

You've heard for years about free radicals, those oxygen-containing molecules that damage your body's cells. Left unchecked, free radicals can cause many illnesses, such as atherosclerosis and cancer, and can contribute to the progression of other diseases, such as rheumatoid arthritis, inflammatory bowel disease, and Parkinson's disease.

Because it's the only antioxidant your body produces, Dr. Delany says, "CoQ10 plays an important role throughout the body" in destroying free radicals and preventing the damage they cause and the subsequent illnesses.

"I commonly use Coenzyme Q10 as one of a group of antioxidants (together with vitamin E, vitamin C, and lipoic acid) that I give to my patients to boost their body's 'antioxidant reserve,'" says Dr. Delany. "In my opinion, the synergistic consumption of a number of antioxidants is sensible preventive medicine."

So Who Should Take CoQ10?

According to Dr. Delany, "People who should be taking CoQ10 regularly would include: (1) any patient who already has an illness known to be associated with free-radical formation, (heart disease, cancer, rheumatoid arthritis, dementia, Parkinson's disease, cataracts, inflammatory bowel disease, smokers, etc.); (2) any patient who is at risk of similar illnesses based on their family history or past medical history (primarily atherosclerosis); (3) patients whose jobs place them at risk of high amounts of free radical formation (e.g. toll booth collectors exposed to the exhaust of automobiles); and (4) patients who consume very little fruits and vegetables, the main source of antioxidants in our food."

In other words, just about everybody can benefit from taking CoQ10. At present, there is no agreed upon dosage, as no side effects have been seen at any level of dosage. Those who swear by the nutrient start their recommended dosages at 100 mg. But many will go as high as 600 mg for those who have advanced heart disease. Some have even hinted that 1,000 mg dosages will be seen in the near future. Most healthy individuals, however, will get plenty of CoQ10 with the standard 100-mg dose. If you think you need more, it would be wise to consult with your doctor before increasing your dosage.

CoQ10 is not without its critics, though. Some studies have not shown conclusive evidence that CoQ10 helps any disease.

Proponents of the nutrient say that most of these studies are flawed in some way. Either they didn't use enough CoQ10 or the people in the study were too sick or the type of CoQ10 was not readily absorbable.

From what I have seen, these complaints about the inconclusive studies have merit and need to be considered. Obviously, the full extent of CoQ10's benefits is not known. But the science is there to support its usefulness, especially in regard to congestive heart failure.

Fighting Cancer

Interestingly enough, Dr. Crane's discovery received its first notoriety in 1961 when it was discovered that blood levels of CoQ10 correlate quite well with certain types of cancer (particularly breast cancer) and the stage of those cancers.

Breast cancer, for instance, is associated with a decrease in the blood levels of CoQ10. In cancers with a bad prognosis, there is a dramatic decrease in CoQ10 levels. *In fact, doctors can fairly reliably determine if you will survive breast cancer by the CoQ10 levels in your body!* The higher your blood levels, the better your chance of survival.

Dr. Karl Folkers, of the University of Texas, Austin, reported on six breast-cancer cases that were treated with CoQ10. The findings were nothing short of amazing: "The overt survival for five to 15 years of six cancer patients, without evidence of cancer, and the complete regression of cancer in five cases, and now a regression of metastases in the liver, are extraordinary...."

Once cancer moves into the liver "it's a prelude to eminent death," said one researcher. So the fact that CoQ10 caused the cancer to leave the liver is indeed a miracle.

This same researcher, Dr. Knud Lockwood, said: "Although in the past, the ethical treatment of breast cancer was based on mastectomy, X-ray treatment, and anti-cancer drugs, this overall treatment rarely, if ever, caused highly significant regressions of the primary tumor and metastases in the liver." He then concluded: "Therefore, our recording of the disappearance of liver metastases in even one patient having breast cancer is extraordinarily salient...."

Although these patients had breast cancer, there is no reason to believe that CoQ10 won't work in other cancers. However, there is still a lot of work to be done in regard to cancer treatment with CoQ10. Unfortunately, we're a long way from having this research done.

How Much and Where to Get It

Because there are no known side effects, we recommend that you take the standard 100-mg dose for cancer prevention and if you have cancer, speak to a doctor who understands this nutrient for a dosage that's appropriate for you.

There is one caveat: CoQ10 cannot be manufactured in the body without the presence of three other vitamins: niacin (B_3), folic acid, and pyridoxine (B_6). Therefore, it's extremely important that you take a good multivitamin (such as Vitality from Women's Preferred or its equal. To order Vitality, call 800-728-2288).

Unfortunately, you won't get enough CoQ10 from most multivitamins, if you get any, so you'll need to take a CoQ10 product separately. CoQ10 dissolves in oil. So if your CoQ10 doesn't come in a wafer that has oil added, you should take cod liver oil capsules or a tablespoon of olive oil with it, or take it with a meal containing fat.

What Is SAMe? Is It Safe?

Whenever a new supplement comes onto the market, we tend to buy and use it, looking for something that will work quickly to effect changes that are difficult to make with lifestyle and dietary changes. Now the hot new kid on the block is SAMe (S-adenosyl-methionine).

SAMe is a synthetic product similar to the natural substance made in your body from the sulfur amino acid methionine (sulfur amino acids are found in cruciferous vegetables like broccoli, cauliflower, brussels sprouts, and cabbage). Your cells use SAMe in many biochemical reactions, like making cartilage, detoxifying the blood, and producing neurotransmitters that counteract depression. So it's being touted as an important nutrient for people with arthritis, depression, and even cirrhosis of the liver. SAMe has been studied in Europe for more than 20 years, and used there successfully with few side effects.

So, if it's natural, something our body makes, and used for decades in Europe, it's safe to use, right? Very possibly — but with a bit of caution, I advise.

SAMe for Arthritis

SAMe appears to work for arthritis, but only if it's osteoarthritis. It not only has been known to reduce pain and inflammation, but it can also stop or slow down cartilage degeneration. Double-blind studies indicate SAMe is as effective as naproxin, a non-steroidal anti-inflammatory prescription drug, without naproxin's side effects. One study used 600 mg of SAMe a day for two weeks, then 400 mg a day. A two-month trial of personal use usually indicates whether or not SAMe is effective.

SAMe and Depression

Depressed people appear to have lower amounts of SAMe than people who are not depressed. SAMe is used to make serotonin, norepinephrine, and dopamine.

Its effects could be even superior to kava and St. John's wort. But again, check this out with your doctor before self-medicating to make sure it won't interfere, or counteract, anything else you're taking. Some people shouldn't take SAMe at all. For instance, if you suffer from bipolar depression, SAMe can trigger a manic episode. SAMe does not seem to work the way other antidepressants do so it should be used with caution and only when it's appropriate. At present, there's still a lot we don't know about the way SAMe effects the brain.

Is SAMe Safe?

Some say there are not enough long-term, random trials on SAMe to assure people of its safety. Dr. Sol Grazi, MD, an assistant professor at the University of Colorado School of Medicine and author of SAMe (S-adenosylmethionine): *The European Arthritis and Depression Breakthrough,* points to more than 20,000

Europeans who have been involved in SAMe studies. The bottom line from all the studies appears to point to its safety.

Still, because it's being used for some serious conditions, we think the most prudent action to take is to bring information on SAMe to your health practitioner and decide, together, whether or not it's worth a try in your case, especially if you're taking medications or herbal antidepressants. Frequently drug-herb-supplement interactions emerge after a substance is used more widely. Interactions that have never been studied can surface. You want to be monitored even when taking a natural substance like SAMe. Although SAMe has few side effects (transient nausea and gastrointestinal upsets seem to occur rarely) it makes significant changes in your biochemistry. This means that SAMe has drug-like effects. Some doctors and researchers believe it should be better regulated and studied more before being used.

How Much SAMe Is Enough?

The dosage for SAMe varies considerably from 400-1,600 mg per day. Like anything — natural or synthetic; supplement or pharmaceutical — you should take just the amount you need, and this amount varies from person to person. Naturopath Michael T. Murray, ND suggests beginning with 200 mg twice a day and increasing to 400 mg three times a day. He then advises reducing the dose back to 400 mg a day. Still, other practitioners find a much higher amount is needed. Good product? Yes. Safe to self-administer? Maybe. But instead of being your own doctor, the best approach might be to become a partner with your doctor.

Calcium D-Glucarate
Protects Against Cancer

Everything has a cause. Cancer often begins with exposure to any of a variety of toxic substances that encourage tumor production. Your risk for cancer and other diseases accelerates when your body can't remove enough toxins. Many of these carcinogenic (cancer-causing) or mutagenic (causing cell mutation) agents start in our diet and environment.

Devra Lee Davis, a professor at the Carnegie Mellon University, found Canadian and Danish studies that show high levels of carcinogenic toxins in women appearing years before their cancer was diagnosed. These toxins, found in cured meat, red meat, plastic wrap, synthetic pesticides, cigarette smoke, and car exhausts are the same cancer-inducing agents removed by the body naturally through a detoxification process called glucaronidation. You may not be able to escape exposure to these toxins, but you can do something to increase the rate at which they're removed by your body.

Increasing Detoxification

Calcium d-glucarate is a natural substance found in fruits and vegetables that actually helps your liver remove carcinogenic chemicals by increasing glucaronidation. Caffeine, cigarettes, and marijuana contain toxins and increase the excretion of glucarate. That means they slow down glucaronidation. The more coffee or colas you drink, the more cigarettes you smoke, the more toxins you accumulate and the more glucarate you lose. Exposures to dietary and environmental toxins or a family history of cancer are two reasons to increase your intake of fruits and cruciferous vegetables (foods high in glucarate). They are also reasons to think about adding calcium d-glucarate to your supplement regimen.

Glucoronidation

This major path of detoxification is basically a chemical reaction that occurs in your liver where a water-soluble substance combines with a toxin, removing it from your cells. This is called glucoronidation. Many of these toxins are known to be carcinogenic, such as those found in some molds or nitrosamines (found in cured meats such as ham and lunch meats). Other tumor promoters, such as steroid hormones (having too much estrogen, for example), can contribute to cancer and are removed through glucoronidation as well.

Remember learning that "every action has an opposite reaction?" Well, this is true with glucoronidation, also. Along with promoting this detoxification, your body produces an enzyme called beta-glucoronidase that stops it. Calcium d-glucarate blocks beta-glucoronidase, allowing greater detoxification. I believe that many people who get cancer, Parkinson's disease, and other chronic health problems have reduced glucoronidation. This means their bodies accumulate toxins at a greater rate than they can eliminate them. Doesn't this make sense? If your body can get rid of harmful substances, they can't stay around and contribute to causing a disease.

What Is Calcium D-glucarate?

Glucarate, d-glucarate, or DGA (for its active ingredient, d-glucaric acid) is a natural substance found in many fruits and vegetables. High levels of DGAs are found in apples, grapefruit, bean sprouts, broccoli, cauliflower, and cabbage. Glucarate binds itself to

Low Thyroid and Zinc Deficiency

A recent Japanese study showed that three-fourths of patients with low thyroid improved after taking zinc supplements for a year. This condition, hypothyroism, happens when the body doesn't produce enough thyroid hormones. The result: such symptoms as fatigue, dull, dry hair and skin, sleeplessness, and numbness and tingling in the hands and feet. These are symptoms that may apply to other imbalances as well. Your medical doctor can easily order thyroid tests. I do not suggest you diagnose yourself or rush out and buy zinc pills. But if you know or suspect you have low thyroid, you may want to include plenty of zinc-rich foods in your diet.

Zinc is particularly high in whole-grains, brewer's yeast, and pumpkin seeds. Essential fatty acids from fish oil can help change a less-active form of the thyroid hormone, T4, into a more active form the body can use, T3. This means including a few meals of fish each week. Turkey, pumpkin seeds, and almonds are also relatively high in amino acid, tyrosine, which has been found to help thyroid function.

Zinc is also an important mineral in the area of infertility. Even a minor deficiency may be responsible for impotence and a low sperm count in men. In women, there may be a loss of libido and a failure to ovulate. Interestingly, these symptoms are also associated with low thyroid function.

some harmful environmental pollutants and other toxins in foods, beverages, and cigarette smoke, as well as attaching itself to excessive estrogen, removing these unwanted materials. Calcium d-glucarate is glucarate attached to calcium. The calcium is a carrier that allows glucarate to be present much longer. Instead of having glucarate remain in your body for one hour, binding it to calcium allows calcium d-glucarate to stay in your body for five hours!

A great deal of research on glucarate has been done over the past 20 years by cancer researcher, Thomas Slaga, PhD. I met Dr. Slaga last year and talked with him for over an hour and was very impressed with his work. In his book, *D-Glucarate: A Nutrient Against Cancer* (Keats Publishing, 1999, $3.95), Dr. Slaga explains how glucarate has been found to be protective against breast, lung, colon, liver, bladder, skin, and prostate cancers by enhancing this detoxification pathway. He reported results of a study on glucarate and breast cancer that showed estrogen levels decreased when calcium d-glucarate was taken. For women worried about having an increased risk for breast cancer from estrogen therapy, glucarate appears to offer a unique form of protection.

How Much Do I Need?

According to Dr. Slaga, 200-2,000 mg of glucarate gives a protective effect. But remember that calcium d-glucarate supports glucoronidation for about five hours. So eat a healthy diet and consider taking calcium d-glucarate supplements two or three times a day.

The amount of calcium d-glucarate you decide to take may depend upon your health, diet, lifestyle, and inherited strengths and weaknesses. If you want some added protection and eat well, don't smoke, and are not exposed to a lot of toxins, 200 mg two to three times a day may be fine. If you want more protection because of past indiscretions or a family history of cancer or Parkinson's, 500 mg twice a day makes sense. That's what I take, even though now my diet is healthy and I live in the country where the air is relatively clean. However, for 30 years, I lived in Southern California and was exposed to high amounts of air pollution, so I want to move any accumulated toxins out of my body. If you've had cancer or been exposed to high amounts of carcinogenic substances, you might want to take 500 mg three times a day. Dr. Slaga has not seen any evidence of toxicity or any side effects with 10 grams (10,000 mg) of any form of glucarate.

Products with glucarate are not being advertised as anti-cancer supplements for a very good reason. They're not. When I speak with oncologists who use nutrition in their practices, these doctors tell me: "There are two steps you need to take. Detoxify and support the immune system. The body does the rest." Glucarate may be a key nutrient in helping us reduce our body's toxic burdens of everything from a lifetime exposure to toxic substances to a course or two of chemotherapy or other drugs.

Since calcium d-glucarate, or glucarate, is a patented nutrient, any supplement you find on the market with this name on it is the real thing. You can safely shop for quantity of the nutrients vs. price and availability and be assured you're getting the same quality ingredient. Are products with glucarate necessary? I don't know. But they do offer good protection, especially if you've ever been a heavy smoker, eaten processed meats, or drank a lot of caffeine.

If you still smoke, you may want to take a more serious look at these products. Just remember that glucarate does not take the place of changing your lifestyle to a healthy one. And it doesn't promise to cure anything. But it could give your body the support it needs to remain healthier longer.

Afterword

A s you have seen, there are no quick fixes. But by taking simple steps and integrating them into your life, you can change the direction of your health. Here are a few suggestions to help you succeed.

Don't try to do too much at a time. If you feel overwhelmed by trying to work an entire program rather than the first step, you'll end up feeling frustrated and a failure. Every step forward counts and will get you where you're going.

Go easy on yourself. Give yourself the same support you'd give your best friend. Instead of being annoyed at what you haven't done, take a break and soak in a hot bath with lavender oil, read a book, take 10 minutes to sit quietly and breathe deeply. Treat yourself gently, with love and compassion. Renew yourself so you can take the next step when you're ready.

Be patient. Don't look ahead at how much you have to do. Instead, occasionally look behind you to see how far you've come. Impatience won't get you to your goals any faster. In fact, I've found there in no fast way. With patience and perseverance, you'll get there. Never give up. You can take breaks from your program whenever you like. After all, it *is* your program. Then, as soon as you're ready, pick up where you left it. It doesn't matter how long it takes you to finish. All that matters is that you do.

I think the most difficult pattern to change is our eating habits. We've had them most of our lives, and suddenly we're faced with reasons to create entirely new habits. It's important to recognize that this is not easy, and that the rewards are greater than the difficulties. Less pain, less illness, more energy, a better quality of life … what more could you ask for?

Congratulations for making the decision to move into better health. I'm so pleased to have been a part of your transformation.

Bibliography

Abraham, Guy E., MD and Harinder Grewal, MD. "A total dietary program emphasizing magnesium instead of calcium: effect on the mineral density of calcaneus bone in postmenopausal women on hormonal therapy," *Journ of Repro Med*, vol. 35, No. 5, May 1990.

Abraham, Guy E., MD. "Nutrition and the premenstrual tension syndrome," *Journal of Applied Nutrition*, September 1984.

Abraham, Guy E., MD. "Nutritional Factors in the Etiology of the Premenstrual Tension Syndrome," *Journal of Reproductive Medicine,* vol. 28, no. 7, July 1983.

Ackerson, Amber, ND & Corey Resnick, ND. "The effects of l-glutamine, n-acetyl-d-glucosamine, gamma-linolenic acid, and gamma-oryzanol on intestinal permeability," Tyler Encapsulations, *Townsend Letter for Doctors,* January 1993.

Aldercreutz, Herman, et al. "Dietary phytoestrogens and the menopause in Japan," *The Lancet,* May 16, 1992, 339:1233.

Alice Lesch Kelly's story comes from an article she wrote in the May 2000 issue of *Health* magazine.

Alternative Medicine the Definitive Guide, compiled by The Burton Goldberg Group, Future Medicine Publishing, 1993.

Alternative Medicine, The Definitive Guide, Future Medicine Publishing Inc., 1993.

Am J Clin Nutr 27(1):59-79, 1974; 60, 1994;129-135.

Am Journ of Nat Med, July/August 1997.

American Diabetes Association, "Consensus statement. Magnesium supplementation in the treatment of diabetes," *Diabetes Care,* 15(8):1065-7, 1992.

American Journal of Clinical Nutrition, November 1996.

"Angioplasty Risks Found for Women," *Boston Globe,* March 9, 1993, p 1.

Angus, Rosalind, et al. "Dietary intake and bone mineral density," *Bone Min,* 88.

Arjmandi, BH, et al. "Dietary soybean protein prevents bone loss in an ovariectomized rat model of osteoporosis," *J Nutr,* 126, 161-167, 1996.

Articles by Mary Shomon from www.thyroid.miningco.com.

Articles from www.lef.org.

Ault, Alicia. "FDA warns on calcium-channel blocker," *The Lancet,* January 3, 1998.

Baltzan, Marc A., et al. "Hip fractures attributable to corticosteroid use," *The Lancet,* vol. 353, April 17, 1999.

Barnhart, K.T., E., Freeman, J.A. Grisso, et al. "The effect of dehydro-epiandrosterone supplementation to symptomatic perimenopausal women on serum endocrine profiles, lipid parameters, and health-related quality of life." *J Clin Endocrinol Metab,* 1999;84:3896–3902.

BBRC, vol. 192, no. 1, 1993.

BBRC, vol. 199, no. 3, 1994.

BBRC, vol. 224, no. 2, 1996.

Beattie, JH, Peace, HS. "The influence of a low-boron diet and boron supplementation on bone major mineral and sex steroid metabolism in postmenopausal women," *Brit Journ Nutr,* 871-84 (1993).

Beutler, Jade. *Flax for Life,* Progressive Health Publishing, Encinitas, CA, 1996.

Biochemical and Biophysical Research Communications (BBRC), vol. 212, no. 1, 1995.

Bioinorganic Chemistry, 1978;8: 303-18.

Birdsall, Timothy C., ND. "5-Hydroxytryptophan: a clinically-effective serotonin precursor," *Alternative Medicine Review,* vol. 3, no. 4, 1998, 271-279.

Bland, Jeffrey, PhD. *Nutraerobics: The Complete Individualized Nutrition and Fitness Program for Life After 30,* Harper & Row Publishing, 1983.

Blaylock, Russell L., MD. *Excitotoxins: The Taste That Kills,* Health Press, Santa Fe, NM, 1997.

Bone, Kerry, B.Sc. "Echinacea: What makes it work?" *Alternative Medicine Review*, vol. 2, no. 2, 1997.

Bone, Kerry, B.Sc. "Echinacea: When should it be used?" *Alternative Medicine Review*, vol. 2, no. 6, 1997.

Bonn, Dorothy. "Haematological neoplasms linked to benzene," *The Lancet,* July 26, 1997.

Brandi, Maria Luisa, MD, PhD. "New Treatment Strategies: Ipriflavone, Strontium, Vitamin D Metabolities and Analogs," *The Amer Journ of Medicine,* Nov 30, 1993; 95 (Suppl. 5A):5A-74S.

Braverman, Eric R., MD, Carl C. Pfeiffer, MD, PhD. *The Healing Nutrients Within,* Keats Publishing, 1987.

British Medical Journal, February 8, 1997.

Brown, Susan E. "Osteoporosis: Sorting fact from fallacy," *Network News,* Nat'l Women's Health Network, July/August 1988.

Brown, Susan E. PhD. *Better Bones, Better Body,* Keats Publishing, Inc., New Canaan, CN, 1996.

Bruner, Ann B., et al. "Randomised study of cognitive effects of iron supplementation in non-anaemic iron-deficient adolescent girls," *The Lancet,* vol. 348, October 12, 1996.

Buhner, Stephen Harrod. *Herbal Antibiotics,* Storey Books, 1999.

Caldu, P., et al. "White Wine Reduces the Susceptibility of Low-Density Lipoprotein to Oxidation," *Am J Clin Nutr 62,* 403, 1996.

Cass, Hyla, MD. *St. John's Wort: Nature's Blues Buster,* Avery Publishing, $9.95, 1998.

Caulin-Glaser, Teresa, MD. "Primary prevention of hypertension in women," *Journal of Clinical Hypertension,* vol. 2, no. 3, 2000.

Chaitow, Leon, DO, ND. *Amino Acids in Therapy,* Healing Arts Press, Rochester, VT, 1985.

Chaitow, Leon, ND, DO. *The Healing Power of Amino Acids,* Thorson's Publishing Group, 1989.

Chenoy R., Hussain S., et al. "Effect of oral gamolenic acid from evening primrose oil on menopausal flushing," *BMI* 308, 1994.

Classen, D.C., et al. "Adverse Drug Events in Hospitalized Patients," *JAMA,* 277 (1997):301-6.

Clinica Chimica Acta, March 15, 1995.

Clinica Chimica Acta, March 31, 1995.

Colditz, G.A., et al. "The use of estrogens and progestins and the risk of breast cancer in postmenopausal women," *New England Journal of Medicine,* vol. 332, 1995.

"Collected reports of adverse reactions to MSG," Truth in Labeling Campaign, May 1, 1996.

Collin, Jonathan, MD. "Treating candidiasis without nystatin, ketoconazole, or diflucan," *Townsend Letter for Doctors,* no. 161, December 1996.

Collin, Jonathan, MD. "Treating candidiasis without nystatin, ketoconazole, or diflucan," *Townsend Letter for Doctors,* no. 161, December 1996.

Collins, Peter, et al. "Cardiovascular Protection by Oestrogen — A Calcium Antagonist Effect?" *The Lancet,* May 15, 1993.

Conversation with Ed Smith, Herbalist and Owner of HerbPharm, October 14, 1999.

Conversations with Luke Bucci, MD, October 1998.

Correspondence with Mark Messina, PhD.

Cowley, Geoffrey. "The Heart Attackers," *Newsweek,* August 11, 1997.

Cox, Cat. "Chocolate Unwrapped: The Politics of Pleasure," The Women's Environmental Network, London, 1993.

Cranton, Elmer, MD, and William Fryer. *Resetting the Clock: 5 Anti-aging hormones that improve and extend life,* M. Evans and Company, Inc, New York, 1996.

Criqui, M.H., Ringel B.L. "Does Diet or Alcohol Explain the French Paradox?" *The Lancet,* 1719-1723, 1994.

Crouse, John R., III. "Gender, Lipoproteins, Diet, and Cardiovascular Risk," *The Lancet,* February 11, 1989.

D'Adamo, Dr. Peter J., Catherine Whitney. *Eat Right 4 Your Type,* G.P. Putnam's Sons, 1996.

Dalton, Katharina, MRCGP. *The Premenstrual Syndrome and Progesterone Therapy,* Year Book Medical Publishers, Inc., Chicago, Illinois, 1977.

Deadly Medicine, by Thomas J. Moore, Simon & Schuster, 1995.

Deal C.L., T.J. Schnitzer, E. Lipstein, et al. "Treatment of arthritis with topical capsaicin: A double blind trial." *Clin Ther.* 1991;13:383–395.

Dept of Agriculture, Agricultural Marketing Service, "Pesticide Data Program: Annual Summary Calendar Year 1993," June 1995.

"Dietary calcium and the prevention of postmenopausal osteoporosis," review from the Nat'l Nutr Institute, Canada, *Nutrition Today,* May/June 1988.

Diethrich, Edward B., MD, and Carol Cohan. *Women and Heart Disease,* Times Books, 1992.

Divi, R.L. and D.R. Doerge. "Inhibition of thyroid peroxidase by dietary flavonoids." *Chem Res Toxicol,* 1996 January/February, 9(1):16-23.

Dreher, Henry. *The Immune Power Personality,* Penguin Books, 1995.

"Drinking Green Tea Every Day May Keep Cancer at Bay," *Healthy Cell News,* Fall/Winter 1997.

Edwards, C.J., et al. "Oral statins and increased bone-mineral density in postmenopausal women," *The Lancet,* June 24, 2000.

Erasmus, Udo. *Fats That Heal, Fats That Kill,* Alive Books, British Columbia, Canada, 1986.

Erdman, Dr. John W, Jr. "Short-term effects of soybean isoflavones on bones in postmenopausal women," Division of Nutr Science, Univ of Ill; "Disease prevention with soy," *HSR Supplement Industry Insider,* November 6-9, 1997, Scottsdale, AZ.

Facchinetti, F., et al. "Oral magnesium successfully relieves premenstrual mood changes," *Postgraduate Medicine,* vol. 90, no. 1, July 1991.

Falck, Jr, Frank, et al, "Pesticides and polychlorinated biphenyl residues in human breast lipids and their relation to breast cancer," Archives of Environ. Health, March/April 1992, vol. 47, no. 2.

Fitzpatrick, Annette. "Calcium-channel blockers may increase breast-cancer risk," *Cancer,* 1997;80.

"Folic acid facts," Wheat Foods Council, 5500 S Quebec, Suite 111, Englewood, CO 80111.

Fugh-Bergman, Adriane. "Wild Yam Cream, Diosgenin, and Natural Progesterone: What Can They Really Do For You?" National Women's Health Network, January/February 1999.

Fuhrman, B., et al. "Consumption of Red Wine With Meals Reduces the Susceptibility of Human Plasma and Low-Density Lipoprotein to Lipid Preoxidation," *Am J Clin Nutr* 61(3), 549-554, 1995.

Gaby, Alan R., MD. *Townsend Letter,* August/September 1995.

Gaby, Alan R., MD. *Preventing and Reversing Osteoporosis,* Prima Publishing, Rocklin, MD 1994.

Gaby, Alan R., MD. "Thiamine improves reaction time," *Townsend Letter,* August/September 1997.

Gartner, C., W. Stahl, and H. Sies. "Lycopene is more bioavailable from tomato paste than from fresh tomatoes," *American Journal of Clinical Nutrition,* 66:116-122, 1997.

General Pharmacology, March 1996.

Ginsberg, Jean. "Environmental oestrogens," *The Lancet,* January 29, 1994.

Goldfarb, John. *The No-Hysterectomy Option,* Wiley Pub., 1997.

Gordan and Genant. "The aging skeleton," *Chrons Geriatr Med,* 1985.

Graedon, Joe and Teresa Graedon, PhD. *Dangerous Drug Interactions,* 1997, St. Martin's Press.

Granato, Heather. "What is the DRI?" *Natural Foods Merchandiser,* October 1997.

Grazi, S. and M. Costa. SAMe (S-adenosyl-methionine): The European Arthritis and Depression Breakthrough, Rocklin, CA, Prima Publishing, 1999.

Haas, Elson M., MD. *Staying Healthy With Nutrition,* Celestial Arts, Berkeley, CA, 1992.

Haris, Susan S. and Dawson-Hughes, Bess. "Caffeine and bone loss in healthy postmenopausl women," *Amer Journ Clin Nutr,* 1994; 60:573-8.

Head, Kathi, ND. *Your Natural Guide to Diabetes,* Prima Publishing, 1999, $6.99.

Hegerfeld, Constance. "Osteoporosis: The pain facts," *Women's Health Connections,* Aug/Sept 1993.

Helzlsouer, K.J., A.J. Alberg, G.B. Gordon, et al. "Serum gonadotropins and steroidhormones and the development of ovarian cancer." *JAMA.*1995;274:1926–1930.

Hernandez, Katie. "The Leaky Gut Syndrome," unpublished paper.

Hickling, Lee. "Antibiotics for the birds: FDA moves to withdraw approval," November 3, 2000, drkoop.com Health News.

Hickling, Lee. "New antibiotic recommended for FDA approval," April 5, 2000, drkoop.com Health News.

"High doses of vitamin C can be harmful-study," (Release at 1800 GMT, Wednesday, April 8) April 9, 1998. LONDON, Reuters (WS) via NewsEdge Corp.

Hobbs, Christopher, LAc. *Medicinal Mushrooms,* Botanica Press, 1986.

Hobbs, Larry S. *The New Diet Pills,* Pragmatic Press, Irvine, CA, 1995.

Holistic Medicine, vol. 4, 145-146.

Hopper, John Llewelyn, PhD, and Ego Seeman, MD, "The bone density of female twins discordant for tobacco use," *New England J Med,* February 10, 1994.

Horowitz, Sala, PhD. "SAMe for depression, arthritis, cirrhosis, and other disorders," *Alternative and Complementary Therapies,* October 1999.

Horton, Richard. "Attacking Heart Disease Among U.S. Women," *The Lancet,* August 27, 1994.

Horton, Richard. "Trials of Women," *The Lancet,* March 26, 1994.

"House Approves Bill to Speed Federal Review of Medicines," *New York Times,* October 8, 1997.

"HSR's Annual Guide to Herbs: St. John's Wort," *Health Supplement Retailer,* December 1977.

Imai, K. and K. Nakachi. "Cross Sectional Study of Effects of Drinking Green Tea on Cardiovascular and Liver Diseases," *British Medical Journal* 1995;310:693-696.

Immaculate Deception II, Suzanne Arms, Celestial Arts, 1994.

International Journal of Clinical Pharmacology and Therapeutics, vol. 36, no. 9, 1998. *Vitamins and Cancer Prevention,* Wily-Liss, NY, 1991.

International Journal of Tissue Reactions, 17(1):199.

Ji H.T., et al. "Green tea consumption and the risk of pancreatic and colorectal cancer," *Int J Can,* 7;253-8, 1997.

Jones, Cindy L.A., PhD. *The Antibiotic Alternative,* Healing Arts Press, 2000.

Jones, Denise M. and Philip S. Weintraub. "Anesthesiologists warn: If you're taking herbal products, tell your doctor before surgery," American Society of Anesthesiologists, Public Education announcement, October 25, 1999.

Joo, S.J. and N.M. Betts. "Copper intakes and consumption patterns of chocolate foods as sources of copper for individuals in the 1987-88 nationwide food consumption survey," *Nutr Res,* 16(1), 41-49(1995). *Intl Clin Nutr,* July 1996, 164-165.

Journal of Aging and Physical Activity, April 1999.

Journal of Surgical Oncology, 15:67-70.

Journal of the American Medical Association, December 25, 1996.

Journal of Women's Health, Fall 1992.

Kamen, Betty, PhD. *Hormone Replacement Therapy — Yes or No?* Nutrition Encounter, Inc. 1993.

Kaslof, Leslie, J. *The Bach Remedies: A Self-Help Guide,* Keats Publishing Co., 1988.

Katan, MD. "Commentary. Fats for diabetics," *The Lancet* 343:1518, 1994.

Katzin, Carolyn, MS, CNS. *Good Eating Guide & Cookbook*, Herbalife, 1996.

Kerrigan, D. Casey, et al. "Knee osteoarthritis and high-heeled shoes," *The Lancet,* vol. 351, May 9, 1998.

Keshgegian, A.A. and A. Cnaan. "Estrogen receptor-negative, progesterone receptor-positive breast carcinoma," *Arch Pathol Lab Med*
  120:970-3, 1966.

Kilbourn, J.P., PhD. "Not all colloidal silver products are created equal!"
  Townsend Letter for Doctors & Patients, October 1996.

Klotter, Jule. "The Individualized Diet Solution," *Townsend Letter for
  Doctors & Patients,* June 1997.

Knekt P., et al. "Antioxidant Vitamin Intake and Coronary Mortality in a
  Longitudinal Population Study," *Am J Epidemiol* 139, 1180-9, 1994.

Kopelman, Peter G. and Graham A. Hitman. "Exploding type II,"
  Supplement to the *The Lancet,* Review 1998.

Kritz H., et al. "Passive Smoking and Cardiovascular Risk," *Arch Intern
  Med* 155:1942-8, 1995.

Kroman, Niels, et al. "Should women be advised against pregnancy after
  breast-cancer treatment?" *The Lancet,* vol. 350, August 2, 1997.

Lahorz, S. Colet, RN. *Conquering Yeast Infections: the Non-Drug solution,* Pentland Press, Inc., 1996.

Lahorz, S. Colet, RN. *Conquering Yeast Infections: The Non-Drug solution,* Pentland Press, Inc., 1996.

Larkin, Marilyn. "Surgery patients at risk for herb-anaesthesia interactions," *The Lancet,* vol. 354, October 16, 1999.

Larkin, Marilynn. "Risk of age-related vision loss wanes with wine,"
  The Lancet, January 10, 1998.

Lee, John R., MD. *Natural Progesterone: The Multiple Roses of a
  Remarkable Hormone,* BLL Publishing, Sebastopol, CA, 1993.

Lee, John R., MD. *What Your Doctor May Not Tell You About
  Premenopause,* Warner Books, New York, 1999.

LeShan, Lawrence and R.E. Worthington. "Personality as a factor in the
  pathogenesis of cancer: A review of the literature," *Brit J Med
  Psychol,* 29, 1956.

Lieberman, Shari, PhD, and Ken Babal, CN. *Maitake: King of
  Mushrooms,* Keats Publishing, 1997.

Lin, David. "Esterified vitamin E acetate and succinate: therapeutically active, preferred — and well documented," *Townsend Letter for Doctors,* January 1993, p. 26-29.

Lininger, Schuyler, W., Jr., DC, editor. *A-Z Guide to Drug-Herb-Vitamin Interactions,* Prima Publishing, 1999.

Liu, Barbara, et al. "Use of selective serotonin-reuptake inhibitors or tricyclic antidepressants and risk of hip fractures in elderly people," *The Lancet,* vol. 351, May 2, 1998.

Liu, Lynda. "Duck liver and chicken soup," WebMD, 1999.

Lock, Margaret. "Contested meanings of the menopause," *The Lancet,* May 25, 1991.

London Daily Telegraph, September 1, 1992.

Love, Dr. Susan. Presentation given at All-Saints Episcopal Church, Pasadena, California, May 1998.

Lukaczer, Dan, ND. "Antioxidants Offer Balance and Protection," *NFM's Nutrition Science News,* August 1996.

Martin, Jeanne Marie, Zoltan P. Rona, MD. *Complete Candida Yeast Guidebook,* Prima Publishing, 1996.

Matkovic, Velimer, et al. "Urinary calcium, sodium and bone mass of young females," *Amer Journ Clin Nutr,* 1995; 62:417-425.

Matthews, Karan A., PhD, et al. "Menopause and risk factors for coronary heart disease," *New Engl J Med,* vol. 321, no. 10, September 7, 1989.

McCarthy G.M., D.J. McCarty. "Effect of topical capsaicin in the therapy of painful osteoarthritis of the hands." *J Rheumatol.* 1992;19: 604–607.

McCarthy, Michael. "New antidepressants no better than old," *The Lancet,* vol. 353, March 27, 1999.

McCarthy, Michael. "COX-2 inhibitors found to impair renal function," *The Lancet,* vol. 356, July 8, 2000.

McCarthy, Michael. "Conflict of interest highlighted in debate on calcium-channel blockers," *The Lancet,* January 17, 1998.

McCarthy, Michael. "FDA bans red yeast rice product," *The Lancet,* vol. 351, May 30, 1998.

McCarthy, Michael. "Guidelines issued for steroid-induced osteoporosis," *The Lancet,* vol. 348, November 2, 1996.

McCully, Kilmer S., MD. *The Homocysteine Revolution,* Keats Publishing, 1997.

McNulty, H. "Folate requirements for health in women," *Proc Nutr Soc* 56, 1977. *Int Clin Nutr Rev,* October 1997, p. 223.

Melina, Vesanto, RD, et al. *Becoming Vegetarian,* Book Publishing Company, 1995.

Menkes, Marilyn S., et al. "Serum beta-carotene, vitamins A and E, selenium, and the risk of lung cancer," *New England Journal of Medicine,* November 13, 1986.

MenoTimes newsletter, Spring 1996.

Messina, Mark, PhD. "The Soy Connection," *J Am Diet Assoc,* 2000.

Miller, Alan L., ND, and Gregory S. Kelly, ND. "Methionine and homocysteine metabolism and the nutritional prevention of certain birth defects and complications of pregnancy," *Alt Med Review,* vol. 1, no. 4, 1996.

Miller, Alan L., ND. "Cardiovascular disease — toward a unified approach," *Alternative Medicine Review,* September 1996.

Miller, Alan, L., ND, and Gregory S. Kelly, ND. "Homocysteine metabolism: nutritional modulation and impact on health and disease," *Alternative Medicine Review,* July 1997.

Moore, Thomas J. *Prescription for Disaster,* Simon & Schuster, 1998.

Mother-Friendly Childbirth Initiative, Coalition for Improving Maternity Services, 1996.

Mowrey, Daniel B., PhD. *The Scientific Validation of Herbal Medicine,* Keats Publishing, New Caanan, CN, 1988.

Murch, Susan J. et al. "Melatonin in feverfew and other medicinal plants," *The Lancet,* November 29, 1997.

Murch, Susan J., et al. "Melatonin in feverfew and other medicinal plants," *The Lancet,* November 29, 1997.

Murray, M.T. *Encyclopedia of Nutritional Supplements*, Sacramento, CA, Prima Publishing, 1996.

Murray, Michael T., ND and Joseph Pizzorno, MD. *Encyclopedia of Natural Medicine*, Prima Publishing, 1998.

Murray, Michael T., ND. "Common Questions about St. John's wort extract," *Amer. Journ of Natural Med*, September 1997.

Murray, Michael T., ND. "Menopause: Is Estrogen Necessary?," *Amer Journal of Natural Medicine*, vol. 2, no. 9, November 1995.

Murray, Michael T., ND. "St. John's wort extract in depression: Over three million prescriptions per year in Germany," *Amer Journ of Natural Med*, December 1996.

Murray, Michael T., ND. *The Healing Power of Herbs*, Prima Publishing, 1995.

Nephron, 1994; 68:197-201.

Ness, Roberta B., MD, MPH, et al. "Number of Pregnancies and the Subsequent Risk of Cardiovascular Disease," *NEJM*, May 27, 1993.

"News in brief," *The Lancet*, April 5, 1977, p. 1002.

New York Times, February 25, 1997.

Nielsen, Forrest H. et al. "Effect of dietary boron on mineral, estrogen, and testosterone metabolism in postmenopausal women," *FASEB Journ*, 1987.

Nutrition Science News, March 1997.

Okumiya, Kiyohito, MD, et al. "Effects of exercise on neurobehavioral function in community-dwelling older people more than 75 years of age," *Journal of the Amer Geriatric Soc*, 1996;44(5):569-572.

P.W. "Vitamin C paper may be flawed," *Natural Foods Merchandiser*, May 1998.

Padus, Emrika. *The Complete Guide to Your Emotions & Your Health*, Rodale Press, 1986.

Pahor, Marco, et al. "Calcium-channel blockade and incidence of cancer in aged populations," *The Lancet*, August 24, 1996. "Calcium-channel blockers: managing uncertainty," editorial *The Lancet*, August 24, 1996.

Palmer, Julie R., et al. "Coffee Consumption and Myocardial Infarction in Women," *American Journal of Epidemiology*, 1995;141(8)724-31.

Parts excerpted from "A Status Report on Osteoporosis: The Challenge to Midlife and Older Women," *Older Women's League,* June 1994.

Pelletier, Kenneth R. *Mind as Healer, Mind as Slayer,* Delacorte Press, 1977.

Personal interview with Richard M. Delany, MD, FACC.

Pike, Malcolm C., Darcy V. Spicer, et al. "Estrogens, progestogens, normal breast proliferation, and breast cancer risk," *Epidemiologic Reviews,* The Johns Hopkins University School of Hygiene and Public Health, vol. 15, no. 1, 1993.

Pini, Pia. "New candidaemia patterns emerge in the U.S.A.," *The Lancet,* vol. 348, August 10, 1996, p. 395.

Piscitelli, Stephen C., et al. "Indinavir concentration and St. John's wort," *The Lancet,* vol. 355, February 12, 2000.

Pizzorno, Joseph, ND. *Total Wellness,* Prima Publishing, 1996.

Plank, Dave. "A new twist on the SAMe story," *Natural Foods Merchandiser,* September 1999.

Press Release, September 10, 1996, The American Society for Bone and Mineral Research.

Press release: Angus Reid Group, Burnsville, MN. (800) 999-4859.

Quincy, Cheri, DO. "Issues regarding menopause ... the politics of estrogen?" privately published (707) 539-3511.

Rapola, J.M., et al. "Randomized trial of alpha tocopherol and beta carotene supplements on incidence of major coronary events in men with previous myocardial infarction," *The Lancet,* 1997; 349:1715-20.

Reaven, G.M. "Dietary therapy for non-insulin-dependent diabetes mellitus. Editorial," *New England Journal of Medicine,* 319(13):862-4, 1988.

Reiss, Uzzi, MD. *Natural Hormone Balance for Women,* Simon & Schuster, 2001.

Rennard, Barbara O., BA, et al. "Chicken soup inhibits neutrophil chemotaxis in vitro," CHEST, vol. 118, no. 4, 2000.

Revised 1990 Estimates of Maternal Mortality, A New Approach by WHO and UNICEF, April 1996.

Rice, M.M., A.B. Graves, S.M. McCurry, L. Gibbons, J. Bowen, W. McCormick, and E.B. Larson. "Tofu consumption and cognition in older Japanese American men and women." *J Nutr* 130: 676S, 2000.

Ricketts, C.D., et al. "Effect of Dietary Caffeine Intake on Serum Lipid Levels in Healthy Adults," *Nutrition Research* 13, 639-647, 1993.

Robbers, James E., PhD, and Varro E. Tyler, PhD, ScD. *Tyler's Herbs of Choice: The therapeutic use of phytomedicinals,* The Haworth Herbal Press, New York, 1999.

Roberts, James, M., MD, "Magnesium for preeclampsia and eclampsia," *The New England Journal of Medicine,* July 27, 1995.

Rogers, Sherry A., MD. *Wellness Against All Odds,* Prestige Publishing, Syracuse, NY, 1994.

Rosen, Clifford J. "A tale of two worlds in prescribing etidronate for osteoporosis," *The Lancet,* November 8, 1997.

Rosenbaum, Michael, MD, and Murray Susser, MD. *Solving the Puzzle of Chronic Fatigue Syndrome,* 1992, Life Sciences Press, P.O. Box 1174, Tacoma, WA 98401.

Ross, Ronald K., et al. "Stroke Prevention and Oestrogen Replacement Therapy," *The Lancet,* March 4, 1989.

Rowe, Paul M. "Housework Recommended for Cardiovascular Health," *The Lancet,* vol. 347, January 13, 1996.

Sack, Michael N., et al. "Estrogen and Inhibition of Oxidation of Low-Density Lipoproteins in Postmenopausal Women," *The Lancet,* January 29, 1994.

Sahelian, Ray, MD. "Author urges caution in DHEA sales," *Nat Foods Merchandiser,* January 1998.

Samuels, Adrienne, PhD. Correspondence, Truth in Labeling Campaign, P.O. Box 2532, Darien, IL 60561, 19197.

Sanchez-Guerrero J, et al. "Postmenopausal estrogen therapy and the risk for developing systemic lupus erythermatosus," *Ann Intern Med* 1995:122:430-433.

Santosh-Kumar C.R., et al. "Unpredictable intra-individual variations in serum homocysteine levels on folic acid supplementation," *Eur J*

Clin Nutr 51, 188-192, 1977. From *Int Clin Nutr Rev,* October 1997, p. 213.

Sardi, Bill. "They're taking the joy out of soy," *Townsend Letter for Doctors & Patients,* October 2000.

Sardi, Bill. "Vitamins vs. veggies, debate continues." *Natural Foods Merchandiser,* May 1998.

Schauss, Alexander G., PhD. "Colloidal minerals: clinical implications of clay suspension products sold as dietary supplements," *Amer Journ Natural Med,* January/February 1997.

Scheffer, Mechthild. *Bach Flower Therapy: Theory and Practice,* Thorsons Publishers, Inc., Rochester, VT, 1981.

Schwartz, G.E. "Disregulation theory and disease: Applications to the repression/cerebral disconnection/cardiovascular disorder hypothesis," *International Review of Applied Psychology,* 32, p. 95-118, 1983.

Schwartz, G.E. "Psychobiology of repression and health: a systems approach," 1990.

Science, January 10, 1997.

Seelig, Mildred, MD and Ronald J. Elin, MD, PhD.,"Myocardial Infarction and Magnesium," *Clinical Pearls News,* January 1996.

Seidler, Susan, "ERT: Drug company sales vs.women's health," *Nat'l Women's Health Network,* March/April 1994.

Selye, Hans. *The Physiology and Pathology of Exposure to Stress,* Montreal:Acta, 1950.

Shields, P.G., et al. "Mutagens from heated Chinese and U.S. cooking oils," *J Natl Cancer Inst,* 1995;87:836-841.

Shrive, E, et al. "Glutamine in treatment of peptic ulcer," *Tex. J. Med.,* 53:840-843, 1957.

Sibbison, J.B. "USA: Women's Health, Women's Rights," *The Lancet,* July 21, 1990.

Spicer, Darcy V. and Malcolm C. Pike. "Hormonal manipulation to prevent breast cancer," *Scientific American Science & Medicine,* July/August 1995.

Stampfer, Meir J., MD, et al. "A Prospective Study of Moderate Alcohol Consumption and the Risk of Coronary Disease and Stroke in Women," *NEJM,* August 4, 1988.

Stampfer, Meir J., MD, et al. "Postmenopausal Estrogen Therapy and Cardiovascular Disease: 10-Year Follow-Up From the Nurse's Health Study," *NEJM,* September 12, 1991.

"Study Finds Bias in Way Women Are Evaluated for Heart Bypass," *New York Times,* April 16, 1990, p. A15.

Survey from The Arthritis Foundation, 2000.

Talley, R.B. "Drug-Induced Illness," *JAMA,* 229 (1974):1043.

te Velde, Egbert R., Huub A.I.M. van Leusden. "Hormonal Treatment for the Climacteric: Alleviation of Symptoms and Prevention of Postmenopausal Disease," *The Lancet,* March 12, 1994.

Teo, Koon K., Yuuf, Salam. "Role of magnesium in reducing mortality in acute myocardial infarction: A review of the evidence," *Drugs,* 1993; 46(3).

"The Best & Worst Dressed List," *Nutrition Action Healthletter*, CSPI, June 1997.

The Carter Center of Emory University, "Closing the gap: The problem of diabetes mellitus in the United States," *Diabetes Care,* 1985; 8:391-406.

"The FDA Approved a Drug. Then What?" *New York Times,* October 7, 1997.

The Lancet, 1983; 2:130.

The Lancet, January 11, 1997.

The Merck Manual of Medical Information, Home Edition, Pocket Books, 1997.

"The PDR Family Guide to Women's Health and Prescription Drugs," *Medical Economics,* Montvale, NJ, 1994.

Traber, M.G., A. Elsner, and R. Brigelius-Flobe. "Synthetic as compared with natural vitamin E is preferentially excreted as alpha-CEHC in human urine: studies using deuterated alpha-tocopheryl acetates," *FEBS Letters,* 1998;437:145-148.

Traynor, Marty. "McGwire supplements Maris' record," *Natural Foods Merchandiser,* October 1998.

Troisi, R.J., Willett, W.C., et al. "Evidence for an oestrogen contribution to the pathogenesis of adult-onset asthma," *Am J Epidemiol* 139 (11), 7S21, 1994.

Truss, C. Orian. *The Missing Diagnosis,* Birmingham, AL, 1983.

"U.S. iron deficiency," *The Lancet,* April 5, 1997, p. 1002.

Vakkanski, L. "Magnesium may slow bone loss," *Med Tribune,* July 22, 1993.

van Papendorp, DH, et al. "Biochemical profile or osteoporotic patients on essential fatty acid supplementation," *Nutr Res* 15(3), 325-334, 1995.

Verhoef, P., et al. "Homocysteine metabolism and risk of myocardial infarction: relation with vitamins B_6, B_{12} and folate," *Am J Epidemiol* 143,1966. From *Amer Journ of Clin Nutr,* April 1997, vol. 17, no 2.

VERIS, Hammond B.R., et al. "Dietary modification of human macular pigment density," *Investigative Opthamol & Visual Science,* 1997;38:1795-1801.

Voss, Andreas, and Paul E. Verweij. "Antibacterial activity of hyperforin from St John's wort," *The Lancet,* vol. 354, August 28, 1999.

Vrazo, Fawn. "FDA Panel Notes Heart Benefits of Postmenopausal Estrogen Drug," *Philadelphia Inquirer,* June 16, 1990.

Wallace, Edward C., ND, DC. "Diabetic Epidemic," *Energy Times,* April 1999.

Walsch, Neale Donald. *Conversations With God,* Hampton Roads Publishing, 1995.

Washington Post, May 13, 2000.

Watts, David L. "Calcium and virus activation," *Trace Elements, Inc. Newsletter,* vol. 3, no. 5, 1989. (P.O. Box 514, Addison, TX 75001).

Weaver, Connie M., et al. "Human calcium absorption from whole-wheat products," *Amer Inst of Nutr,* May 3, 1991.

Weeks, Nora. *The Medical Discoveries of Edward Bach, Physician,* The C.W. Daniel Co, Ltd., Ashingdon Rochford Essex, England, 1940.

Wei M., et al. "The Impact of Changes in Coffee Consumption on Serum Cholesterol," *J Clin Epidemiol* 48(10), 1189-1196, 1995.

Weiner, Michael A., PhD. *Maximum Immunity,* Simon & Schuster, Inc., 1987.

Wenger, Nanette K., MD, et al. "Cardiovascular Health and Disease in Women," *NEJM,* vol. 329, no. 4, July 22, 1993.

Werbach, Melvyn R., MD. *Nutritional Influences on Illness,* Second Edition, Third Line Press, 1996.

Werbach, Melvyn R., MD and Murray, Michael T, ND. *Botanical Influences on Illness*, Third Line Press, Tarzana, CA 1994.

Werbach, Melvyn R., MD. *Nutritional Influences on Illness,* CDRom 1998.

"What about soy?" *FDA Consumer,* May-June 2000.

Wheatley, Carmen. "Vitamin trials and cancer," *The Lancet,* June 21, 1997.

Whitaker, Julian, MD. *Is Heart Surgery Necessary?* Regnery Pub., 1995.

White, L.R., H. Petrovitch, G.W. Ross, K. Masaki, J. Hardman, J. Nelson, D. Davis, and W. Markesbery. "Brain aging and midlife tofu consumption." *J Am Coll Nutr,* 19: 242-255, 2000.

Whitehead, et al. "Effect of Red Wine Ingestion on the Antioxidant Capacity of Serum," *Clin Chem* 41:32-5, 1995.

Willett, W.C., et al. "Weight, Weight Change, and Coronary Heart Disease in Women," *JAMA* 273, 461-465, 1995.

Willett, Walter C., et al. "Intake of Trans Fatty Acids and Risk of Coronary Heart Disease Among Women," *The Lancet,* March 6, 1993.

Wilson, Peter W.F., et al. "Postmenopausal Estrogen Use, Cigarette Smoking, and Cardiovascular Morbidity in Women Over 50," *NEJM,* October 24, 1985.

Wolf O.T., O. Neumann, D.H. Hellhammer, et al. "Effects of a two-week physiological dehydroepiandrosterone substitution on cognitive

performance and well being in healthy elderly women and men."
J Clin Endocrinol Metab. 1997;82:2363–2367.

Wolff, Mary, "Blood Levels of Organochlorine Residues and Risk of
Breast Cancer," *Journal of the Nat'l Cancer Institute* 85, 8, April
21, 1993:648-52.

Wong, Conroy A., et al. "Inhaled corticosteroid use and bone-mineral
density in patients with asthma," *The Lancet,* vol. 355, April 22,
2000.

Wyngate, Pamela. "The science behind SAMe," *Natural Foods
Merchandiser,* September 1999.

Yance, Donald R., Jr., CN, MH, AHG. *Herbal Medicine, Healing &
Cancer,* Keats Publishing, 1999.

Zang, E.A. and E.L. Wynder. "Differences in lung cancer risk between
men and women: Examination of the Evidence." *J Natl Can Inst*
1996;88:183-91.

Zeb, Shahid and N. Lawrence Edwards. "Osteoarthritis: nonpharmaco-
logic therapy," *Clin Rev,* Summer 14-17, 1998.

Zhou, J.R., E.T. Gugger, T. Tanaka, Y. Guo, G.L. Blackburn, and S.K.
Clinton. "Soybean phytochemicals inhibit the growth of trans-
plantable human prostate carcinoma and tumor angiogenesis in
mice." *J Nutr,* September 1999, 129(9):1628-35.

Index

B